COMMUNITY MENTAL HEALTH NURSING

COMMUNITY MENTAL HEALTH NURSING
NEW DIRECTIONS IN THEORY AND PRACTICE

Dixie Koldjeski, Ph.D., R.N., F.A.A.N.
Professor
Graduate Studies in Nursing
Community Mental Health Nursing
East Carolina University
Greenville, North Carolina

A WILEY MEDICAL PUBLICATION
JOHN WILEY & SONS
New York • Chichester • Brisbane • Toronto • Singapore

Cover design: Wanda Lubelska

Library of Congress Cataloging in Publication Data:

Koldjeski, Dixie.
  Community mental health nursing.

  (A Wiley medical publication)
  Includes index.
  1. Psychiatric nursing. 2. Community mental health
services. I. Title. II. Series. [DNLM: 1. Community
mental health services—Nursing texts. 2. Psychiatric
nursing. WY 160 K81c]
RC440.K6 1984   610.73'68   83-14768
ISBN 0-471-04442-3

Printed in the United States of America

10 9 8 7 6 5 4 3 2 1

PREFACE

The purpose of this book is to present professional nursing students and clinicians with a concept of community mental health nursing that offers some new directions in theory and practice. One new direction is the elaboration of a model of community mental health nursing and the identification of its rationale by using a synthesis of nursing concepts and principles, a social psychological perspective of human behavior with relevant concepts from other sciences, and the ideology of community mental health. The model developed from these sources suggests some new emphases for clinical nursing practice. A second direction is an emphasis on preventions with adaptive or healthy families to promote and maintain positive mental health as an area of clinical practice.

Specific objectives are the following: (1) to present a general model of community mental health nursing that may be used to organize and guide preventions and interventions with population groups having different mental health needs; (2) to define the conceptual and clinical bases of the model; (3) to. apply the model in the less well-developed area of prevention to demonstrate its utility and general adaptability; and (4) to stimulate interest in developing other models of nursing practice that unify and consolidate many concepts, special theories, research, and clinical experiences to advance the development of the science base of community mental health nursing.

The conceptual and clinical practice bases that are identified may differ in a number of respects from some of the more familiar bases grounded in psy-chodynamic and behavioral theories. Theories about mental health, mental illness, and the distinctions between community mental health nursing, mental health nursing, and psychiatric nursing offer clarifications about conceptual and practice bases. A theme throughout is that man and environment are in constant interaction—which leads to an emphasis on interrelationships and connections between primary socialization and daily living groups and community net-works, organizations, and activities in communities. Groups of patients in a variety of mental hospital settings are considered in this framework as special group experiences organized to provide corrective life experiences for people experiencing emotional and mental health problems.

An attempt to consolidate and unify a variety of concepts and theories that are commonly used as the basis for community mental health nursing practice is a formidable task. Add to this difficulty the belief that a holistic concept of nursing is an integral part of all nursing practice and the idea that there does not seem to be "one single thread" that indicates or predicts mental health or illness in either families or individuals, then the complexity of the task begins to be appreciated as a challenge of considerable proportions! It will, no doubt, take a number of years of work in this field before diverse models of nursing theory that would have particular applicability to the problems and concerns of community mental health nursing can be developed. All mental health disciplines share some knowledge and practice bases, but each discipline uses and shapes this shared knowledge in ways that make it possible for each to make unique contributions to mental health care.

It is hoped that the ideas presented in this book will be of use to clinicians in their clinical practice and will encourage both scholars and clinicians in the field to accelerate their efforts to develop more comprehensive models and related applications. The need to move forward in this effort is great. Advances have been made in community mental health nursing over the past four decades of which nurse clinicians can be justifiably proud. It is a good time to try to advance the conceptual bases of community mental health nursing in order to assist in the expansion of and new directions in this special area of nursing practice. Through such efforts, community mental health nurses will increase their already considerable contributions to the mental health of the citizens of the nation.

D.K.

ACKNOWLEDGMENTS

I wish to acknowledge my debt to my husband, Ted, who provided encouragement and unwavering support during the years of writing this book. He shared and often assumed many of the responsibilities for our daily living so that I could have uninterrupted time for thinking and writing.

Obviously, I am also indebted to the many pioneers in psychiatric, mental health, and community mental health nursing as well as contemporary colleagues for many insights about my chosen field of clinical nursing practice. My teachers and colleagues in sociology and nursing have been both stimulating and encouraging in the effort to think differently about the conceptual and practice bases of community mental health nursing.

Special acknowledgment is due to my manuscript typist, Mrs. Iris O'Dell, whose commitment to the book had a great deal to do with the speed with which she returned drafts.

D.K.

FOREWORD

A psychiatric–mental health clinical nurse specialist and renowned educator offers a fresh perspective for community mental health nursing practice and research. A rich background in nursing on the national scene at NIMH as well as on state and local levels has undoubtedly influenced Dr. Koldjeski's thoughtful prescriptions for research and practice for the future. She has clearly differentiated the nature of practice in community mental health nursing, mental health nursing, and psychiatric nursing—a herculean task that was long overdue.

The growth of psychiatric nursing in the past two decades has highlighted the need for a clear elaboration of the clinical and conceptual bases of community mental health nursing. Dr. Koldjeski's social-psychiatric model of mental health and mental illness and her conceptual base for community mental health nursing clearly answer this need. With its emphasis on prevention and preventive counseling including indicators for assessing the mental health of communities, her work has profound implications for nursing. The author's scholarliness in the selection and documentation of relevant authoritative sources further enhances the quality of this book, which should prove highly useful to students, teachers, researchers, and practitioners in nursing.

M. Leah Gorman, Ed.D., R.N.
Professor of Nursing
School of Nursing
Emory University
Atlanta, Georgia

CONTENTS

TABLES

PART ONE

CONCEPTUAL AND CLINICAL BASES OF COMMUNITY MENTAL HEALTH NURSING

OVERVIEW

In this part of the book, the conceptual and clinical practice bases of community mental health nursing are identified and discussed. Important conceptual bases from which clinical frameworks are developed include nursing, community mental health, theories and concepts relating to mental health and mental illness, basic sciences, and the psychiatric sciences.

There are four chapters in this part. Each chapter focuses on an important aspect of community mental health nursing. A social psychological perspective is emphasized throughout and serves as the integrating thread in the models of mental health and mental illness that are presented.

Chapter 1 describes the rationale for community mental health nursing, which differs from those of mental health nursing and psychiatric nursing. Distinctions supporting this position are presented. Community mental health nursing practice involves small social organizational systems in which milieus are created that are highly intense learning environments for people throughout their lives. Principles of community mental health nursing interrelate concepts and principles of mental health and clinical practice. The roles of the generalist and specialist nurse are considered.

Chapter 2 considers relationships between the conceptual bases of community mental health nursing and nursing in general. The structure of nursing is identified in terms of a number of unique aspects which should be present in community mental health nursing practice. Some influences on the basic structure of nursing in community-based mental health care are discussed. The difficulties of identifying the role of the professional nurse generalist in a specialized system of mental health are noted.

Chapter 3 considers some of the evolutionary changes that have occurred in concepts of mental health and mental illness and the relationships of these to models of community mental health nursing. Assumptions about mental health and mental illness using basically a social psychological perspective are established and used to define mental health and mental illness as two distinct life experiences. Social psychological models of mental health and mental illness are shown. The implications of these for clinical practice in this subspecialty of nursing practice are noted.

Chapter 4 relates the conceptual bases of community mental health nursing to the policies and ideology of mental health care initiated at the national level. Traditional and contemporary factors that have influenced the development of community mental health as a concept for organizing services are identified. Current issues focus on changes in policy at the national level in relation to support for continued education and training and an emphasis on biomedical and neuroscientific research with a diminution of monies for social, psychological, and behavioral research. A decline in the number of nurses being recruited in the field is cited as a grave national concern of the profession.

CHAPTER 1

COMMUNITY MENTAL HEALTH NURSING: BASIC CONCEPTS AND PRINCIPLES

INTRODUCTION

A conceptualization of community mental health nursing that uses primarily a social psychological framework embodies the idea of man and environment in interaction. This orientation is based on a principle of social ecology holding that all living things are interrelated and influence one another in the process of adaptation to daily living. In community mental health nursing emphasis on this principle is reflected in an explicit concern about the interactions of four important things: (1) the mental health of individuals; (2) the small social groups in which individuals live, work, and play; (3) community and social networks; and (4) situational contexts in which the interactions and emotions of people are expressed and help give meaning to experiences.

Lancaster (1980) described the man–environment perspective as a framework that health care providers can use to look at total human experiences. This approach is based on the recognition that a person's health status results from the dynamic interplay between two ecological universes: one's own internal environment and the external multienvironments in which one exists (Hanlon, 1969).

The principle that humans and environment must interact in order for adaptation to occur orients the clinician in community mental health nursing to consider both mental health and mental illness as more than the psychological responses of individuals. Adaptation refers to the modifications in social life that are necessary to join physical and social environments with individual needs for growth, development, and self-actualization. The mental health of people depends in large part on the kind and quality of interrelationships occurring between and within the different social systems in which they are members. Mental health also depends on family and primary group support as well as the availability of needed resources vital to the enhancement of emotional, personal, and social growth.

Community mental health nursing uses concepts from a number of sources: nursing, ecology, social psychology, psychophysiology, psychology, and related basic health sciences. An organizing framework using knowledge from these areas is necessary in order to make explicit the key interrelationships between people in groups, community networks, and the social settings in which they live.

Nursing preventions and interventions may be applied to one or more levels of relationships that are created as people interact in environments. Such relationships may be of various kinds: social, interpersonal, family, and group. Clinicians in community mental health nursing have to address relationships and linkages between people in social groups and between these groups and community networks and activities. This focus is necessary to understand what, if any, changes are needed to promote and improve the mental health of families, individuals, and communities in which they live.

3

Perspectives of man and environment in interaction consider humans as only one system, albeit the most important one, that is constantly in interaction with many other systems of different sizes and complexity. Putt (1978) described the pattern of increasing complexity and size of different kinds of systems in the social development of people in the following way. First, a two-person family joins with other nearby families to form villages; then come towns, cities, and countries: and finally, countries unite to form such organizations as the United Nations. In all these systems, the social, cultural, physical, and psychological dimensions of relationships are basic to the development of common goals and a sense of identity for individuals, families, and country.

Inherent in the view of man and environment in interaction is the assumption that the mental health of individuals and families is not separate from or independent of the social settings and contexts in which socialization of children and adults occurs. Common features of all socialization, irrespective of the kind and structure of settings in which it occurs, are the patterns of emotional, mental, and cognitive responses learned in particular settings in order to cope, adapt, and develop an organization of the self. This complex learning process may be explained by using many conceptual frameworks. For example, Wilson and Kneisl (1979) use concepts from social psychological and systems theories. This conceptual approach emphasizes social interactions that influence the development of both mental health and mental illness.

Community mental health nursing is assumed to be different in a number of respects from mental health nursing. Both subspecialties differ in other respects from psychiatric nursing. These differences are important because they influence the selection of phenomena about which the community mental health nurse seeks information. They affect the relative emphasis given to selected data and its use for making clinical decisions, the selection of appropriate preventions and interventions for clinical applications, and the identification of desired behavioral outcomes in the client.

In this chapter, differences between community mental health, mental health, and psychiatric nursing are identified. Issues relating to these distinctions are noted. Characteristics of community mental health nursing, mental health nursing, and psychiatric nursing highlight distinctions. Six basic principles of community mental health nursing are discussed. The role of clinical nurse generalists and specialists in community mental health nursing is examined.

COMMUNITY MENTAL HEALTH
NURSING: DISTINCTIONS AND ISSUES

The assumption that there are conceptual and clinical practice distinctions among community mental health nursing, mental health nursing, and psychiatric nursing is a view about which clinicians in this subspecialty have honest differences of opinion. It is recognized that any one of the three terms may be used to identify this subspecialty of nursing practice. This interchangeable use of terms continues for many reasons, two of which are tradition and lack of clarity about conceptual and practice bases.

The assumption that differences exist among community mental health nursing, mental health nursing, and psychiatric nursing has been evolving for some years among clinicians. One of the first in this respect was Osborne (1970) who cited two kinds of practice: community mental health nursing and community psychiatric nursing. He suggested that each kind of clinical practice touched two fundamentally different bases of theory and addressed two different kinds of population groups. Community psychiatric nursing was identified as the community management of clients who had considerable psychopathology of mental disorder, the community treatment of such disorders, and the psychiatric nursing care of these individuals in curative and rehabilitative aspects. Community mental health nursing is based on mental health theories and focuses on well populations. The goal of community mental health nursing was cited as the lessening of incidence and prevalence of mental and emotional disorders. Underwood (1980) has proposed that the knowledge bases and clinical competencies needed to provide nursing care to hospitalized mental patients differ from those needed by therapists for clinical management of clients experiencing emotional and mental health problems and being maintained in community settings.

The rationale for assuming that there are major differences in the three subspecialities of clinical nursing in mental health is based on several points. First, theory and research available today show distinctions not heretofore discerned. Second, theories and related research about mental health and mental illness have over the past decade been developed from a number of different perspectives. These perspectives have highlighted some of the different ways mental health and mental illness may be conceptualized and experienced. Many of these concepts emphasize social and cultural factors and relationships in mental health and mental illness and the influence of social and community networks and activities. Last, research in social ecology has provided knowledge of the impact that small group settings and situations, as highly intense learning environments, have on behavior and attitudes (Moos, 1976).

Early in the community mental health movement, there was a need for the new practice area of community mental health nursing to identify and use traditional psychiatric nursing theories and practice to provide mental health services in community-based settings. In time, these bases were also used to expand roles and help clinicians to identify new roles that needed to be developed in community mental health nursing. The situation today is quite different. With the knowledge and research that has accumulated from nursing and other major science areas, it is possible to consider different clinical nursing models and to test these with different population groups both to promote and maintain mental health and to provide more enlightened clinical nursing management in hospital and community settings. For example, Kuntz and co-workers (1980), in their review of the literature of one nursing journal in community mental health, found that in the last half of the 1970s there was an emphasis on integration of theory adapted from other fields into clinical practice, and tests of these theories. This finding is indicative of a general shift in the advanced practice of nursing in mental health from that of application of traditional models of nursing to more scientifically based models derived from a wide range of theories and research. It is a major reason why it is now possible to consider conceptual distinctions in clinical practice that were not possible two decades ago.

Distinctions in conceptions of mental health nursing, psychiatric nursing, and community mental health nursing have been confounded by the interchangeable use of all three terms in the language of clinical practice and of theoretical formulations (Mereness and Taylor, 1978). Various combinations of concepts have also been paired together or hyphenated; however, distinctions associated with a particular concept have not been clear (ANA, 1966; Deloughery, Gebbie, & Newman, 1971; ANA, 1973; Kalkman and Davis, 1976; Burgess and Lazare, 1976; Burgess, 1981). Some of the confusion surrounding the three practice areas is exemplified by the following incident.

The nursing student in the front row of the class looked perplexed. She had been listening intently to the nurse instructor lecture on the theory and practice of psychiatric nursing. In concluding her remarks, the instructor assured the students that they would like their clinical experiences in community mental health nursing. She commented that mental health nursing would be a unique experience.

At this point the student in the front row appeared more perplexed and asked in a plaintive voice, "How can I like something when I don't even know what it is? Is there a difference between psychiatric nursing, community mental health nursing, and mental health nursing?" The instructor looked startled, then smiled brightly and said, "You will understand the answer to your questions when you get to the clinical setting and talk to some patients."

In relation to the questions raised by the puzzled nursing student, the instructor could have made several clarifications. She might have pointed out that no differences in meanings were intended. Or she might have noted that the meanings of the concepts depend in large part on the theoretical perspective of mental health and mental illness held by the mental health professional. And she might have pointed out that there are differences in the concepts but the theoretical bases for each are in the process of being more clearly refined. Such clarifications are important in order to help clinicians recognize distinctions in clinical nursing practice.

Conceptions of clinical nursing practice in community mental health nursing in conjunction with those held about mental health and mental illness make up an important clinical orientation for the community mental health nurse. This orientation guides the selection of concepts and theories on which to base clinical practice. It influences the kind and scope of assessment, evaluation of data, and elaboration of clinical inferences. From these data, a rationale is developed to guide the selection of therapeutic interventions and preventions, evaluation of their effectiveness and therapeutic use of self. The degree of warmth and the expressions of concern and caring that the community mental health nurse wants to convey in interactions with families, clients, and significant others are important parts of this rationale.

COMMUNITY MENTAL HEALTH NURSING: CHARACTERISTICS AND FOCUS

Community mental health nursing is characterized by a unique clinical process based on a synthesis of concepts from nursing, mental health, health, social psychology, psychology, community networks and organization, and the basic sciences. The clinical process is applied in a systematic way to families and other kinds of primary socialization groups to promote and maintain high levels of functioning that are related to positive mental health of members. Adaptive family systems with high levels of functioning provide the kind of highly intense learning environments and use of resources that promote mental health, prevent mental illness, and reduce the stress of daily living. Family systems are major behavior settings in which close and continued human relationships occur over long periods of time and through socialization influences the mental and emotional health of members from birth throughout life.

In community mental health nursing, the nurse assists all kinds of primary socialization groups, such as families and school and work groups, to help members develop a personal organization of the self, strengthen their abilities to adapt and cope, achieve selfhood, and maintain independence and autonomy in their relationships. Primary socialization groups help members identify their strengths and promote the use of these to realize the promise of achieving and maintaining optimal levels of social, mental, and emotional health. A major concern is to help family systems develop in their members basic social competencies and problem-solving skills that are necessary to achieve satisfactory interactions and working relationships.

Community mental health nursing considers the social, psychological, and situational aspects of life and living that influence the emotional health and mental health of people. Its clinical practice orientation takes into account social and cultural factors involved in creating and maintaining mental health and mental illness. Thus, a focus of clinical practice is to strengthen the small social systems such as families and other kinds of primary groups in which socialization of children and adults takes place across the life span. Clinical practice takes place in part in natural settings in communities. It may also be conducted in designated sites in the community that provide mental health care and services (Koldjeski, 1981).

Major theoretical orientations are derived from theories stressing the interrelationships and influences on behavior that are created in system settings. An important characteristic of these interrelationships is that clients are expected to be responsible for and participate in activities that promote and maintain mental health. Clients are not expected or encouraged to adopt the sick role.

The focus of community mental health nursing differs from that of mental health nursing and psychiatric nursing in several significant ways. Clinical practice is characterized by emphasis on the following:

- Mental health of families rather than the mental health of individual clients
- Promotion and maintenance of mental health rather than clinical management of mental illness and various kinds of social and psychological pathologies
- Primary socialization groups as small systems in interaction rather than individuals as independent entities
- Patterns of interaction and roles of individuals in small group settings in terms of the impact that these patterns have on the development of mental health and self-actualization of members rather than individual behavioral manifestations as expressions of uniqueness of individual clients
- Community, family, and group interrelationships as key influences on the mental health of individuals rather than early childhood experiences that are presumed to have caused unresolved inner conflicts that are expressed in behavior
- Social psychological, cultural, and situational determinants of mental health rather than intrapsychic ones
- Conceptual frameworks that synthesize a body of knowledge focusing on the development and maintenance of the mental health of small groups and populations rather than ones emphasizing psychopathologies of individual clients

The conceptualization of community mental health nursing in this presentation is based on a synthesis of theory, research, and experience that emphasizes a nursing and social psychological perspective. The complexity of this conceptualization can be made more explicit by a glance at the concepts used to develop this perspective:

- Unique aspects of nursing
- Nursing theory
- Community mental health nursing theory
- Mental health theories
- Community mental health ideologies
- Community aspects of mental health
- Social and cultural theories of mental health

- Family, systems, and social organizational theories
- Small group theories
- Social interactional and interpersonal theories
- Personality theories
- Situation theories
- Institutional influences on behavior
- Social and community network theories
- Human growth and development theories

The synthesis of concepts and principles from many theoretical bases is difficult but essential to develop the comprehensive theoretical base necessary for community mental health nursing. The advancement of the field depends in large part on how well clinicians develop and use such frameworks to test models of clinical practice.

Mental Health Nursing

Mental health nursing is more akin to community mental health nursing than community mental health nursing is to psychiatric nursing. Mental health nursing is the application of a clinical process that is based on a synthesis of nursing and basic science concepts applying to the development, promotion, and maintenance of the *mental health of individuals*. Emphasis is on helping a person to achieve optimal levels of functioning in handling stress to develop a mature selfhood, and to become an autonomous person while remaining a caring one. It focuses on promotion of *personal and interpersonal relationships* as these relate to a person's feelings and expressions of behavior. Interpersonal processes may be examined in order to understand how and why one person relates to another by using particular relationship patterns. These patterns may either facilitate or impede understanding of communications and development of relationships.

Mental health nursing is concerned with the personal, psychological, and social interactions and the lasting relationships that relate to the development of the personal organization of the self, or ego. Interpersonal relationships are examined as they evolve in one-to-one situations. Therapeutic interventions are designed to examine and change characteristic patterns of interactions and communications that people use. Selected social and cultural aspects of living may be considered as they relate to interpersonal behavior. The emphasis, however, is to try to make interpersonal relationships more effective, to extend the use of social problem-solving skills to more varied relationships and opportunities, and to encourage the person to develop into a caring and fulfilled human being. These efforts require the development of good communication skills and learning to test reality in ways that promote growth. Successful use of such competencies provides the feedback from others that is a necessary concomitant to self-growth and development of a positive concept of self.

Mental health nursing is also concerned with helping people develop and use more satisfying social and interpersonal relationships by understanding how they express anxiety. It is necessary for a person to learn that anxiety at different levels of intensity influences the perceptions one holds about what happens in interpersonal relationships.

Therapeutic activities in mental health nursing are usually interventions in a one-to-one relationship involving a professional mental health nurse and a client. Stress management and crisis theory are applied as needed. Some behaviors such as those associated with addictive life styles may be changed through behavior modification or resocialization approaches. The focus of clinical practice is to help individuals gain understanding and insight about the ways in which they relates to others, how these relationships are perceived by self and others, and the impact that such perceptions have on the concept of self. The process of one-to-one therapy offers a unique opportunity for a person to try out new ways of relating to a significant other in a nonjudgmental setting.

In mental health nursing, clinical practice settings are usually clinics and centers offering mental health services or a combination of health and mental health services. Clinical services are also provided in private practice settings. The important concept, however, is the use of the dyadic relationship to establish a therapeutic learning environment. Such a relationship can be established in many kinds of settings so long as privacy can be assured to allow the two participants to focus on what is happening *within* the ongoing relationship.

Major theoretical orientations are derived from theories stressing the psychological growth and development of the personality of an individual. Of major concern are the problems developing in cognition, emotions, and behavior because of conflicts within the structure of the personality and in interpersonal relationships. Clients are not encouraged to develop the sick role; however, therapists may encourage the development of a dependency relationship as a means of working through unresolved conflicts about a significant other.

Psychiatric Nursing

As a subspecialty in nursing, psychiatric nursing is much older than either mental health nursing or community mental health nursing. Early textbooks describe two major roles for psychiatric nursing: (1) to provide physical and protective nursing care to patients who are mentally ill and (2) to assist the physician in administering somatic treatments, such as insulin and electric shock, and executing medical orders (Steele, 1937). The psychotherapeutic role of psychiatric nursing was developed for the first time in the mid-1950s and focused on therapeutic nurse–patient relationships (Peplau, 1952).

Psychiatric nursing is defined as the clinical practice of nursing that uses a synthesis of psychiatric nursing theory including its unique aspects, social and psychopathology theories, social milieu concepts, social psychology, and interpersonal theories for its theoretical bases. This clinical framework is applied through social and psychotherapeutic interventions to *patients* who experience mental, emotional, and social disorders to a degree that mental hospitalization or other kinds of institutional living arrangements are necessary. Psychiatric nursing is the science and art of providing protective, therapeutic, supportive, physical, and social care to people too ill to be completely responsible for management of their own behavior. For patients in mental hospitals and other institutional settings, the psychiatric nurse is the primary health care provider and is, in fact, a primary mental health care nurse.

The overall goal of psychiatric nursing is to assist patients to learn to become productive members of society and to reach as full a potential of their assets as possible. This goal may be oriented toward a long-term stay in a mental hospital or other domicilliary setting and toward preparation for returning to the family and community.

In achieving the goals that psychiatric nurses must undertake with patients, patients must have opportunities to develop more positive self-concepts and to relate to others in productive and satisfying ways. Patients must also learn in interaction with psychiatric nurses the identification of patterns of behavior they use in expressing and managing anxiety. This process is facilitated by structuring informal social relationships in the ward milieu setting and through formal nurse–patient relationships to permit the introduction of change strategies. The continuing nurse–patient relationship is an important therapeutic event because it provides the patient with opportunities to test new patterns of interaction and different ways of relating to another person.

Psychiatric nursing is also concerned with establishing therapeutic milieus for patients and staff in mental hospital settings. In such milieus, patients and staff relate around daily living experiences. In these contexts, a considerable amount of learning occurs as a result of role modeling by staff of appropriate ways of relating to individuals and groups. In essence, a therapeutic milieu provides support and learning opportunities to maintain and improve physical, psychological, and social health of patients through management of the environment.

In psychiatric nursing, therapeutic interventions cover a range of strategies: one-to-one relationships, group therapy, humane custodial care, milieu therapy, behavior modification approaches, psychopharmacological therapies, and assistance with various somatic therapies. These therapies may be provided in clinical practice settings in the psychiatric units of general hospitals, mental hospitals, psychiatric units in prisons, and special psychiatric settings. To some extent, each of these settings operates on the principles of a total institution.

Major theoretical orientations for clinical nursing practice are derived from a variety of theories about mental illness and mental disorders, therapeutic modalities associated with various theories, and social cultural influences on behavior. An important aspect of these orientations is an inherent assumption that patients adopt the sick role. The adoption of this role has profound implications for the relationships that the patient subsequently develops with staff in the mental hospital, maintains with spouse, and continues with friends, family, and peers.

A considerable amount of the mental health care provided by nurses in community mental health centers and clinics is, in conception, mental health nursing. This is evident when the distinctions between community mental health nursing, mental health nursing, and psychiatric nursing are examined. A summary of these differences is shown in Table 1.1.

Six major distinctions characterize these three areas of nursing practice. One or two characteristics may be similar for a couple of areas; however, what is important is that the sum total of the pattern of characteristics for each area of nursing in mental health is different.

RELATIONSHIP BETWEEN COMMUNITY MENTAL HEALTH NURSING AND SOCIAL ORGANIZATIONAL SETTINGS

A social psychological perspective of community mental health nursing is linked to the social organizational systems in which daily living occurs. Concepts from organizational, socialization, and small group theories may be used to rank different kinds of social settings in terms of their potential to provide supportive milieus that enhance the development and maintenance of the mental health of families and their members. This is an important relationship existing between community mental health nursing, social systems, and the positive mental health of people in such systems.

Concepts of social organizational systems and community mental health nursing need to be linked in an orderly way. Such systems may be organized as to level, kind, and degree to which close and intimate relationships are fostered. Where such relationships are possible, these systems are known as highly intense learning environments. Using

Table 1.1
Characteristics of Community Mental Health Nursing, Mental Health Nursing, and Psychiatric Nursing

Characteristics	Community Mental Health Nursing	Mental Health Nursing	Psychiatric Nursing

Populations	• Primary socialization groups
	  Adaptive and healthy
	  Stressed } Responses
	  Distressed
	• Peer groups
	• *Families*
	• *Groups*
		• Individuals
		  Healthy and adaptive
		  Stressed } Responses
		  Distressed
		• *Clients*
			• Mentally and emotionally ill individuals
			  Disturbed } Responses
			  Disabled
			• *Patients* who have been medically or legally labeled to have mental illness

Goals of clinical practice	• Promote and maintain mental health of family systems and their members through prevention counseling and use of interventions • Maintain and increase the potential of primary groups to use their strengths to provide essential competencies for social, personal, and cognitive growth that relate to positive mental health behaviors for members • Teach families and members in primary groups to recognize tensions, coping, and communication patterns that have an adverse impact on members and to learn new ones • Help families and members of primary groups recognize that behavior has social, cultural, and situational aspects and the influences these have on group functioning and member behavior • Teach families and members to	• Promote and maintain mental health of individuals through prevention, actualization, and intervention counseling • Help clients to develop more satisfying and productive interpersonal relationships and competencies related to positive mental health • Assist clients to learn through interpersonal and personal experiences coping patterns that promote or retard reaching personal goals • Help individuals recognize the impact of social, situational, and cultural expectations on their personal responses of coping and adaptation • Encourage personal responsibility and accountability for own health and mental health; teach to monitor mental health and general health • Use self-care	• Provide healthy group and interpersonal relationships to learn new ways of relating and new behaviors through use of role modeling and socialization • Help patients develop awareness and understanding of how unresolved interpersonal, personal, and familial conflicts influence current behavior with other people and groups • Assist patients to recognize the influence of anxiety on behavior and learn how to use this to foster new learning in interpersonal and group relationships • Use patient and staff groups organized around daily living in a specialized community to develop personal responsibility and control over one's behavior and acceptance of some responsibility for helping others control their behavior • Prepare patient for living in family or community in terms of being a

Table 1.1
(Continued)

Characteristics	Community Mental Health Nursing	Mental Health Nursing	Psychiatric Nursing
	monitor their mental health and that of their communities • Use self-care		productive citizen and resuming social and personal roles and relationships; teach to monitor mental and general health • Use self-care
Sick role	• *Not adopted* by members in families and in other kinds of primary groups	• *Not adopted* by individuals	• *Adopted* by patients
Clinical practice settings	• Natural community settings • Community-based health and mental health settings • Primary groups settings: families, groups in schools and workplaces, leisure and other special groups in communities	• Community-based health and mental health settings • Outpatient clinics • Crisis clinics • Community-based homes and halfway houses • Private practice settings	• Mental hospitals • Psychiatric units in general hospitals • Special care settings such as retreats and homes for inpatient psychiatric care and treatment • Special psychiatric units in penal systems

Major focus of interventions	• Prevention counseling
	• Community mental health nursing
	• Therapeutic intervention
	  Crisis management
	  Therapy with distressed families
	• Group process and counseling
	• Transitional counseling
	• Mental health education and teaching of self-help and self-monitoring activities
	• Stress management of daily living stresses and tensions in family systems
	• Prevention and therapeutic activities with targeted groups at risk for
		• Individual counseling
		• Nurse-patient relationship therapy
		• Crisis intervention
		• Mental health education about indicators of mental health self-monitoring approaches
		• Stress management of personal tensions and behavior
		• Prevention and intervention activities relative to the client's personal and social needs
		• Resocialization activities based on personal problems of client and individual needs
		• Behavior modification for selected
			• Psychiatric nursing relationship therapy
			• Behavior modification
			• Group therapy
			• Custodial care
			• Psychotherapy
			• Education about the kinds of behaviors and expectations needed posthospitalization
			• Therapeutic nurse-patient relationships that focus on impulse control and anxiety-driven behavior; how to minimize and manage so learning will occur
			• Psychiatric nursing care and

mental health problems and interventions with distressed families
- Socialization activities that use the potential of families and primary groups to maintain and promote the mental health of child and adult members

Major models of practice
- Holistic nursing (wellness)
- Community mental health nursing
- Social psychological
- Socio-cultural
- Systems (small)
- Interactional
- Developmental
- Transactional
- Group
- Family

problems
- Pharmacologic therapies (on medical orders)

- Holistic nursing (wellness)
- Mental health nursing
- Psychological
- Developmental
- Psychodynamical
- Interpersonal
- Behavioral
- Biochemical
- Self-actualization

management when patient needs external controls in managing his or her behavior
- Milieu therapy as a major resocialization activity, behavior modification, and interpersonal relationships
- Humane custodial care environments where needed
- On medical orders assist with
  Pharmacologic therapies
  Somatic therapies

- Holistic nursing (illness management oriented to wellness)
- Nurse-patient relationship
- Biochemical
- Psychological
- Social milieu
- Behavioral
- Interpersonal
- Medical illness
- Custodial

social organizational and small group theories as a basis, a frame-work is shown in Table 1.2 using these concepts. Systems are organized as small or micro systems, middle or mezzo systems, and large or macro systems (Mullen, Dumpson, et al., 1972).

Small Social Organizational Systems

Small social organizational systems are the primary group systems in which much of living occurs. The smallest system is the individual as an entity and as a self-system. Other small organizational systems are primary groups of different kinds—such as two-party groups, families, and groups found in school, employment, and recreational settings.

Small organizational settings are characterized by face-to-face, warm, supportive relationships and direct interactions. Communication lines are direct and immediate feedback is possible from member to member. These primary group settings are very influential on a day-to-day basis in stabilizing the concept of self and enhancing the development of essential social and interpersonal competencies necessary for positive mental health.

In small groups, members usually know one another rather well and develop relationships based on trust, mutual concern, and affection for one another. Roles and functions evolve that complement the group's functioning and encourage the development of a sense of cohesion and belonging. A great deal of learning occurs in the give-and-take of interactions. In such milieus where intimacy and caring are possible, people become human and social, learn about themselves, and, in doing so, learn to be concerned about and responsible for others .

Primary groups of various kinds are important social organizations in the life of people. A person is born in a group, lives in a group, and dies in a group. This means that the group is an important source of learning and social support through all of the great crises of life.

As small systems in interaction, primary groups usually have considerable freedom and autonomy to carry out their goals and functions. Authority is usually set forth in the form of rules, traditions, and expectations. Considerable leeway is allowed in the way in which this authority is interpreted and applied to meet individual needs and address specific kinds of experiences. In these milieus, basic social competencies and problem-solving skills are developed and routinely used.

The family as a small social system is the major social organizational setting for the socialization and humanization of the young in society. As a primary group, the family is like other such groups in some ways. It differs, however, in some very important respects. Families are usually held together by affective bonds, whereas other primary groups are organized and remain together on the basis of common interests, needs, and goals. Families have special interrelationships, roles, kinship ties, memories, and historical origins. These intimate experiences create deeply held values and relationships. Families are unique living and dynamic interacting systems in which the reproduction of the young occurs and the stabilization of adult personalities is an ongoing process. These kinds of experiences cannot be replicated vicariously in other kinds of primary groups, thus making the family a special kind of primary group.

In families and other kinds of primary groups in which child and adult socialization is a major purpose, preventions and interventions for the promotion of mental health and prevention of mental illness may be provided. The family has long been considered an interacting social unit. The family as a system has long been used by mental health professionals as an area in which to apply intervention strategies for many kinds of

Table 1.2
Schema for Organizing Levels of Systems and Strategies Useful for Each System Level[a]

Levels of Systems	Examples of Systems	Strategies for Different Systems
Large-level systems (macro systems)	Systems of national scope National health and human service systems National political systems State political systems Regional political systems Human service systems (local, state) Local political systems	Hold membership in special interest organizations Contacts with national representatives Provide information related to issues Influence policy and philosophy by participation on boards, in political process, etc. Advocacy Special interest group actions Candidacy for public office
Middle-level systems (mezzo systems)	Community health settings Hospital systems Leisure activity settings Employment settings Religious systems/networks School systems Community (groups with community identity) Neighborhoods (social/community networks)	Corrective health care settings: assess services, philosophy, economics, etc.; provide information Environmental stress inventory Peer group participation Map networks, services, and organizations, goals, philosophy Community mapping Epidemiologic study of health and illness concerns Social, cultural values, norms Patterns
Small-level systems (mini systems)	Primary groups (living, work, peer) Families (interacting systems) Interpersonal (dyads) Individual (one individual conceived of as a group of systems in interaction)	Group meetings; group dynamics, and counseling; and self-help approaches Family counseling or family therapy Interpersonal relationships, strategies, and counseling Individualized care strategies Self-actualization efforts Self-help approaches

[a] Arrows denote flows of interactions between and within system levels.

problems and pathologies. An important task of community mental health nursing is to develop preventions and related strategies that will promote and maintain a family's mental health and to continue to develop more effective and innovative approaches for working with families who are stressed and families who are distressed by major mental problems of members.

Subcultural values and beliefs can be very pervasive in families and small groups because of the person-to-person relationships, emotional ties, and direct lines of communication. These values and beliefs can be stressed through persuasion and giving advice and suggestions. They are used to control behavior. Social and physical exclusion from the family or group is always a possibility if strongly held values and beliefs are violated by any member. Such an action may be initiated by a member or exclusion may occur by the collective action of members.

As small social systems, families tend to experience rather intensely the subcultural influences and values common to the communities in which they live. For example, families develop their own systems of values and norms and these are usually related to community values and norms. Community values and norms relate to some degree to regional and national cultural values and norms. There may be, however, considerable variation and conflict between what a family holds as guiding values and beliefs about an issue or problem and the values and beliefs held by the larger society.

The individual as a system has an organization of self that is made up of biological, psychological, genetic, social, and interpersonal factors and experiences. These are unique in many respects and common to all humans in other respects. At the individual level of organization, relationships and interactions between external and internal environments are a major concern to physical and mental health. Traditionally, mental and emotional problems experienced by people have received psychological, pharmocological, and somatic interventions. Personality theories usually focus on the dynamics of what goes on *within* the psychic infrastructure of a person. The assumption is that these inner forces determine coping and adaptation responses. In this model of mental functioning, the therapist focuses on changing the feelings and cognition of patients experiencing conflict rather than trying to effect changes in the social organizational systems in which they live, work, and play.

Middle-Level Social Organizational Systems

Social organizational systems between small and large ones encompass a range of organizations and networks. These systems, such as hospitals, schools, and local governmental service agencies, have been organized for specific purposes. Employment organizations are major systems at this level and are important because, in these, the world of work, cultural work ethic, environmental conditions, and social relationships come together to form daily experiences that have both positive and negative consequences on the stabilization of personality and concept of self.

Middle-level systems, such as schools and hospitals, experience subcultural and cultural influences that may be both positive and negative in terms of the goals of these institutions. At this level of social organization, one community group's neighborhood values, norms, and desires may coincide with those of other community groups so that a general consensus on issues and actions may be reached. On the other hand, conflicts between community groups over local and regional values are highly probable. For example, there is often conflict between groups of parents in communities and between parents and school officials, and between both of these groups and state educational goals about the inclusion of sex education in the curricula of public schools. Where a consensus is reached, it often becomes strained, if not broken, over issues relating to what is to be taught and who is to do the teaching.

In middle-level systems, peer groups are a major concern for the community mental health nurse. It is in such groups associated with institutions and places of employment that a considerable amount of socialization of children, young adults, and adults across the life span takes place. These groups have a high potential for controlling and shaping the attitudes and behaviors of people who live and work in these systems on a daily basis. Satisfactions achieved by group members relate to their emotional and mental health. Groups at the middle level are not primarily organized for socialization of youths and adults. Usually, their main purpose is an essential function such as education and employment. These settings, however, socialize people in the process of meeting their special goals.

Peer groups in educational and employment settings may be formally or informally organized. In either case, they can be identified. For example, informal groups may be identified through sociometry techniques by asking employees or students questions about who they would go to for advice and assistance, borrowing money, and finding answers to personal problems. Formal and informal groups may act in accord to accomplish a common goal or they may act in conflict with one another. Formal groups may try to carry out the official goals of the organization, whereas informal groups may try to thwart the realization of such goals by using various blocking actions. Informal groups may have independent goals that members try to meet that are inimical to the official goals of the organization. An example of such a situation is one that is all too familiar to parents. They find that their children in school have become allied with peer groups who rebel against the demands of an education and accept membership in groups that support the use of drugs and adopt the values of the subculture of drug users and pushers.

Middle-level organizations include mental hospitals, psychiatric units in general hospitals, and psychiatric units in prisons. These organizational settings all have special structures and functions that relate to institutional goals.

Large Social Organizational Systems

Large social organizational systems have a wide scope of influence touching the lives of many people and populations. They are organized as a rule for the development and implementation of policies and regulations that have both a direct and an indirect authority over the actions of people.

Community mental health nursing has a role at the large social system level. It is primarily one of participation—promoting education about mental health needs—rather than applying preventions and interventions. The nurse has to help such organizations promulgate policies and procedures addressing the mental health needs of citizens. This process is greatly facilitated when nurses are appointed or elected to key advisory boards and policy-making groups.

Large social system organizations may cross national boundaries and be international in scope. At this level, cross-cultural, cultural, and national influences merge to become a potpourri of values, beliefs, and meanings. This mix of values and beliefs usually conflicts in many respects and may make it very difficult to obtain a consensus about controversial issues and problems.

Policies and decisions made at the macro system level resonate through the middle and micro levels. This happens because systems at the three levels are open and interconnected by cultural values and beliefs, social norms and expectations, and policies and regulations. The community mental health nurse has to recognize these interconnections and identify additional ones that may be having a particular impact on the micro group level.

In Table 1.2, systems on the basis of size are identified with strategies that are useful for different system levels. Systems are open and indicated by broken lines. Major strategies for interventions are identified.

From an epidemiologic perspective, community mental health nursing has to be concerned about the mental health of populations and groups with whom activities can be focused. In the coming decade, activities associated with health promotion and primary prevention will be major challenges for the field. The development of a repertoire of strategies that will be effective in promoting mental health with diverse population groups is an exciting and pioneering effort in which community mental health nursing has a major role.

The schema presented for organizing social organizational systems is consistent with a social psychological and systems perspective of community mental health nursing. It is one way in which linkages between systems can be identified in a consistent and orderly manner. It orients the community mental health nurse to translate to a holistic clinical approach many of the relatively abstract ideas and concepts associated with community mental health nursing and community mental health.

PRINCIPLES OF COMMUNITY MENTAL HEALTH NURSING

Consistent with the conceptual framework that has been presented, six principles of community mental health nursing are identified. These principles are used by the community mental health nurse to apply theory in clinical practice.

> *Principle 1: Community mental health nursing is distinguished by a unique conceptual framework, clinical process and intervention strategies.*

The framework for community mental health nursing is a synthesis of concepts, theory, and research from nursing, mental health, and related sciences. This synthesis is unique in that it consists of a special set of concepts that addresses the diverse multidimensional aspects of community mental health nursing. Concepts include the primary groups in which child and adult socialization takes place, the organization of the self, or personality of each person, community networks, social and cultural factors involved in mental health and mental illness, and the contexts in which behavior occurs and is given meaning.

The principle assumes that the unique aspects of nursing are included in the synthesized theoretical base for the practice of community mental health nursing. This is an important assumption because it relates to whether or not the nurse practices community mental health nursing or applies general concepts of mental health as a nurse. This latter approach to clinical nursing practice occurs when the nurse adopts the conceptual frameworks, therapy models, and perspectives developed by other mental health disciplines and applies these by using associated strategies and roles. When therapy models including the role and behavior of the therapist are borrowed from other disciplines and used without reconceptualization to include nursing theory and concepts, then the nursing aspects of community mental health are greatly diminished or absent.

The individual and group models of therapy that are used today by most mental health professionals focus on a relatively narrow range of human experiences. These models use perspectives of mental health and mental illness that particular disciplines other than nursing have developed. However, community mental health nursing has to focus on a wide range of human experiences. These experiences occur in quite diverse settings and under both usual and unusual circumstances and go beyond traditional models of therapy. A comprehensive theory base is necessary for this purpose.

The principle also assumes that when conceptual frameworks are comprehensive and adequate for the nurse to organize assessments, collect data, formulate clinical inferences, select interventions, decide about therapeutic use of self, and evaluate interventions, then the clinical nursing process that is generated is distinct. This is so because the content of the clinical process, the nursing process, and the role of nurse in therapeutic use of self as an almost universally accepted helping person, all blend into a rare combination of interactions.

This principle can be illustrated by using the example of a cake. Basically, cakes all have a core of similar ingredients: eggs, flour, sugar, milk, and shortening. By making variations in these ingredients, a variety of cakes can be baked that taste different, look different in appearance, and, in fact, are different. By adding some new ingredients, such as chocolate, to the cake batter or icing, a different kind of cake is created. This analogy is akin to what happens when community mental health nursing uses concepts from other mental health disciplines and basic sciences. When the special concepts of nursing theory and research are added to this mix something special is created: a unique conceptual base for the practice of community mental health nursing (Leininger, 1980).

An experience common to community mental health nurses is an observation by mental health professionals from other disciplines that the clinical process of assessments and therapeutic functions generated by community mental health nurses are somehow different. And they are. A comparative analysis of clinical data collected over several years from nurses and other mental health professionals and from personal observations shows differences in the clinical process (Koldjeski, 1974). These data revealed that nurses performed the following:

1. Used a holistic orientation for collection and evaluation of data that covered multiple aspects of a person's life and included personal, interpersonal, physical, social, cultural, familial, and psychological experiences.

2. Investigated interrelationships between physical, mental, and emotional health in greater depth and covered a wider range of possibilities than nonmedical mental health professionals.

3. Integrated immediately assessment data and used cues generated from the ongoing interaction process to branch out to consider different kinds of information and relationships that otherwise might not have been considered.

4. Conveyed a more expressive, warm, and empathic use of self in the interaction process.

5. Assumed an active role with clients and families in the clinical process and shared with them the possibility for problem identification, problem solving, and goal setting.

6. Recognized that clients and families identified with the nursing role because they shared intimate personal data that was part of the presenting emotional and mental problem.

7. Established a sense of trust and confidence with clients and families that indicated that the nurse therapist was really concerned about them and was available.*

---

* Helen D. Koldjeski. *Unique Characteristics of Clinical Nursing Practice in Community Mental Health Nursing.* Unpublished working paper. Greenville, NC: East Carolina University, 1974.

Although it was possible to analyze and identify these distinctive aspects, the community mental health nurses themselves were usually not able to identify what made their clinical practice different. However, most of the nurses interviewed thought that such differences existed.

The conceptual bases of mental health and mental illness are consolidated in a common core of knowledge and practice used by many mental health professionals. This core includes theories of psychopathology, psychodynamics of the personality, behavior, and other theories of mental functioning. Basic intervention modalities include individual, group, and family therapies, behavior modification, and crisis intervention. These theoretical bases and the techniques for applying such strategies are mastered and used by people with quite diverse professional and educational backgrounds. However, nonmedical mental health professionals do not have the special and unique knowledge, skills, and perspectives that are needed to assess and manage the complex social, organizational, and psychophysiological health and mental health problems that are experienced by clients and families and the factors that promote and maintain positive mental health. This health–mental health linkage is important because it relates the total health experience of people. Community mental health nurses must more clearly emphasize these aspects of the mental health care they provide.

Intervention strategies in community mental health nursing primarily address (1) promotion of mental health of well populations, (2) primary prevention activities of populations at risk, and (3) secondary prevention activities with families and other primary groups in family, community, social, employment, and school settings who experience stress and adaptation problems in daily living activities.

Strategies that address the promotion of mental health of well populations at the present time are the most difficult for the community mental health nurse to undertake. There are few, if any, mental health systems that have organized programs assigned to address the mental health of well populations by working with small groups and middle level organizations to change systems or to make selected ones more effective in promoting and maintaining the mental health of people.

Typically, community mental health centers have provided prevention services such as case consultation to other health professionals, program consultation to educational systems, and health education relating to mental health. An example of the latter is the list of warning symptoms of emotional and mental health problems that have been disseminated to the general public.

Mental health promotion of well populations has often been conceived on a grand scale, that is, programs have been designed to reach large population groups over regional, state, and national levels. Evaluations of the effectiveness of such programs by measuring the incidence and prevalence of mental illness at different points in time have been attempted. However, it has been difficult to determine their effectiveness. This approach is based on epidemiologic principles of prevention pioneered in public health. This type of prevention model has been difficult to apply in mental health because the causes of mental illness are too diverse to define, and it does not address social, cultural, and situational components of emotional and mental problems (Shamansky & Clausen, 1980).

Community mental health nursing based on a nursing and social psychological model addresses mental health promotion from a different perspective. Mental health promotion includes various kinds of activities related to mental health education and prevention counseling in direct interactions with concerned groups. A major activity is to teach families and groups how to identify characteristic patterns of interactions and to assess the impact of these on the adults and children who spend much of their time in

these groups. Families need to be taught what positive mental health is, crisis intervention strategies, and applications of change theories in order to have alternative ways
to bring about changes in patterns of adaptations and resolution of role conflicts. Responses to stress must be made real for people by showing them their behavior on
television or by using kinds of audiovisual media, role modeling, or simulations. Families can learn to identify the coping strategies they use to handle recurring stressful
situations. Members can learn to participate in identifying the way in which coping
patterns affect their concept of self and feelings toward other members (Santopietro &
Rozendal, 1975). It also involves teaching people alternative approaches for coping and
relating to others in less stressful ways than those they are using. The promotion of
mental health helps to remove some of the mystique about basic human relationships
and facilitates an understanding of using knowledge in ways such that people learn to
help themselves and others.

Primary prevention activities are defensive efforts used with targeted population
groups who are already at some risk of mental or emotional problems because of some
particular set of circumstances. Such activities are easier to implement than health
promotion activities because targeted populations at risk are usually known to social
and human welfare agencies. The concept of targeted population groups orients the
community mental health nurse to identify the kinds of life experiences that put members
at risk (Burgess & Lazare, 1976). It also helps to establish boundaries about significant
group memberships (Surgeon General's Report, 1979, 1980).

Prevention counseling is an important activity in community mental health nursing
and is quite effective in family and peer groups. An example is counseling with groups
of people who are anticipating retirement to prevent postretirement role conflict, depression, and an increase in drug use, particularly sleeping pills. In counseling, major relationships are examined, particularly those that relate to the retiree and her or his
spouse, peers, and significant others. Anticipatory guidance is provided to understand
some of the things that are going to happen as disruption or cessation of work relationships occur when a person retires. New roles and relationships have to be established and these usually change existing roles and functions in the home. Such changes
can cause severe stress in the close relationships that the newly retired person has with
others. For example, the newly retired businessman may decide to use his organizational
know-how and talents to reorganize the way in which his wife manages the housework
and cooking. Such reorganization can reach the point where there is role reversal with
the husband taking on both housewifery and chef roles. In this process, the man res-
tructures his expectations about his wife's role while she undergoes a dislocation process that disenfranchises her from usual roles and satisfactions. The outcome of such
changes, unless directed in constructive ways, causes considerable stress for the wife,
for the husband in carrying out the activities he has assumed, and for peers and friends
who find the situation both amusing and confusing.

> *Principle 2: Social settings and situational contexts in which families,
> groups, and members experience the stresses and problems of daily
> living must be considered in terms of their potential for the promotion
> of mental health and prevention of mental illness.*

Social settings are the specific social contexts in which behavior occurs and where there
are interrelated roles, positions, and statuses for the people in roles. For example, some

of the roles, positions, and statuses attached to the role of mother, father, son, and daughter have specific relationships and meanings in the context of family systems. But when these roles are applied in other social settings, they change considerably in their meanings. The role of baby in a family is usually accorded to the youngest child. When the role of baby is applied to a woman in a love relationship, it takes on quite a different meaning because the role of lover, social setting, and situation have all changed, thus changing the role of "baby." Specific roles have to be considered in particular contexts that influence the sequences of interactions occurring between people occupying the roles. In such situations, both content and process of interactions have to be considered (Lennard & Bernstein, 1969).

Situational contexts represent the immediate events that impinge on people in specific social settings. The nature of such events and the influence they have on behavior are quite variable. It is this uncertainty about events that makes such contexts an important factor in their own right if a sense of their special contributions to behavior is to be obtained. For example, Fillenbaum (1979) found that residents in institutional settings are less able to assess their own health status than residents in community settings. He thinks that this difference is due to the situational context, which gives different meanings to the criteria of health.

The social contexts in which behavior takes place have considerable influence on the meanings given to behavior (Mischler, 1979). Mischler questioned whether there is any meaning to experiences other than in contexts. He stated that science has not yet discovered universal laws of behavior that operate irrespective of the contexts in which such behavior occurs. Human action can be understood only within its own context of socially grounded rules for defining, categorizing, and interpreting the meaning of conduct.

Mischler (1979) also described a process which he calls "context-stripping," which is based on the assumption that the contexts in which behavior occur are unrelated to the behavior and the meanings given to it. Bronfenbrenner (1977) compared different research studies in developmental psychology and found that many findings on cognitive and social development were in fact context specific. This finding has raised questions about the generality of much research in this and other areas of study.

The consideration of contexts in which behavior occurs is very important for community mental health nursing. There is a considerable body of research in mental health on the influence of situational contexts on behavior, yet all too often it is not used in clinical practice in mental health services that are community-based. For example, one of the seminal pieces of research in mental health is the work of Tudor (1952), who showed that staff and patient interactions mutually influence the emergence and use of particular behaviors by patients in mental hospital ward settings. Comparative studies of parent–child interactions in laboratory settings have shown that substantial and systematic differences occur between these contrived experiences and experiences observed in natural settings in the home (Bronfenbrenner, 1977). In community mental health nursing, it is necessary to observe and assess group and family interactions in both natural community and organized health care settings.

The family is an important social setting because it is where the young begin learning attitudes, social roles, and rules of behavior. It is in this milieu that the young child learns how to cope with the social processes of competition, cooperation, respect for authority, use of discipline, and ways to master aspects of the environment. In this setting basic interpersonal processes are experienced and learned in dynamic contexts. A person comes to know what love and respect for others means. Interactions and feedback from family members help each member develop a sense of individuality and self-identity. Through patterns of interactions within the family and between its members, adaptation processes and coping patterns are learned. These coping patterns help families as a group and each member to learn to cope and manage in often stressful and ambiguous situations.

Social groups function in the context of daily living and have a degree of stability and constancy. However, not all systems in which people spend a lot of time exert the same kind and amount of influence on daily relationships and efforts to cope and adapt. For example, the family system exerts more influence on toddlers and very young children about the kinds of behaviors they learn and their meanings than school or peer groups. By the time the teenage years are reached, the influence of the family on the adoption and use of norms, standards, and rules of behavior by young adolescent members is likely to be considerably less. Peer group systems tend to become major reference groups for teenagers. These groups are very influential and powerful in their ability to socialize members to adopt standards and kinds of behavior, some of which are usually in conflict with parental values.

Social settings and situational contexts have a considerable influence on people's behavior by the way they are organized and structured. The following case history illustrates this point as well as the potential for learning both nondeviant and deviant behavior.

Case History

A former mental patient was discharged from a large state mental hospital where he had been a patient for the past 10 years. His new residence was a rooming house for transients. The social organization of this milieu influenced the pattern of daily living activities and interpersonal relationships of the new resident in several ways. First, the resident had to be responsible for his personal care and make arrangements for securing food and other basic necessities. Some arrangements had been made for hot meals but the resident had to assume responsibility for presenting himself to the proper place at mealtimes. When human contacts and communications were established and maintained, some efforts had to be made by him to meet other people. In order for this resident to use social and community resources, he had to organize his activities and efforts to make contacts and attend to necessary procedures.

Contrast the above milieu and its expectations about behavior with a ward milieu in a mental hospital in which this resident lived for many years as a mental patient. In this special social setting, ward routines revolved around daily living activities that were long ago established to permit the expedient management of large groups of patients. Patients had little or nothing to say about such routines. Interpersonal contacts between nurses and patients in this ward milieu might be initiated by the patient, but if they were not, the staff arranged for interpersonal contacts. Opportunities for social interventions were scheduled as were other aspects of living. Consequently the mental patient had little choice, responsibility, and control over the daily events in which he was expected to participate.

What is different about these settings is that in natural social settings, an individual is expected to assume responsibility for activities of daily interpersonal and social living. The satisfying of basic needs and the obtaining of human companionship are powerful motivating factors. When a person will not or cannot assume these responsibilities, it is likely that she or he will be returned to a total institution or be placed in a more sheltered and protective milieu where many of the aspects of his or her life are decided by others.

In social settings, the interactions of families and members are shaped by the stresses of daily living, the strengths of the family, its organization, and the resources available. Values and beliefs help in the process, including those held about mental health and mental illness. Beliefs may include stereotypes as they are pervasive in our society and incorporated in our belief systems so easily that most of us are unaware of how much they influence our evaluations and expectations about what is mental health and mental illness behavior. For example, Olmsted and Durham (1976) studied the stability of attitudes toward mental health and found these similar to ones reported two decades earlier. The college students and members of the public participating in the survey had perceptions and attitudes about mental health and illness arising from a common social and cultural belief system.

Both mental health and mental illness are known to have social, situational, and cultural components as well as psychological and physical ones. Although there is little agreement among mental health professionals about the relative importance of such factors, they do need to be explicitly considered in community mental health nursing practice. A focus on the problems of individuals in their psychological dimensions lessens the likelihood that social settings and contexts are adequately considered in either preventions or interventions in mental health.

> *Principle 3: Community mental health nursing uses a holistic approach that relates the concept of wholeness to life experiences.*

Holism is a perspective that looks at the wholeness of experiences of individuals, the social groups in which they are members, and situational contexts. This view contrasts with a perspective that selects one or two components of the total human experience to focus on when addressing the mental health of families and individuals. Social, psychological, and cultural factors influencing the interactions of individuals in social settings and situational contexts are an integral aspect of this perspective. These factors are sometimes in harmony and sometimes in conflict when different levels of social systems interact. Holism involves trying to understand and identify what the whole experience is and how it influences the growth, development, and mental health of people.

For the community mental health nurse, a holistic perspective can be a special way of looking at people in interaction in groups in their natural environments. This perspective orients one to look for a wholeness to organization of relationships and interacting sequences and patterns. Each component cannot be handled separately and then "added up" to make a whole. However, if this is done, the nurse uses an assumption that the individual and the milieu are a sum total of separate parts, an assumption not consistent with a holistic perspective. Holism holds that all the interacting component parts are *more than* the sum total of the parts. In clinical practice, the nurse finds that incongruent and conflicting information does not always fit together to make a whole, but the search for connections and interrelationships is essential. In this process, the nurse often discovers that information can be obtained by asking different questions and exploring different avenues. With additional and new information, more coherent patterns of experiences are identified. Ellis (1968) noted that holism requires one to be concerned with any factor, be it physiological, racial, or any other, that affects a patient's health, and these factors must be treated in combination—not isolation.

The holistic perspective differs in respects other than consideration of the wholeness of experiences as compared to fragments of experiences. It differs from the traditional view of a mind and body dichotomy that has been a major factor in the organization of most of medical, psychiatric, and nursing services in this country. In psychiatry, a dominant view of human behavior emphasizes psychodynamic forces above all others. Emotional and mental illness are supposed to be caused by conflicts within the personality structure of the individual. Such conflicts are assumed to be ever-present between the unconscious (id), the conscious (ego), and the conscience (superego) aspects of the personality and generate intrapsychic tensions that become the major determinants of behavior. Although social and cultural influences have long been recognized as factors in mental behavior, the belief that an individual's behavior can be determined in large part by external influences runs counter to the dominant psychodynamic theories of behavior. These theories rely heavily on the belief that early childhood psychosexual traumas, which have been repressed in the unconscious, are the main determinants of behavior.

In contrast to a holistic approach, Heine (1972) described the approach that has been used in the development of psychology as a discipline. He noted that virtually from its inception as an empirical science, psychology has dispersed its investigative efforts over a wide range of small specialized areas of inquiry. These efforts include intense work on learning, cognition, motivation, perspection, sensation, and other standard problems in psychology. Such studies have been undertaken to illuminate some subassembly of the human species as a laboratory animal rather than to explain the behavior of the human functioning in natural and social environments. Heine concluded that psychology is a sprawling marketplace comprising boutiques of every shape and size.

> *Principle 4:* Community mental health nursing provides a special kind of mental health care because the social and professional roles of the nurse converge to make possible a mix of humanistic and caring relationships and scientific approaches.

Social and professional roles of the community mental health nurse provide access to and grant the privilege of participating in a broad range of human concerns relating to health and illness. These roles make it possible to provide nursing and health care to people with a wide variety of social, personal, psychological, and physical conditions that are inimical to the growth, development, and actualization of the human potential. Nurses are situated in direct care roles in all health care services and systems. Their presence and accessibility to clients, families, and group systems make nurses the key group of professionals who provide compassionate and humanistic caring and application of scientific knowledge.

In community mental health, in interpersonal, family, and group models of therapy, the therapist's role usually has special behaviors that place personal and social distance between the therapist and the clients or groups seeking help. It is not unusual for therapists to try to maintain a more or less neutral role in the therapeutic process. The norm in the therapists' behavior is to be rational and objective in the therapeutic use of self. To some extent, these models have aspects that are inconsistent with the caring, expressive, and humanistic concerns that are at the heart of nursing. The community mental health nurse needs to recognize that these models and related therapeutic strategies minimize or suppress many of the caring aspects of nursing. Yet, these are the aspects of relationships that human beings need in both wellness and sickness. A major role of nursing is to address the humanistic needs of the people requiring professional health care services.

Humanism holds that every individual possesses both dignity and freedom and has the right to have respect from others and a chance to develop individuality. The effort to achieve these rights is always in the context of the often coercive and opposing forces in society. The well-known dehumanization of health care systems has taken a toll on the respect and dignity of individuals and families who use such services. The professional nurse, who is often the first health care professional to see the client and provide health care, sets a standard and a model for seeing that humanistic concerns are an integral part of mental health care.

Humanism is for everyone and that includes the nurse. Just as the client, families, and group members deserve respect, dignity, and the exercise of basic rights, so does the nurse. In some situations, nurses may have to become assertive about their rights, but if they allow themselves to be dehumanized, then it is difficult for them to address the humanistic concerns of others.

In community mental health nursing a judicious mix of humanistic concerns and scientific principles in the delivery of mental health care has an added significance. Thompson (1980) described the role of the nurse as a synergist who uses humanism and scientism as the basis for clinical practice, participation in health planning and policy making, and activation of system change. Such a role is essential because of the complexity of the myriad factors involved in mental health. The mental health of individuals and the social groups in which they live, work, and play takes place in natural living environments. Individuals, families, and peer groups function even when under stress and try to adapt to both stressful and nonstressful aspects of their natural physical and social environments. In providing services, the nurse is able to observe and bring together personal, interpersonal, and social aspects of mental health care so that clients and patients are not dehumanized and are provided quality professional health care.

> *Principle 5: The concept of community in community mental health nursing means that targeted populations and social and community networks are a primary concern.*

Community mental health is conceptualized in a general sense as the mental wellness of targeted population groups in a particular community. Social and community networks are an integral aspect of the community and link its people.

Unfortunately, the development of community mental health programs has not always reflected the concept of mental health for populations. Mental health services have for the most part focused on treatment of individuals who are emotionally upset or mentally ill. Promoting and maintaining the mental health of targeted groups or populations has not been an emphasis. Instead of finding new and more effective ways of assessing, evaluating, and changing the social environments and minimizing adverse factors that directly and indirectly affect the mental health of citizens in a designated area, most community mental health professionals provide services within the mental health service center's walls and focus on changing the behavior of individuals who voluntarily ask for services or are referred by service agencies or other professionals.

The lack of clarity about what is meant by a *community's mental health* is evident in the ways in which it has been defined in community mental health nursing (Evans, 1976; Burgess & Lazare, 1976; Grace, Layton & Camilleri, 1981; ANA. 1966). One way in which the community aspect of community mental health nursing has been described is in the most recent *Statement on Psychiatric and Mental Health Nursing* (ANA, 1976). It described settings and arrangements for practice and identified setting as "more than the physical surroundings and makeup of the clinical facility. This implies that there is an aggregate of both the physical arrangements and those philosophical influences that give the practice environment special character. The sum total consists of the emotional climate, ideology, conventions or governance, finances, and purposes, whether planned or implicit."

The concept of community in mental health needs to be defined in its own right. There are a number of ways in which this may be approached. One way is to map out basic indicators, networks, and resources essential for a quality of life conducive to good mental health of the citizens. Social networks linking citizens into key support groups are a part of the community. Patterns and trends of relationships in a community and with related communities can be identified. These are not readily apparent when the focus is on an individual or even one family in a case-by-case context. Other indices of community mental health are demographic data involving health and illness patterns. Unusual as well as usual behavioral and coping styles of citizens in cultural and sub-cultural settings may be examined. The impact of social and economic policies on the lives of citizens in a community may also be used to consider the community's potential for fostering the mental health of its residents.

A major use of information from demographic and epidemiologic sources is to identify populations at risk. Such high-risk groups are prime targets for prevention activities. These include such activities as consultation and liaison activities to community groups and organizations. Leadership may need to be provided by the nurse to highlight social and community changes needed to make a community more responsive to the mental health needs of citizens.

> *Principle 6: Community mental health nursing focuses on interrelationships formed in group contexts as people interact in daily living activities.*

A distinctive aspect of community mental health nursing is that it focuses on *something more* than the problems of an individual. The "something more" includes the interactions generated between the social units in which an individual holds membership and the many factors that influence coping and adapting in daily living. It includes in these interactions a host of sociocultural factors and attitudes about self, family, mental health, mental illness, authority, and one's place in the world of his or her community. The dreams, aspirations, and economic factors that facilitate or hinder a family and its members in achieving their goals are important.

In trying to determine interrelationships between people and their community, the nurse seeks to find answers to questions such as the kinds of social networks of kith and kin individuals and families have to rely on for emotional and other kinds of support; dominant values and attitudes a family holds about the worth and value of each one of its members; and roles and responsibilities family members have been socialized to accept. These and other realities of family, group, and community life contribute to the mental health of people and of community.

A major contribution of community mental health has been to identify social and cultural aspects of mental health and mental illness. This emphasis has led to an increase in both research and theory development from a variety of perspectives. It has had the effect of helping to expand the scope of nursing practice in community mental health nursing from the traditional focus on the nurse–patient dyad model to a focus on small social systems in action, such as families and groups in community and organizational contexts.

It is recognized that social milieus, or environments, in which human beings live and work contribute to the promotion and maintenance of mental health as well to the incidence and prevalence of mental illness. What is not clearly understood is why or how given factors in a particular milieu operate in a noxious way for a particular family or member. The importance of being concerned about systems in interaction cannot be overstated in community mental health. It is difficult for families and individuals who have been able to make desired changes in behavior through counseling or other therapeutic activities to maintain such behavior if the major systems in which they live and work continue to operate in the usual manner and support the resumption and retention of less adaptive behaviors.

Consultation to middle-level organizations and agencies about the impact of their services on the mental health of clients and families continues to be needed. Too often, mental health workers assume that needed services, when provided, are sufficient in and of themselves, and they do not overly concern themselves with the social consequences services may have on clients. These consequences may be so emotionally stressful for clients that the ability of the family and its members to cope is strained. A case history is cited to show some of these strains for one family.

Case History

The client was a 20-year-old man, with a large body build, unkempt appearance, and surly manner. This young man lived with his mother, a widow of many years, in a small farming community. He had entered college the previous fall. At college, the client undertook a heavy course of study in the hope of completing work in three years. He also worked part-time in the college library. Co-workers in the library began to notice around Easter that the young man talked to himself, hid in the stacks, and argued with students about borrowing books. After several disruptive episodes with students, college officials requested that the young man see a psychiatrist. After examination, the psychiatrist diagnosed the young man as suffering from schizophrenia and recommended that he be sent home to his family. This action was taken. The mother made an appointment for her son to see someone at the mental health center. She drove her son and accompanied him inside. The son seemed remote, uncommunicative, and placed himself in a chair well away from everyone, including his mother. The mother told the mental health professional that she was afraid of her son and had a difficult time getting him to come for the appointment.

In the initial interview, as information was provided about the family, the mother got the distinct impression that she was being blamed for her son's illness. By the time she had been interviewed by several different people, this impression became even stronger. When one of the professionals informed the mother that she probably needed therapy as well as her son, the mother began to feel anxious and did not understand what was happening to either herself or her son. As the mother and son left the mental health center, the mother was informed that someone would come to the home to assess the family situation.

In due time, after assessments of various kinds were conducted, the mother was informed that the mental health center recommended that her son be referred to a day care rehabilitation center and that she enter therapy.

Meanwhile, back in the small town in which the family lived, it became gossip that mother and son were both having major mental health problems. This information was conveyed to the mother by a neighbor who had seen the worker from the community mental health center visit the home. When the mother returned to the mental health center for the next appointment, she was angry and concerned about what had happened to her and her son since first seeking help. She told the therapist about her experiences and feelings toward the staff. She stated that she felt that the staff blamed her for her son's problems and she was concerned about how to handle changes in relationships that were occurring with her neighbors and friends. The therapist did not help the mother examine these issues and she left quite anxious, angry, and frustrated.

The outcome of this experience was that the mother sought private psychiatric care for her son. She was invited to join a group of parents who had children with emotional and mental health problems. Her participation in this group was a major learning experience. The experiences and relationships these parents had in the community with friends and strangers helped the mother handle her own relationships in more positive ways. Before the year was over, the son had returned to college and was doing well.

Without making judgments on the quality and appropriateness of the mental health care provided, the case history is an example of professionals providing mental health services and failing to acknowledge interrelationships between the family and the community. The impact of seeking mental health services in a small community can have many unanticipated consequences, some of which can be minimized if not avoided. A major problem in this case was the lack of awareness by the staff that mental health services to clients and families are simply not discrete activities delivered in a social vacuum.

Six principles of community mental health nursing as an applied professional practice discipline have been presented. These principles relate to the organization of the clinical or nursing process, substantive content, and directions of mental health care for community mental health nursing. They may be used to structure the application of preventions and interventions to clients.

ROLE OF THE NURSE GENERALIST

The nurse generalist is the first-level professional practitioner in nursing. This means that in community mental health nursing, the nurse is expected to be able to manage with competency and efficiency many of the stresses and traumas experienced by families and their members in the process of daily living. Daily living events create the need for various kinds of coping responsibilities on the part of families, groups, and individuals. These patterns of coping may develop in productive and growth-promoting ways or in destructive ones.

It is not anticipated by manpower planners that there will ever be enough mental health specialists in this country to provide adequate mental health care and services to people who need help managing emotional and mental health problems. At the same time, it is now recognized that a great many such problems do not need the attention of mental health specialists. This means that the generalist professional nurse practicing in mental health needs to have certain basic competencies and certain kinds of knowledge bases, and must be able to provide particular kinds of prevention and intervention strategies. Moreover, it is crucial that the professional nurse generalist be able to assess mental health as well as mental problems with considerable accuracy in order to refer promptly and appropriately those persons who require the skills and knowledge of a mental health specialist.

Nurse generalists are the most widely placed professionals in the health care system. They provide both physical and mental health care. In this respect, they have to be able to conduct comprehensive community mental health assessments, make clinical decisions based on data, and provide certain kinds of therapeutic interventions (Koldjeski, 1978). Such assessments include but go beyond the traditional mental status examination to cover the community, social, cultural, and organizational aspects of daily living. There needs to be an examination of coping patterns and a determination of whether they are effective and under what conditions. Nurse generalists sort and synthesize a set of complex interacting factors that are of particular importance to a current situation for particular families and individuals.

Community mental health nursing provides opportunities for the nurse in mental health to function in preventions, interventions, and rehabilitation activities. For example, a strategic population group is aftercare patients—those patients discharged from mental hospitals. Alternative community placements in homes and other domiciliary arrangements for this group of citizens have yet to be developed to any extent in most communities. Therefore, the nurse in community mental health nursing is the logical professional to monitor the health status, to make referrals when needed, to provide social and psychological support and counseling as necessary, and to serve as the constant health professional during acute crises as well as during rehabilitation activities.

ROLE OF THE CLINICAL NURSE SPECIALIST

In community mental health nursing, the clinical nurse specialist provides mental health care and services through the use of specialized knowledge and strategies. These advanced, prepared specialists provide direct services to clients and patients, serve in consultant and liaison roles to nurses and other professional and citizen groups, and serve as educators, administrators, and supervisors. An important function is to serve as a patient-care consultant to the generalist nurse and be available for referrals of patients or clients who experience emotional or mental health problems that need a level of expertise beyond the knowledge and competency of the generalist professional nurse.

A considerable amount of energy has been expended by educators and clinicians in community mental health nursing to become competent in the application of mental health treatment modalities common to the field. Clinical specialization in community mental health nursing has now developed to the point where attention can be focused on testing clinical applications using different conceptual frameworks. In this process, new roles will evolve, such as the primary mental health nurse (Koldjeski, 1979, 1980). This task is increasingly important because the clinical specialist in community mental health nursing has to justify third-party payments and other financial arrangements in terms of the effectiveness of therapeutic interventions *as a nurse* rather than as a generalist mental health worker. The relationship between generalization and specialization has recently been discussed in a social policy statement (ANA, 1980).

Up to now, it has been difficult to legitimize the role of the clinical specialist nurse for the public, third-party reimbursers, and other mental health professionals (Woodrow & Bell, 1979; Barrett, 1979). Clinical specialists in community mental health nursing have to convey more clearly to the public and other interested parties the unique kinds of services they provide even though they appear similar to services provided by other mental health professionals. There is a need to correct the notion that the "nursing component" of mental health is only giving medications and following medical orders. For career advancement, many clinical specialist nurses accept positions in functional roles of coordinator and director. Although significant contributions can be made in such positions, the clinical role of nursing tends to become deemphasized. Clinical specialists occupying such positions have a special responsibility to provide a milieu in which community mental health nursing can be practiced to its fullest potential and to develop new nursing models.

One example of such potential is the model of the community nursing care for chronic psychiatric patients proposed by Krauss (1980). A network of services is identified that consists of five basic functions: (1) maintaining a stable level of adjustment; (2) meeting the patient's dependency needs; (3) assisting the patient to cope with crisis; (4) providing social and vocational rehabilitation opportunities; and (5) coordinating all networks. All these functions have been provided in community settings in one way or another for many years. What is different about this model is that it identifies a role for the community mental health nurse as a coordinator of the health and mental health care components in order to integrate these in ways that provide the kind and variety of services a person needs.

It has been difficult to develop models of community mental health nursing in the community mental health center setting. One factor that has contributed to this difficulty has been the limited role-sets held by mental health professionals and by nurses themselves about role expansions. Another factor has been the emphasis on all mental health professionals using a core of general therapeutic modalities and this has promoted diffusion and blurring of roles. In fact, this emphasis has often produced considerable role confusion. Distinctions in role and functions of different mental health professionals have been downgraded and minimized community mental health service settings. Nursing should be very much aware of the implications the generic model has on its scope of practice and the nature of its practice. If nursing is to achieve and demonstrate its potential in mental health, a more comprehensive model that includes the *community and unique aspects of nursing* must be emphasized in both nursing education and clinical practice. The clinical specialist is the key person to spearhead this advancement in community mental health nursing.

SUMMARY

Community mental health nursing as a practice area is different from mental health and psychiatric nursing. These differences relate to populations to which mental health services are provided, settings in which services are delivered, focus of clinical nursing practice, major orientation of interventions, models of mental health or mental illness, adoption of the sick role, and the clinical nursing process.

Community mental health nursing emphasizes the interactional effects of social, cultural, psychological, physical, and situational factors on mental health. These effects are considered in the contexts of family and other small group systems. Family systems are especially important because they are primary socialization systems that are intense learning environments and what is learned and how it is used have a direct relationship to positive mental health and to development of mental and emotional problems.

Social organizations are important settings for human interaction. As such, these may be organized in levels in order to have a framework to guide clinical applications in community mental health nursing. Families and other kinds of primary groups, at the small-group level of organization, are behavior settings in which clinical preventions and interventions may be directly and effectively applied to promote positive mental health.

Principles of community mental health nursing identify the multiple dimensions of living that are involved in clinical practice. The contributions of the nurse generalist and the nurse specialist complement each other by providing distinct aspects of professional nursing care.

REFERENCES

American Nurses' Association, Congress for Nursing Practice. *Nursing: A Social Policy Statement.* Kansas City, MO: American Nurses' Association, 1982.

American Nurses' Association, Division on Psychiatric and Mental Health Nursing. *Statement on Psychiatric and Mental Health Nursing Practice.* Kansas City, MO: American Nurses' Association, 1976, p. 7.

American Nurses' Association, Division of Psychiatric and Mental Health Nursing Practice. *Statement on Psychiatric and Mental Health Nursing Practice.* Kansas City, MO: American Nurses' Association, 1966, pp. 5–6.

Barrett, Jean. Administrative factors in development of new nursing practice roles. *Nursing Digest* 6(4):27–31, Winter, 1979.

Bronfenbrenner, Urie. Toward an experimental ecology of human development. *American Psychologist* 32:513–531, 1977.

Burgess, Ann W. *Psychiatric Nursing in the Hospital and the Community,* 3rd ed. Englewood Cliffs, NJ: Prentice-Hall, 1981, pp. 24–36.

Burgess, Ann W., and Lazare, Aaron. *Community Mental Health: Target Populations.* Englewood Cliffs, NJ: Prentice-Hall, 1976, pp. 93–272.

Burgess, Ann W., and Lazare, Aaron. *Psychiatric Nursing in the Hospital and Community,* 2nd ed. Englewood Cliffs, NJ: Prentice-Hall, 1978, p. 510.

Deloughery, Grace W., Gebbie, Kristine M., and Newman, Betty. *Community Mental Health Nursing.* Baltimore: Williams & Wilkins Company, 1971, pp. 17–36.

Ellis, Rosemary. Characteristics of significant theories. *Nursing Research* 17:217–222, 1968.

Evans, Frances M. Carter. *Psychosocial Nursing.* New York: The Macmillan Company, 1976, pp. 124–125.

Fillenbaum, G. G. Social context and self-assessments of health among the elderly. *Journal of Health and Social Behavior* 20:45–51, March, 1979.

Grace, Helen K., Layton, Janice, and Camilleri, Dorothy. *Mental Health Nursing: A Socio-Psychological Approach,* 2nd ed. Dubuque, IA: Wm. C. Brown Company, 1981, chapters 1–4.

Hanlon, John. An ecologic view of public health. *American Journal of Public Health* 59:4–10, 1969.

Healthy People. Surgeon General's Report. Washington, DC: Department of Health and Human Services, 1979.

Heine, Ralph W. Foreword. In Maddi, Salvatore, and Costa, Paul, eds. *Humanism in Personality.* N.Y.: Aldine-Atherton, 1972.

Kalkman, Marion E., and Davis, Anne J. *New Dimensions in Mental Health-Psychiatric Nursing,* 5th ed. New York: McGraw-Hill Book Company, 1976, pp. 11–26.

Koldjeski, Dixie. Primary health care nursing: The psychosocial component. In Burgess, Ann, ed. *Psychiatric Nursing in the Hospital and the Community.* Englewood Cliffs, NJ: Prentice-Hall, 1981, pp. 637–647.

Koldjeski, Dixie. Primary care and future directions. Presented at *Perspectives in Psychiatric Care for the 80's,* Philadelphia, May, 1980. Audiotapes available from Concepts, Inc., Wakefield, MA.

Koldjeski, Dixie. Mental health and psychiatric nursing and primary health care: Issues and prospects. *Proceedings of the Fourth National Conference on Graduate Education in Psychiatric and Mental Health Nursing.* Kansas City, MO: American Nurses' Association, Division of Psychiatric and Mental Health Nursing Practice, 1979, pp. 30–34.

Koldjeski, Dixie. *Primary Care and the Psychiatric Mental Health Nurse.* Keynote address of workshop given by American Nurses' Association Division on Psychiatric and Mental Health Nursing Practice, Pittsburg, October, 1978. Kansas City, MO: American Nurses' Association, 1978.

Koldjeski, Dixie. The mental health role of the primary health care nurse. *Journal of Clinical Child Psychology* 7(1):37–39, Spring, 1978.

Krauss, Judith. The chronic psychiatric patient in the community—A model of care. *Nursing Outlook* 28:308–314, 1980.

Kuntz, Sandra, Stehle, Joan, and Marshall, Ruth. The psychiatric nurse specialist. *Perspectives in Psychiatric Care* 18:90–92, March–April, 1980.

Lancaster, Jeanette. An ecological perspective in community mental health nursing. In Lancaster, Jeanette, ed. *Community Mental Health Nursing: An Ecological Perspective.* St. Louis: C. V. Mosby Co., 1980, p. 10.

Leininger, Madeleine. Caring: A central focus of nusing and health care services. *Nursing and Health Care* 1:135–143, October, 1980.

Lennard, Henry L., and Bernstein, Arnold. *Patterns in Human Interaction.* San Francisco: Josey-Bass, Inc., 1969, pp. 8–40.

Mereness, Dorothy, and Taylor, Cecilia. *Essentials of Psychiatric Nursing,* 10th ed. St. Louis: C. V. Mosby Co., 1978, pp. 6–7, 489–490.

Mischler, Elliot G. Meaning in context: Is there any other kind? *Harvard Educational Review* 49:1–19, February, 1979.

Moos, Ralph. *The Human Context: Environmental Determinants of Behavior.* New York: John Wiley & Sons, Inc., 1976, chapters 1–5.

Mullen, Edward J., Dumpson, James R., et al. *Evaluation of Social Intervention.* San Francisco, Josey-Bass, Inc., 1972, chapters 1 and 3.

Olmsted, Donald W., and Durham, Katherine. Stability of mental health attitudes: A semantic differential study. *Journal of Health and Human Behavior* 17:35–44, 1976.

Osborne, Oliver. A theoretical basis for the education of the psychiatric-mental health nurse. *Nursing Clinics of North America* 5:699–712, 1970.

Peplau, Hildegard. *Interpersonal Relations in Nursing.* New York: G. P. Putnam, 1952, pp. 43–70.

Promoting Health, Preventing Disease. Washington, DC: Department of Health and Human Services, 1980.

Putt, Arlene. Living systems in interlocking hierarchy. In Putt, Arelen, ed. *General Systems Theory Applied to Nursing.* Boston: Little, Brown, & Company, 1978, pp. 17–18.

Santopietro, Mary Charles, and Rozendal, Nancy A. Teaching primary prevention in mental health. *Nursing Outlook* 23:774–779, 1975.

Shamansky, Sherry I. and Clausen, Cheri L. Levels of prevention: Examination of the concept. *Nursing Outlook* 28:104–108, 1980.

Steele, Katherine. *Psychiatric Nursing.* Philadelphia: F. A. Davis, 1937, p. 41.

Thompson, John D. The passionate humanist: From Nightingale to the new nurse. *Nursing Outlook* 28:290–295, 1980.

Tudor, Gwen W. A sociopsychiatric nursing approach to intervention in a problem of mutual withdrawal on a mental hospital ward. *Psychiatry* 15:192–217, 1952.

Underwood, Patricia. *Psychiatric and Mental Health Nursing Practice in the 80's: Directions for Patient Care.* Presentation at the Council of Psychiatric and Mental Health Nursing, American Nurses' Association Convention, Houston, 1980. Kansas City, MO. American Nurses' Association.

Wilson, Holly S., and Kneisl, Carol R. *Psychiatric Nursing.* Menlo Park, CA: Addison-Wesley, 1979, pp. 19–42.

Woodrow, Mary, and Bell, Judith A. Clinical specialization: Conflict between reality and theory. *Nursing Digest* 6(4):22–28, Winter, 1979.

CHAPTER 2 | COMMUNITY MENTAL HEALTH NURSING: INTERRELATIONSHIPS WITH NURSING

INTRODUCTION

The social psychological framework of community mental health nursing presented in this book integrates the unique and general concepts of nursing and the general and special concepts of mental health. Community mental health nursing is a subspecialty in nursing; thus, a large part of its conceptual and clinical practice bases is anchored in general nursing theory and practice.

Students in nursing have often expressed difficulty identifying and integrating general nursing concepts with the special concepts from mental health that form part of the conceptual basis for community mental health nursing. This difficulty may have been unintentionally increased by a focus on social, psychological, and psychiatric concepts commonly used in clinical applications in the mental health field. Such concepts and applications in clinical specialty practice have been developed for the most part independently of clinical nursing practice, and special efforts have always been necessary to interrelate nursing's distinct conceptual bases. The common conceptual base that is grounded in the psychiatric and psychological sciences and used by all mental health professionals in the management of emotional and mental health problems has been a great advantage in advancing specialized clinical practice. At the same time, emphasis on this aspect of practice has often obscured the nursing aspect of community mental health nursing.

The professional nurse generalist is expected to have mastered a core of knowledge common to a range of health and illness experiences. Clinical competencies using this knowledge include a number of basic nursing interventions that may be applied to many different kinds of emotional and mental health problems occurring in different practice settings. The application of such strategies assumes a level of competency in conducting comprehensive health and mental health nursing assessment, family and interpersonal counseling, crisis intervention, and group counseling, and the ability to analyze factors in social and organizational milieus that influence the health and mental health of people as they engage in the daily living activities of life, work, and recreation.

The knowledge base that the nurse generalist is expected to have includes concepts and principles of nursing as they relate to mental health and emotional and mental illness. This knowledge must be synthesized in ways that emphasize the unique aspects of nursing. These unique aspects are important because they characterize the constants, or universals, of clinical nursing practice. They make the roles and functions of community mental health, mental health, and psychiatric nursing different from those of other mental health professions. This is true because the synthesis of the major knowledge and experience bases from nursing, from mental health, and from the basic sciences and humanities creates a clinical practice framework and process that is different in content, purpose, dynamics, and interactional data.

The clinical process in community mental health nursing may show that concepts, rationales, and strategies for therapeutic use of the self are based more on mental health–related concepts and modalities than on nursing ones. This is easy to understand because community mental health nursing in the past has had to do a considerable amount of "interprofessional borrowing" of concepts and clinical interventions from other mental health disciplines in order to form adequate theoretical bases to support clinical nursing practice. In this process, roles and role components, role expectations, and related behaviors have also been borrowed.

The interprofessional borrowing of roles and related clinical strategies among the mental health disciplines has had an influence on the organization and delivery of community-based mental health services. On one hand, such borrowing increased the rate of development of the nation's pool of mental health manpower on the assumption that a general core of therapeutic treatment modalities could be delivered by all kinds of mental health professionals. On the other hand, this assumption over the years has had the effect of creating considerable confusion and uncertainty about roles and identity among the various mental health professionals. Community mental health nurses, like other professionals, have experienced these ambiguities. Some of these uncertainties continue to influence roles and functions in community mental health nursing today.

Extensive borrowing of theories, strategies, roles, and role models from one profession to apply in another has a number of consequences. First, there is an acceptance of these on the basis of the authority of the profession from which the borrowing occurs. A danger of this practice is that the theories, principles, generalizations, and applications of principles that are borrowed may be untested, yet come to be accepted as dogma on the basis of the authority of the discipline from which they are borrowed rather than on scientific evidence. Second, interprofessional borrowing causes confusion about professional identification of the clinicians who use the borrowed roles, strategies, and theories (Coyle, 1958).

Distinct nursing roles and functions and an identity as a nurse in community mental health can be more clearly identified and supported when they are related to the unique aspects of nursing as an integral part of the community mental health nursing process. In this respect, there is a need to interpret more clearly the roles and functions of community mental health nursing not only to community mental health nurses but also to patients, clients, employers, and other mental health professionals. The ability to describe the unique aspects of nursing and show how these make a difference in community mental health care enhances the development of professional nursing identity. These differences make possible the communication of an identity by nurses to other nurses and serve as the basis for expanded roles. These tasks are not easy but they are ones that community mental health nursing will need to address more specifically in this decade.

Burgess (1981) identified three questions that need answering in relation to the role of the psychiatric nurse: In contemporary roles, are nurses different from social workers, psychologists, or psychiatrists? Is there an "essence" to psychiatric nursing regardless of role? Should psychiatric nursing retreat to a unitary, more clearly defined role? As a profession, the answer to the first two questions is an unqualified "yes," the answer to the third one is an unqualified "no." The clinical practice of nursing in mental health *is* different from the clinical practice of other disciplines simply because of the "essence" that Burgess mentions. Part of this essence includes the unique aspects of nursing applied in community mental health nursing. At the same time, holding this belief does not mean that there is one nursing role in community mental health nursing. The adoption of a position that there is a unitary role would unduly constrain the evolution of new roles just at a time when there is a need to develop new ones that will more effectively address the quite diverse mental health needs to which nursing can make a significant contribution.

In community mental health nursing, there has been of necessity a major role transfer from other mental health disciplines. This transfer includes the shift from the more clearly defined role of the psychiatric nurse in the mental hospital to the less clearly defined role of the community mental health nurse in community-based mental health services (Davis & Pattison, 1979). There is little doubt that this role transfer has contributed to some of the difficulties experienced by nursing students and community mental health nurses in trying to clearly define their roles, functions, and self-identity in community-based mental health services.

Nursing, the key health profession, has unique aspects that are often not clearly identified in descriptions of nursing practice. These unique aspects, in concert with the professional, social, and legal aspects of nursing roles and functions, merge in clinical nursing applications in ways that influence the scope, directions, and process of nursing. Identification of the unique aspects of nursing and the influence of these on community-based mental health care will assist the nurse in developing conceptual frameworks in community mental health nursing that include these aspects.

In this chapter, some of the unique aspects of nursing are identified. They are examined in the context of community-based mental health care. If community mental health nursing is to advance its clinical practice base and roles in mental health, there is a need to understand more clearly some of the issues that have to be addressed. Several of these concern the interrelationships between the concepts of nursing and the application of these concepts in community-based mental health care. There is some urgency to this task because of current and proposed changes in relation to the delivery of mental health services in this country. Changes in the service system of community-based mental health care will have an impact on the roles and functions of both nurse generalists and nurse specialists in community mental health nursing. A change already taking place is the expectation that the nurse generalist, as the key professional in primary health care, will provide a considerable amount of mental health care to citizens in this country (Koldjeski, 1978, 1981).

THE STRUCTURE OF NURSING: UNIQUE ASPECTS OF CLINICAL NURSING PRACTICE

The structure of nursing consists of specialized knowledge and stable patterns of helping relationships. Within this structure, the independent, interdependent, dependent, and unique functions of nursing are organized and provided to individual clients, groups, and families in diverse social and institutional settings. At least five aspects of the structure of nursing contribute to the special essence that makes clinical nursing practice unique: (1) the nursing perspective; (2) the special character of the nurse–patient or nurse–client relationship; (3) the privilege of access; (4) the special mix of humanistic, scientific, and nursing concepts in the practice base of nursing; and (5) the multiple dimensions of health and illness care that are the domain of professional nursing practice.

The unique aspects of clinical nursing practice are present in all nursing roles and functions because they are universals. That is to say, they exist in nursing practice to some extent under all conditions. These unique aspects are generated in the nursing process through the application of nursing, health, mental health, and basic sciences. When synthesized, they form a framework on which preventions, interventions, and therapeutic use of self are based. The unique aspects of nursing transcend the various subspecialties of nursing practice and the settings in which nursing care is provided. That is not to say, however, that all of the unique aspects of nursing operate in every nursing situation with equal force to achieve the same outcomes. The five unique aspects of nursing that contribute to the development of a special quality of nursing care are examined.

The Nursing Perspective

The nursing perspective influences the very nature and process of nursing care. More specifically, this perspective is defined as the mental view, or picture, of the special caring process that nurses provide to people in relation to health and illness experiences as these occur in the context of daily living. The nursing perspective provides a focus to nursing process and shapes the roles and functions that define the scope of professional nursing practice. The fact that it exists indicates that there is a body of knowledge and beliefs about human relationships and human rights in relation to health and illness that nursing as a profession values and implements in clinical nursing practice.

The nursing perspective includes humanistic and caring aspects of care as well as scientific and technological bases of nursing. It orients the profession to explore different kinds of roles that nurses can use to provide health care to all people. This perspective helps nurses to focus on the kinds of questions they should ask and the answers they should seek. It guides them in the selection of specific data from all of the data available in a situation and the relationships from which to explore vital connections and patterns of interactions and modes of coping. The nursing perspective shapes the clinical hypotheses nurses formulate from nursing theory and research. This shaping, in turn, gives meaning and direction to the leads and cues nurses use to branch out to ask different kinds of questions, obtain additional data, and conduct clinical problem solving.

To a large extent, the nursing perspective structures the routine daily relationships of nurses: nurse–patient, nurse–client, nurse–family, nurse–physician, and nurse–nurse. In short, the nursing perspective orients nurses to have a special way of viewing and caring about human beings, of forming helping relationships with people in relation to health and illness experiences, and of providing essential services to individuals with respect to their dignity and rights.

The Special Character of Nurse–Client Relationships

There is a special character to nurse–client and nurse–patient relationships. This special character has several distinctions that are not evident in the professional relationships of other health professions. Society, law, and the nursing profession believe that the essential purpose of nursing is the provision of care to the ill, health promotion, primary prevention of illness, and maintenance of the health of individuals and families at the most optimal levels possible. This purpose legitimizes the nature of nurse–patient and nurse–client relationships in a number of ways. These distinctions in turn influence the scope and complexity of professional relationships in nursing practice. Five of these distinctions are identified and discussed.

Therapeutic Use of Self by Nurses

The therapeutic use of self in the conduct of nurse–patient relationships is usually diverse and flexible. The freedom to exercise diversity and flexibility is greater for nurses than that accorded other health and human services professionals.

Professional nurses have the freedom to decide how to use themselves therapeutically in different ways because of the different kinds of health and illness care problems they are presented with in the course of their nursing practice every day. Such health care problems may arise in many different kinds of settings, cover the entire age span, and range from minimal to catastrophic.

The "script" for nurse–patient and nurse–client relationships is open and interactional in nature. Nurses obtain and process data and impressions from the ongoing relationship. In these interactions, nurses may be expressive in communication and caring or more controlled in their communications and emotional involvement. Communication may be initiated with patients and clients for many reasons. This communication may range from comforting words to more collaborative problem-solving efforts.

The degree of flexibility and diversity in the therapeutic use of self accorded to nurses can be looked at another way. Other health professionals tend to have more prescribed role and relationship models that cover a narrower range of health care concerns. Communications are restricted and focus on the range of concerns that a particular profession takes to be its domain of human experiences for which it will provide special services.

Differences in the therapeutic use of self by two kinds of mental health professionals are illustrated in the following case history.

Case History

A young woman was escorted to the mental health center by a policeman who reported that she was upset and acting strangely on the street. The policeman had approached the woman and asked her if she would like to be taken to the mental health center. She indicated that she didn't care, so he took her there.

A psychologist was summoned and asked to assess the client's mental status. He stated the client was having an acute psychotic episode with disorientation and hallucinations. He recommended that the client be taken to the local emergency room where a psychiatrist could examine her because he believed she needed immediate hospitalization. When this information was provided to the young woman, she became more visibly upset. The psychologist then requested that the nurse in the clinic get a medical order for "something to quiet the patient."

The community mental health nurse approached the young woman. The nurse had the distinct impression that the client was terrified and did not understand what was happening to her. She sat down and invited the young woman to sit beside her. Speaking in a soft voice, she told the client that she was a nurse, gave her name, then asked if there was anything she could do to help. On hearing that the person sitting beside her was a nurse, the young woman looked at her closely, picked up her hand, and said, "Thank God there is somebody here that I can trust."

They sat quietly for awhile. Then the nurse asked the client if she could talk about what had happened to her on the street. The client, showing evidence of considerable anxiety, told the nurse that earlier in the day she had been to her doctor for the report of her "woman's" checkup. She had been informed by the physician that she had a suspicious Pap test reading. He had recommended consultation with another physician and told her that it was possible she might have to have a hysterectomy. The client, not understanding what all this meant, had fled the physician's office in panic. In her anxiety, she had walked the streets, begun to cry, talked to herself, and looked for someone to help her. It was this behavior that the policeman had observed and resulted in his bringing the woman to the community mental health center.

The community mental health nurse explained to the young woman what a Pap test is and what the implications of a test result such as hers might mean. The woman listened carefully. She asked several questions, then indicated that she understood more about the situation. She asked the nurse to call her physician to see if she could go back to see him. The nurse called the physician and explained to him how panic-stricken the client had become about the information that had been provided to her.

Later, the client's physician called the community mental health nurse and asked her if she could provide some follow-up counseling and support to the client. They discussed some approaches that might be considered if the client had to undergo surgery. When surgery became necessary, the nurse provided therapeutic counseling before and after the experience. The client did not experience any more panic during all the traumatic events that occurred to her. Today, she is gainfully employed in a responsible position and seems relaxed and happy.*

The role of the psychologist in providing mental health care to a client such as the one described in this case history is limited by the legal scope of the practice of psychology. Where there are major health problems interacting with emotional and mental problems, the psychologist is neither legally authorized nor socially sanctioned to provide those aspects of health care. Equally important is the knowledge that an assessment base for making decisions about the mental status of people that does not fully consider the interactional effects of mental, physical, and social aspects of health can lead to clinical decisions that may not be conducive to proper management of a person's health status.

Community mental health nurses, on the other hand, have a number of roles that may be used within the legal and social mandates governing the clinical practice of nursing. The choice of role and how it will be enacted depends on a comprehensive health assessment of the patient or client and the contexts in which usual and unusual daily experiences occur. From a number of possibilities, nurses may choose to be supportive caring people who initiate crisis intervention activities, or they may decide that active support from several sources is needed to help a person or family regroup to the point where assumption of responsibilities is possible. Nurses clearly recognize that obtaining information only about a client's mental or physical status is not an adequate base from which to make clinical decisions about therapeutic nursing interventions in community mental health nursing. Rather, communication and interactional data from people seeking health care are essential if a holistic approach to organizing such care is to make a difference in outcomes.

Compassion and Intimacy in Nurse–Patient Relationships

Compassion and a special kind of intimacy are created when certain kinds of caring functions are provided to sick people. This feeling and these activities create a special

* Dixie Koldjeski. *Case History Data*. Unpublished data from a clinical project in which the author was involved. Greenville, NC: East Carolina University, 1976.

quality in nurse–patient relationships. The kind and scope of such functions potentiate the development of this special quality.

In nurse–patient relationships, the nurse has to deal with events, feelings, and thoughts involving the most intimate personal, interpersonal, and familial aspects of human experiences. Experiences routinely include major life events associated with birth, daily living, illness, survival, and death. These experiences all include physical, psychological, social, economical, and spiritual aspects. These blend to integrate into feelings and behavior about the people who provide care, support, and assistance at the time when they are needed. The nurse is the major health provider who is usually present and counted on to provide professional nursing that addresses the needs of people at such times. People are terribly vulnerable during such experiences and the nurse fills a special role by respecting this vulnerability. In the helping process, maintaining the integrity of people and helping them to keep a sense of reality in order to cope as well as they can require a delicate balance between compassionate caring and helping the family or individuals to solve problems and to learn.

In the process of attending and monitoring functions of the body and caring for a person who has received injury or insult, a very special kind of interpersonal awareness and feeling is generated between the nurse and the patient. The nurse must assure that the patient's integrity, privacy, and sense of self are maintained during sensitive and intimate experiences involving the self and the body. The provision of nursing care to people during such experiences creates a hard-to-define but qualitative aspect in the professional nursing relationship. This special aspect involves a sense of togetherness and a trusting bond between those who need care and those who provide care. This closeness alters the quality and process of the nurse–patient relationship in ways that make it unlike any other professional–patient or professional–client relationship. The feelings developed under these circumstances between nurse and patients tend to generalize to other interpersonal situations.

Nursing roles and functions set the structure in which other special qualities can develop in nurse–patient and nurse–client relationships. Caring is the most important of these. It is a universal quality in nursing and is a special and precious thing. Engel (1980) calls caring the essence of nursing and states that as a profession, nursing has perfected the science of caring. Diers and Evans (1980) identify caring as the aspect creating excellence in nursing and assert that excellence cannot be present in nursing if caring is missing. Diers (1978) has also pointed out, quite correctly, that giving tender loving care is exquisitely difficult. She notes that nursing, practically alone among human service professions, deliberately tries to train and educate its young in empathy, sensitivity, and compassion.

Professional nursing emphasizes personalized caring as an integral part of the clinical process in maintaining wellness and providing care during illness. Nursing care is conceptualized in a holistic framework. This includes individuals in their families and their community and cultural groups. Such scientific caring is based on tested or verified knowledge. It refers to those judgments and acts that consider humans and environment in interaction and uses a helping process. It is based upon philosophic, phenomenologic, and objective data and subjective feelings, all of which are used to assist the nurse in the provision of nursing care. Caring is the central focus of nursing and has both scientific and humanistic bases (Leininger, 1980, 1977; Watson, 1979).

Other health professionals cannot and do not replicate the complex set of circumstances and relationships in the provision of professional services that cause the qualities unique to the nurse–patient relationship to develop. Nursing models incorporating the special qualities of the nurse–patient or nurse–client relationship are as appropriate in community mental health nursing as in other areas of nursing. These special qualities should not be attentuated or discarded in favor of models that are based on psychological and psychiatric concepts and principles of mental health developed by other professions to highlight the unique aspects of their practice—but not those of nursing practice.

The Use of Touch

The use of touch is a distinctive aspect of nursing. Nurses have a unique professional and social sanction to lay on hands in order to provide personal services and nursing care to people in health and illness. This sanction is not given to any other health professional except the physician and physician assistant. Nurses have the freedom inherent in professional autonomy to decide the most appropriate use and kind of touch needed by patients and clients. They assume the responsibility for its use in the implementation of health care functions and interpersonal relationships.

Nurses can address basic personal needs involving physical contact in ways that would be questioned if engaged in by other health professionals, with the possible exception of the physician. For example, the nurse is expected to provide back care including back rubs to patients, particularly those confined to bed for long hours. Back rubs are usually administered by rubbing the surface of the back with some type of solution to cool the skin and administering comforting strokes to relax the muscles of the back. If this commonplace nursing function were to be conducted by a psychologist or social worker, questions would be raised, and rightly so, about the ethical and legal aspects of such an action.

The Influence of Time

Time has a considerable influence on the structure, content, and process of nurse–patient and nurse–client relationships. Nurses have the freedom to decide the length of relationships based on the goals to be achieved. This freedom makes nurse–patient and nurse–client interactions flexible helping situations. Of all health professionals, nurses characteristically spend the most time with patients, clients, and their families. Within this context, there are no set rules for how much time a usual ''helping'' relationship should take. Nurses have the freedom to make decisions about this on the basis of interactional data evolving as the relationship progresses. Helping relationships may range from brief to long-term arrangements. In the former, brief supportive communications and the visibility and presence of nurses may be all that is needed. In the latter, the nurse–patient or nurse–client relationship may be used to explore and work on a number of patient, client, and family needs, problems, and concerns.

The openness of nurse–patient or nurse–client relationships is in contrast to those established by physicians. The medical practice model of the physician–patient relationship promotes the use of time-limited, focused, and impersonal relationships with patients. In psychiatry, various therapy models are based on a set amount of time that the therapist spends with the patient or client. This time may range from a brief encounter to an hour.

Nurses have the flexibility to determine the amount of time needed to develop a helping relationship. Usually, decisions take into account the purposes, the condition of the person or family seeking help, and the context in which life events are occurring. Nurses can also make rapid changes in priorities concerning any and all of these factors if emergent data suggests that there is a need to do so.

The Accessibility of Nurses

Nurses are more immediately accessible to patients, clients, and families throughout the day and night than any other health professional. They are the only professionals in most inpatient care settings on the scene 24 hours a day, seven days a week.

The accessibility of nurses in institutional care settings has contributed to the acceptance by nursing of responsibilities that are directly, indirectly, and remotely related to the provision of nursing care simply because nurses are "there." To nurses falls the responsibility for providing essential and support services that patients need *as well as* the decision-making and management activities that are necessary to maintain continuity of care and services in the institution. For example, if a patient spills coffee on the floor and the janitor is not around to mop it up, nurses have to locate someone to do it or do it themselves because of the safety hazard it poses.

If the business office closes for the weekend or is staffed with insufficient help, the nursing supervisor has to make the necessary arrangements for unscheduled arrivals and departures. Such maintenance and organizational functions have for years been so demanding in hospitals and other institutional care settings, nursing care has had to be delegated to nonprofessionals or conducted by professional nurses under conditions of intense frustration.

The situation of nursing in hospitals has been described by Anderson (1978) in her portrayal of a nurse's day by noting that because there is no agreement about what a nurse is, there is obviously no limit to responsibilities. Furthermore, a nurse's role tends to be whatever other people decide it should be.

"Being there" is not the best way to develop nursing roles and functions and this has to be examined in relation to "being used." In this respect, and with tongue in cheek, attention is called to the Law of the Sun that operates in hospitals and other kinds of inpatient facilities. Basically, this law has two operating principles: as the sun rises in the east to herald the day, the range of administrative skills and clinical expertise of the nurse wanes and as the sun sets in the west to herald the approach of evening and night, the range of administrative skills and clinical expertise of nurses waxes to full bloom! The application of this law is self-evident. It can be readily observed in any hospital that between the hours of 9:00 A.M. to 4:00 P.M., the need for an extensive cadre of health care professionals and hospital administrators, complete with full supporting staffs, is absolutely essential for patient care and management of the institution. But as the day wanes, nurses are expected to handle the same administrative problems and functions that during the daylight hours other health care professionals feel only they can handle. Jones (1981) described a problem that repeatedly occurs when nurses try to define nursing: the not-so-obvious-limits to nursing. This description aptly describes the daily expansion and contraction of the scope of nursing practice in hospitals.

The role and functions of nursing have been unduly warped and shaped in institutional settings by other professionals who select the services they will provide and the hours and conditions under which these will be provided. Too often major decisions involving the allocation of institutional resources for nursing services and management of nursing care are made by hospital and medical administrators on the basis of *their* professional judgments and unrealistic economic projections about staff needs. It is not unusual to find that many nursing administrators do not participate in decision making about resource allocation for the nursing services that they accept the responsibility to provide.

The "care, cure, and coordination" aspects of nursing defined by the American Nurses' Association have not proven to be particularly helpful in arriving at clearer definitions of nursing that might have been used to set boundaries on professional nursing (ANA, 1965). At the time of publication, this major position paper had little relevance to ambulatory care settings and there were soon questions about its relevance to institutional care settings (Sarosi, 1968). Some of the questions raised over a decade ago have never been adequately addressed and continue to be relevant today. The concepts of care, cure, and coordination have been questioned in terms of their ability to stimulate the development of new theory and research. Moreover, questions have been raised about whether the concepts have had the unanticipated consequences of contributing to perceptions that nurses have little or no professional autonomy and have little claim to being intellectuals in the professional community. The question of whether the care, cure, and coordination concepts have advanced the development of frameworks promoting the potential of nursing in general and mental health nursing in particular has been raised (Zahourek & Tower, 1972).

Many factors other than the ones identified contribute to the fact that nursing is the only health profession permitting its unique and general services to be identified, defined, controlled, and downgraded by other professions and organizational and situational demands. What is important is that this problem continues to be part of the everyday reality in too many health care settings. Thus, the negative consequences of such practices for the continued development of nursing as a profession will continue if its professionals continue to meet the demands of others rather than meet the health care needs of clients, patients, and families. If demands from other professionals and institutional managers continue chronically to deflect nursing from its main reason for being—the provision of quality health and sickness care—conflicts will continue to exist between organizational expectations and the ability of modern nursing services to provide professional nursing care. In this situation, nursing roles and functions will continue to be defined and shaped in ways that are not conducive to the development of professional nursing. Nursing resources will continue to be deployed in ways that are not supportive of the development of autonomy in nursing practice. More important, the "being there" quality of professional nursing, which should primarily benefit people in need of health or sick care, cannot be used to the fullest potential to meet the primary reason nurses are readily accessible to patients, families, groups, and clients.

Five distinctive aspects about the character of nurse–patient and nurse–client relationships have been identified. These distinctions all focus on the nurse as a special helping professional who provides a special kind of help to people who need a special kind of health care: quality professional nursing care.

The Privilege of Access

The privilege of access granted nurses is unique. Nurses have an exceptional degree of access to individuals, families, and community groups in both usual and unusual situations and circumstances in homes, schools, institutions, and industries. This access is virtually unparalled when compared to that accorded other health professionals. Nurses are rarely questioned about access to settings or social groups when there is a need to provide health care.

This unusual privilege of access, granted to nurses by society, is deeply rooted in the historical role of women as caretakers of the ill and feeble. The nurse, like the physician, is closely linked to the helping, caring, and healing aspects of sick care. This helping and caring ethic of nursing comes from a tradition that is as old as civilization. An integral part of it is the nonjudgmental value associated with the provision of health care. This is to say, a person is entitled to receive health care irrespective of individual circumstances, race, color, creed, ability to pay, or the contexts or situations in which illness occurs. For example, a victim of a gunshot wound is given the best nursing and medical care possible, and, if needed, so is the person who pulled the trigger.

Professional nurses, characteristically, have had social, cultural, educational, and economic backgrounds not too dissimilar from the people they serve. Similarities in background and interests have tended to reduce the social distance between the nurse as provider of health care and the client as recipient of such care. For example, nursing is not considered by the public to be an "elite" profession such as medicine and law. This similarity in background contributes to the acceptance of nurses as helping people.

The privilege of access is one that nurses should guard with care and zeal. Other health and human services professionals as well as law enforcement officers may request the assistance of nurses to gain access to homes and other kinds of settings from which they have been refused admission. Nurses should not, except in extreme circumstances, allow themselves to have privilege of access so used. The implications of such an action need to be examined in terms of both short-range and long-range consequences for the public trust inherent in this privilege.

Special Mix of Humanistic, Scientific, and Nursing Concepts Guiding Practice

There is a special mix of humanistic, scientific, and nursing concepts in the conceptual frameworks of nursing that guides clinical practice. This mix is unique among the health professions. Emphasis on humanism in nursing has been identified not only as a matter of doing but also as a matter of being (Paterson & Zderad, 1976). These nurses state that humanistic nursing "requires being and doing in a situation and subsequently setting the experienced reality at a distance (that is, objectifying reality) and entering into relation with it." Nurses experience, value, reflect, and conceptualize information. They are available with their total being to the nurse–patient relationship.

The humanistic aspect of nursing practice is present in the nursing process and across all specialties and subspecialties. This is one aspect of nursing that every nurse must face and resolve in terms of her or his own humanness with well and sick people. In some subspecialties, such as intensive and coronary care nursing, or where psychopharmacologic or somatic treatment activities are provided, the technophysiologic aspects of nursing care are critical for survival of the patient. But these aspects of nursing care can assume a primacy that excludes, to a large extent, the humanistic aspects of nursing. When this happens, a necessary and vital aspect of nursing care is not provided and the patient experiences this loss. Although it is difficult to document objectively the differences that humanistic aspects of nursing care make to patient care, comfort, and recovery, a great deal of anecdotal and experiential data are available to support the need for these aspects to be present.

A description of the humanistic aspect of the nursing process may be illustrated in an actual nursing situation. The data are from an anecdotal report of activities of a head nurse in her work situation on a busy medical ward (Kramer, 1975). The head nurse, the patient's physician, an intern, a resident, and a nurse researcher who acted as an observer visited the patient, a very sick woman. The patient had had a battery transplant for a heart condition. She continued to be hypotensive but was allowed out of bed with assistance. During the visit, there was considerable discussion about the patient's condition with the patient listening and answering questions. The nurse frequently translated to the patient the essence of what was being discussed in a way that was understandable to the patient. After the physicians left the room, the nurse and the observer remained. The following description of interactions then occurred between the nurse and the patient.

Case History

Kelly (the head nurse) had been standing at the foot of the bed and as the physicians left she moved in and stood directly next to Mrs. M [the patient]. She put her hand on Mrs. M's arm and repeated her instructions that Mrs. M was not to get up without help. Then she said to Mrs. M, "You look as though you are feeling kind of blue this morning." Tears welled up in Mrs. M's eyes almost at once, and she said, "Yes, I thought I would be feeling better by now." Kelly said, "You aren't having any more pain, are you?" The patient said, "Oh, no, not at all like it was before surgery," and then repeated, "I thought I would be feeling better by now." Kelly said, "Do you mean anything other than the fact that you are still dizzy and weak?" The patient said, "No, that is what I mean." Kelly then sat down on the bed and took the woman's hand in her hand and went on, in the most beautiful way I have ever heard, to describe exactly what the surgery was, how the implant was done, and she explained that it would be 6 to 10 days before the battery could be hooked up. I was watching the woman's face during this explanation, and she had the most trusting look in her eyes. I don't know whether the woman felt better afterward, but it was apparent to me [Kramer] that she was physically more relaxed. I noticed her other hand, the one lying on the bed. It had been somewhat clenched before; in fact I had noticed that her hand was clenched all during the discussion with the physicians, but now it began to open up and was just lying there in a very relaxed position. She was still smiling (she had been smiling before), and patted Kelly's hand and said, "Thank you, dear." Kelly and I left. (Kramer, 1975)

This vignette of an actual nursing interaction describes poignantly what Paterson and Zderad (1976) must have meant when they said that nurses must be available to their patients with their total being in the nurse–patient relationship. In this case history, the situation described the head nurse's concern for her patient and this was expressed by addressing technical, physical, psychological, and humanistic aspects of the experience that the patient was living through and with which she was trying to cope. Kelly, the nurse, experienced, valued, reflected, and evaluated information and observations, and synthesized all of these to decide how to handle the patient's anxiety and how to use herself in a therapeutic way. The outcome of this process was that the head nurse provided professional nursing care, in both its scientific and humanistic aspects, in meeting the patient's mental and physical health care needs.

Traditionally and to the present, nursing has been a profession dominated by women. Certain characteristics of the nursing process, and the methodology by which nursing practice is organized, are related to this feminine influence. Most notable of these are expressivity, warmth, and willingness to be physically and psychologically close to patients and clients when they are needed. Nursing is unique among health professions in that it tries to plan for the judicious mix of humanistic and scientific concepts as an essential part of nurse–patient relationships.

Multiple Dimensions of Health and Illness Care

Health and illness care are the domain of nursing. Professional nursing takes as its professional and social mandate the provision of health care in its many dimensions, thus giving nursing practice a wide scope. This scope covers the health and illness care of individuals, families, and groups as well as services that range from primary prevention to rehabilitation. Such services are provided both in hospitals and in the contexts in which daily living occurs in order to understand and change some of the factors influencing health and illness.

Within the general scope of nursing, different dimensions of health and illness have to be considered as care is provided to various people and groups. Of particular concern in community mental health nursing are the dimensions related to social, cultural, and situational aspects of both mental health and mental illness. Such factors are known to be associated with much of the behavior that gets labeled as mental illness and they are also involved in judgments about what constitutes positive mental health. Providing mental health services to people in community settings means that these factors have to be given special attention because of the direct impact they have on behavior.

Models of community mental health nursing have to be organized so that the social and cultural aspects of mental health and the contexts of human experiences can be systematically and routinely considered. Many behaviors thought to indicate mental and emotional illness have no direct and specific causes. Rather, in daily living experiences, it is the interactional effect of many such experiences that joined together to make a difference. Once such effects are set into motion, it is almost impossible to sort out one or two of them to cite as causes of a particular emotional or mental health problem.

The relationship between poverty and mental health is a case in point. This relationship is real as well as complex. Poverty in and of itself probably does not cause mental illness. But, in poverty, people exist hour to hour, day to day, under considerable stress and conditions that provide for survival but little else. Coping patterns learned under these circumstances are often accompanied by a high level of anxiety. Consequently, such patterns are not the most adaptive for less stressful social situations.

Patterns of coping and survival influence the organization of the self. The concept of self developed by people under chronic stress tends to be characterized by a lack of self-worth, low self-esteem, and a sense of powerlessness. These influences are accentuated because in poverty, educational, economic, social, and cultural opportunities available for personal and professional growth, development, and advancement may be relatively meager. Where such opportunities do exist, a person may have educational and experiential deficits of such magnitude that it is impossible successfully to overcome these.

Many health problems today have mental health consequences even though no specific causes can be isolated. Such problems tend to be complex and are little understood in their interrelated social, biological, physical, emotional, and chemical dimensions. The contribution that any one dimension makes to a particular health problem usually cannot be stated with any precision. Smoking and obesity are two examples of health problems that fall in this category. Generally, public health education has been directed toward reducing incidence and prevalence by emphasizing the deleterious effects of smoking and overeating on general health status. Despite these efforts, both problems continue to be a national concern.

Many factors of both smoking and excessive eating interact to make it very difficult to change attitudes and actions associated with these health-threatening activities. Various forms of behavior modification and biofeedback have been used to try to curb smoking and excessive eating. Both of these approaches focus on therapy that does not try to identify underlying motivations related to why people smoke and overeat. Each approach has been successful for some people but neither has been effective for most people. A major reason for this lack of success is because social, situational, and emotional factors interact in different ways as "triggers" for using the undesired behavior. This problem is confounded because assessment tools and other kinds of measurement devices are not able to sort out exactly what factor or factors may be most important for a particular person.

It is known that situational contexts charged with "cues" to encourage people to eat and smoke in order to be sociable and do the "in" thing have an impact on the ability of people to resist smoking and excessive eating. However, it is not known how to predict resistance to such cues or what helps people to be successful resistors. Until a broad range of social, cultural, and environmental aspects are taken into consideration in programs designed to change personal health care practices, it seems likely that the effectiveness of such programs, based on selective aspects of behavior, will continue to be successful for a relatively small number of people.

The importance of social and environmental factors in causing and maintaining illness has been recognized in nursing for many years. However, the collection of such information and the use of it as the basis for clinical problem solving have not been developed to optimal potential. One reason for this is the emphasis nursing has placed on the process and content of the nurse–patient relationship as the focus of nursing actions and interventions. Patients or clients are conceived of as unique people with unique needs, as they in fact are. This framework, however, orients the nurse to minimize the social and environmental factors influencing both the unique aspects of each person's behavior and the social aspects of living that contribute to the ways in which unique characteristics of behavior are expressed. It is difficult, if not impossible, adequately to address a person's health concerns if relevant familial, social, and environmental aspects are not adequately considered. Engel (1977) discussed this problem in relation to psychiatry and its use of medical disease models for the treatment of mental illness. He called for a new model, a biophysical one that also considers the psychosocial dimensions of health and illness in a systems context.

INFLUENCES OF COMMUNITY-BASED MENTAL HEALTH CARE ON THE STRUCTURE OF NURSING

The unique aspects of the structure of nursing have to be considered in ambulatory and community settings if these qualities of professional nursing are to be an integral part of community mental health nursing. Community-based mental health care and services have had a profound influence on the structure of nursing and its unique aspects of practice.

The placement of mental health services in community settings affected the structure and relationships of both community mental health nursing and mental health nursing. This influence has been extensive because of the way in which basic structures and relationships were affected.

The "bold new approach," that is, community-based mental health care, had as its cornerstone the movement of mental health care and services from state mental hospitals to community-based mental health centers. This change in the location of services was instrumental in altering to some extent the roles, functions, and clinical process of all the core mental health disciplines. Nursing, however, experienced more changes in these basic areas than other mental health disciplines.

The change from hospital-based psychiatric nursing to community-based mental health nursing also created the need for major conceptualizations and changes in clinical nursing practice. Some time had to pass before nurses could assess their experiences in community-based mental health services. Thus, the task of reconceptualizing the theory base for community mental health nursing and translating new concepts into expanded roles and functions lagged behind experiences. The way in which integration of theory, roles, functions, and experiences in community mental health nursing occurred in the early years of community-based mental health care had implications for definitions of nurse generalist and nurse specialist roles in community-based mental health centers and services.

The clinical nurse generalist has had a more difficult time than the clinical nurse specialist integrating changes in concepts in clinical practice and adopting new roles in community mental health settings. As noted, many professional nurses have expressed this difficulty by comments that "community mental health nursing is different." Part of this concern seems to be the lack of clarity about where the nurse generalist fits into the mental health structure, a structure established on the principle of specialized services. Because generalist nurses are not prepared to provide the specialized therapies used in mental health, their role in community mental health has, sadly, come to be defined around a small core of technical functions.

Basing community mental health nursing in community settings has had a number of consequences for clinical practice. Some understanding of these, because they continue to operate, may help the nurse to establish and maintain the integrity of the nursing role in community mental health nursing practice.

Nurse-Patient Relationship Models Not Valued

The relationship models developed in nursing were never particularly valued in community mental health. Valued models of mental health care have been those developed and used by psychiatry and psychology. The distinctions that make nursing models effective have, generally, been altered to incorporate distinctions of the generic therapy models of mental health. Where distinctions of nursing models have been retained, clinicians have had to incorporate these as best they could in the therapy models developed by other disciplines for their clinical process and practice.

General models of mental health therapies, such as individual and group modalities, are based on a core of knowledge about mental health, mental illness, and personality development. Their use has been enhanced by the assumption of community mental health ideology that this core of knowledge, supported by appropriate therapeutic activities, could be safely and effectively performed by many kinds of mental health professionals and paraprofessionals. This assumption has proven to be true in many cases.

The assumption that a number of different kinds of mental health professionals could provide quality therapeutic modalities to people suffering from mental and emotional problems helped to advance the development of community mental health, mental health, and psychiatric nursing. Nurses in these subspecialty areas, trained as specialists, have come to be recognized by clients, patients, and other professionals as expert clinicians. This recognition, in turn, has led to the acceptance of the professional nurse specialist as one of the four core mental health professions (Stokes et al., 1969; DeYoung & Tower, 1971; President's Commission on Mental Health, 1978).

Emphasis on generic models of therapeutic modalities in mental health has had other effects. One in particular is that the development and use of nursing models relating to mental and emotional health have been minimized in clinical practice. Most models used by nurses in mental health are not primarily based on nursing models. Rather, therapist roles, therapist behaviors during therapeutic process, criteria for selection of therapeutic modalities, communication patterns, length of therapy sessions, and the conditions under which therapeutic activities are conducted are based for the most part on experiences and traditions of clinical practice developed by other mental health disciplines. It is unfortunate that social psychological models of nurse–patient relationships have not significantly altered basic therapy models in mental health. Alterations, for the most part, have been the other way: the unique aspects of nurse–patient relationship models have not been maintained and highlighted in terms of their special qualities.

Early in the community mental health movement, models of nurse–patient relationships were available in which concepts from other therapy models could have been incorporated. Although these nursing models were developed for use with hospitalized mental patients, they were general enough to have been modified for use in community mental health nursing.

Foremost among nursing models is the one developed by Peplau (1952). Based on interpersonal, learning, and nursing theories, it provide a clinical framework for nursing practice in many kinds of settings and with people in general. Another model, though not as well developed as the interpersonal model, was proposed by Orlando (1961). In this model, mental health principles guided nursing practice with the purpose of helping patients maintain or restore their sense of adequacy or well-being in stressful situations associated with their illness. Orlando noted that whereas other fields develop theory and practice, there are marked and important differences between the principles of nursing and the principles derived from other fields that have their own distinct aims and responsibilities. This position is similar to that of interprofessional borrowing, that is, when concepts and principles from other disciplines are used as a basis for nursing practice without a reconceiving of these to include nursing principles that include the unique aspects of nursing. The third example of a nursing relationship model is that proposed by Mellow (1968). This model explicitly addressed two kinds of data: that which arises in the experiences of the nurse and patient in the ongoing care process and that which comes through theory from other disciplines.

Many unique aspects of the nurse–patient relationship are in conflict with the psychiatric models of therapy used in mental health. A number of examples can be cited. Data on health and illness that nurses traditionally obtain from patients are usually not dealt with in a holistic and interactive way in psychologically focused therapy. The use of touch is viewed as suspect by many mental health professionals. The length of time to be spent with the patient or client is regulated by the concept of a "therapy hour" or some other external control. Therapeutic relationships in both number and kind may be geared to organizational demands and needs requiring the therapist to see a particular number of patients per day in order to make services cost-accountable, thus reducing the flexibility of structuring the nurse–patient relationship to meet client needs. Community and home contacts with families and community groups may be limited because of costs and philosophic beliefs that only the target patient needs to be dealt with. Case findings may be limited because of an underlying assumption held by many mental health professionals that people should be self-motivated to seek treatment. Impersonal use of self during therapist–patient or therapist–client interactions is emphasized. The empathic and expressive use of self that is a characteristic of nurse–patient relationships is questioned by other professionals in terms of appropriateness and whose needs are being met. The nurse finds that her presence or availability to patients and clients is controlled to a large extent by organizational and economical factors. The range of social and environmental data that the nurse characteristically collects may not be considered relevant or used in a meaningful way. These and other factors have caused the nurse–patient relationship model, valued in other health care settings, to undergo major changes in structure and function in mental health settings. The community mental health nurse may not be aware that these changes have occurred and continue to occur.

The generic model of mental health therapy has, however, had some positive effects on community mental health nursing. The assumption that a common core of knowledge and clinical expertise could be taught and used effectively by mental health professionals from many disciplines was a revolutionary idea in 1960. This experience has had the effect of tearing away many of the myths associated with providing psychological therapies and made possible opportunities for nursing to demonstrate just how effective its clinicians can be in providing professional mental health care.

Another positive impact of the generic model has been the expansion of community mental health nursing services through consultation and liaison activities to other areas of nursing practice. These activities have sensitized nurses and helped them address social and psychological dimensions of health and illness as an integral part of the human experience.

Still another positive impact has been the election and appointment of mental health and psychiatric nurses to health and mental health policy-making bodies. The ability of nurses to articulate a nursing perspective that includes expanded roles and functions has resulted in an increase in opportunities for participation in decision making and expansion of roles.

But there have also been some unexpected consequences of the ideology of mental health that maximized the common core of clinical knowledge and practice while minimizing the unique aspects of each discipline's contributions. A major consequence concerns the development of professional identity and self-identity of nurses in mental health. In this respect, Lego posed the question of whether nurse psychotherapists differ from other therapists (1973). In her classic analysis, she emphasized that the knowledge and skills a nurse brings to the practice of psychotherapy are uniquely different from those possessed by the psychiatrist, psychologist, and social worker. Such differences are the holistic approach that orients nursing practice, an orientation for dealing with crisis situations, and a knowledge of general health matters. However, there seems to be considerable variation in the extent to which these differences are emphasized by nurse therapists. Unfortunately, there is little research to show what, if any, differences the use of the unique aspects of nursing have on the outcomes of therapy conducted by nurses, although clinicians report positive changes. Ujhely (1973) identified another problem related to professional identity of nurses in mental health: the "disowning" of nurse psychotherapists by colleagues in other areas of nursing and by some in psychiatric nursing. This suggests that nurse psychotherapists may not be considered to be nurses—a grave intraprofessional identity problem.

Concerns about nursing identity relate to the nature of nursing practice and the roles used by nurses to implement concepts and principles of nursing. Nurses who use models of practice developed from and identified with other disciplines to provide clinical services in mental health may have a self and professional identity quite different from nurses who take such models and reconceptualize these to incorporate concepts and principles from nursing for clinical practice in community mental health. Therapeutic interventions and preventions are the means through which nursing applies principles and theories from nursing and the mental health sciences. Mental health interventions that are solely based on models used by all mental health professionals should not unquestionably be accepted to the point that the essence, focus, and theories of nursing are overlooked or simply not considered.

Generalized Nursing Practice in Specialized Mental Health Services

The scope and organization of general nursing practice have been difficult to implement in community mental health centers because these were organized to provide specialty mental health care. The professional nurse generalist is prepared to provide a wide array of general services to clients for many different kinds of health concerns, but she or he is not prepared to provide such specialized modalities as individual, group, and family therapy. The conceptual bases on which general nursing practice is based are also different from the underlying basis of the special therapeutic modalities.

The philosophic basis of general nursing practice has also added to the difficulty of defining a clear practice role for the nurse generalist in community mental health. For example, the holistic perspective orients nurses to look at interconnections between situations, events, and personal experiences in health and illness (Brallier, 1978). Nursing, as a profession, advocates the preparation of a professional nurse generalist prior to specialist education. The generalist is prepared to address a number of illness and wellness concerns over the life cycle of people, and clinical nursing covers a wide range of experiences in both institutional and community settings.

The ability of professional nurse generalists to provide a wide range of clinical nursing services is based on their ability to generalize a common core of concepts and principles about health and illness to people who experience many diverse kinds of health problems in different kinds of situations. This generalist approach prepares a nurse who can provide health care to well people, sick people, and families over extended periods of time. Nursing process includes assessing, monitoring, and intervening to maximize prevention of illness and minimize the immediate and cumulative impact of illness. An integral aspect of general nursing is the maximization of the potential of environments for the promotion and maintenance of general health.

Theory and clinical strategies directly relating to the application of therapeutic interventions in mental health are grounded for the most part in psychiatric and psychological knowledge of diseases rather than in research and theory about mental health and wellness. Clinical data are collected that focus on psychiatric and psychological content, processes, and pathologies. This means that a data base about mental health needs to be established because such experiences address a different slice of life than psychiatric and psychological data.

Some of the problems relating to the integration of basic concepts from the mental health sciences and community mental health nursing theory and practice are due in part to differences in developmental phases of the various disciplines. Such problems are also related to the degree to which other mental health professions have developed and researched their theoretical bases for practice. Different kinds of mental health modalities have been developed at different times in the history of psychiatric care and treatment. For example, the one-to-one therapy model was developed by Freud early in this century for the treatment of emotional problems he thought resided within the psychic structure of an individual's personality. The process and strategies used in treatment came to be known as psychoanalysis and are based on psychoanalytic theories of psychic functioning. Current models of family therapy have developed over the past two decades and are based in large part on a social systems perspective. This perspective focuses on the family as a small social system in interaction. By contrast, nursing therapy models tend to be of more recent origin, even though some of these began to be developed over three decades ago. All, however, need clinical tests of their effectiveness. Nursing is a relative newcomer in testing out its practice models.

Scope and Speed of Change in Mental Health

The scope and speed of change in mental health have been contributing factors in the limited adoption of nursing models of practice in community mental health. These changes, along with the actual change in locus of providing and putting into place a system of mental health care, created revolutionary changes in key traditional nursing roles and functions. When community mental health centers first became a reality, few nurses had had experiences in community management of people suffering from mental and emotional problems in their home or community settings. By contrast, many psychiatrists, psychologists, and, to some extent, psychiatric social workers had such experiences in their private practices and from employment in community agencies. Traditionally, the role of psychiatric nursing had been to provide care to both acute and chronic mentally ill patients *in mental hospital settings*. Consequently, nursing roles, functions, strategies, and relationship models had been developed over years to include nurturance and technical care, ward and patient management, and selected therapeutic activities with psychotic patients. When community-based mental health care was instituted, this body of knowledge and clinical expertise had to serve in large part as the basis for new roles and expanded functions in contexts that were radically different from the mental hospital settings and with population groups who experienced emotional problems of a different kind and degree than the severe problems experienced by hospitalized mentally ill patients.

Community mental health centers were established in a relatively short time under the stimulation of a federal mandate that included generous financial support. The rapid establishment of these centers created the need for nurses accustomed to practice in mental hospitals to use in the best way possible the known roles and clinical practices that were developed and successful in psychiatric nursing. The need to reconceive and expand these roles was soon recognized by community mental health nursing clinicians but their ability to address this need was hampered by the small amount of nursing research and theoretical conceptions available.

During the first decade of community mental health, there seems to have developed an assumption that community mental health nursing and psychiatric nursing were one and the same, or very nearly so, in terms of the conceptual bases and therapeutic strategies associated with clinical practice. This assumption can no longer be justified, if it ever could, and needs to be critically examined if theory and practice concepts in community mental health nursing are to be further advanced.

Impact of Community-Based Mental Health Care on Structure and Practice of Nursing.

There has been a tendency in nursing to underrate the impact that community-based mental health services has had on the practice of nursing in these settings. One reason has been a general lack of knowledge about the influence of settings on clinical practice. For many years, nurses had to focus on learning many new competencies, different knowledge bases, and new roles. In meeting these challenges, the effects that the new community-based mental health settings were having on the nature and direction of the clinical practice of community mental health nursing were not of primary concern.

From a different perspective, the focus that nursing has given to the patient or client as a unique person with unique needs and who requires specially planned nursing care has also minimized the impact that social settings and contexts has had on the structure and practice of nursing. Engelke (1980) identified several variables operating in ambulatory settings that influence the clinical role of nurses: the development of an "ambulatory care nursing identity," ambulatory care nursing leadership, control of the budget, development and recognition of increasing clinical responsibilities, support services that are appropriate, and interdisciplinary approaches to patient care. The important point made by the author is that settings influence the way in which the six variables operated to influence the delivery of nursing care. A focus on people and their families without due consideration for the influence of settings in which nursing care is provided limits the potential effectiveness of nursing interventions.

Family therapy has come to be a major treatment modality in community mental health. In 1975, Smoyak pointed out that community mental health centers might be "over-focusing" on the family as the unit to work with in providing therapeutic services. The family as a case, like the individual as a case, can orient clinical practice and interventions in ways that social situations and contexts are not adequately considered in terms of the factors helping to cause the behavior that the nurse observes in clients.

It is paradoxical that data from social situations and contexts in community-based mental health care have been used so marginally in making clinical decisions. For example, it has been recognized for years that the social structure and relationships on wards in psychiatric hospitals have been important factors in generating the behavior of both staff and patients. Such knowledge has probably best been used in therapeutic communities. These are social organizations in which the relationships of everyone in the community and the structure of daily living activities are designed to reduce ambiguity in expectations, communications, and interactions between people in the community. Participation in the achievement of community goals, set by members of the community, include accountability for one's own behavior and helping other members control their behavior. Assuming responsibility for achieving such goals is an integral part of this form of social psychological therapy for clients.

Few mental hospitals have transformed their structure, relationships, and functions into therapeutic communities because of the difficulties encountered in trying to change staff and patient roles. Concerns about status, relationships, privileges, and authority of various professionals in mental hospitals have minimized the use of this form of therapy. Furthermore, the knowledge gained through such experiences in therapeutic communities has not been generalized to any extent to community mental health settings and used to understand how settings influence the clinical practice of the mental health disciplines.

The structure of organization in mental hospitals influences the clinical practice of the mental health profession. The organization of most mental hospitals is a bureaucratic hierarchy. The physician occupies the top place in the treatment hierarchy, and other mental health professionals and paraprofessionals are arranged in levels one below the other. Psychiatric nurses have traditionally been ranked at or near the bottom of this staff hierarchy. They tend to be perceived by higher ranked mental health professionals as the group that provides certain kinds of functions to help better qualified mental health professionals carry out their roles and responsibilities; who keep order on wards; who care for patients when they are too ill to be treated by special psychotherapeutic activities administered by other mental health professionals; who carry out physician's orders; who assist the physician in giving somatic and psychopharmacological treatments; and who provide services to patients 24 hours a day, 7 days a week, throughout the year. Several of these functions continue to make up the content of community mental health nursing in community mental health settings.

The issue of how the structure of organizations affects the practice of community mental health nursing deserves more attention than it has received. Until the nursing profession gains some measure of control over the settings in which clinical nursing practice is performed, it will continue to be difficult to establish milieus in which professional nursing can be practiced. Such changes need to consider the much broader perspective of man and environment in interaction in order to include essential sociocultural, environmental, and situational factors, along with the more traditional ones, in the professional practice of community mental health nursing.

SUMMARY

The interrelationships between nursing and the subspecialty of community mental health nursing are grounded in common conceptual and practice bases, unique aspects of nursing, and the social and professional roles of the nurse. The structure of nursing is unique in terms of its perspective, the special character of the nurse–patient relationship, the privilege of access, the special mix of humanistic, scientific, and nursing concepts in the conceptual base, and the multiple dimensions of health and illness that nursing includes in its scope of professional practice.

Community-based mental health care has had a profound influence on the structure of nursing. Community mental health services were organized on a principle of providing specialized mental health care to clients on first contact. Community mental health centers and services have been established to carry out this mandate by using the services of specialists in mental health more than those of generalists. This organization of community mental health services has had the consequences of making the role of the professional nurse generalist very difficult to define.

In general, nursing models of care that nurse generalists use have not been valued in community mental health settings. Generally, nurses have been urged to learn nurse specialist roles and competencies. Where this was neither desirable nor possible, nurses all too often have found clinical nursing defined as a relatively narrow technical role.

The challenge in community mental health nursing today is for nursing clinicians, both generalists and specialists, to make a more concerted effort to redefine the role and functions of nursing in community-based mental health settings. In this process, nursing models, with their principles of care, need to be considered in relation to existing mental health models of therapeutic activities.

REFERENCES

American Nurses' Association. *A Position Paper.* New York: American Nurses' Association, 1965, pp. 1–6.

Anderson, Peggy. *Nurse.* New York: St. Martin's Press, 1978, p. 31.

Brallier, Lynn W. The nurse as holistic health practitioner. *Nursing Clinics of North America* 13:643–655, December, 1978.

Burgess, Ann W. Psychiatric nursing: The state of the art. In Burgess, Ann W., ed. *Psychiatric Nursing in the Hospital and the Community,* 3rd ed. Englewood Cliffs, NJ: Prentice-Hall, 1981, pp. 36–51.

Coyle, Grace M. *Social Science in the Professional Education of Social Workers.* New York: Council on Social Work Education, 1958, pp. 12–13.

Davis, Ellen D., and Pattison, G. Mansell. The psychiatric nurses' role identity. *American Journal Of Nursing* 79:298–299, 1979.

De Young, Carol D., and Tower, Margene. *The Nurses' Role in Community Mental Health Centers: Out of Uniform and into Trouble.* St. Louis: C. V. Mosby Co., 1971.

Diers, Donna. A different kind of energy: Nurse-power. *Nursing Outlook* 26:51–55, January, 1978.

Diers, Donna, and Evans, David L. Excellence in nursing. *Image* 12:27–30, June 1980.

Engel, George L. The need for a new medical model: A challenge for Biomedicine. *Science* 196:129–136, April, 1977.

Engel, Nancy S. Confirmation and validation: The caring that is professional nursing. *Image* 12:53–56, October, 1980.

Engelke, Martha K. Nursing in ambulatory settings: A head nurse perspective. *American Journal of Nursing* 80:1813–1815, October, 1980.

Jones, Judith N. The not-so-obvious limits of nursing. *Nursing and Health Care* 2:64–66, February, 1981.

Koldjeski, Dixie. Primary care nursing: The psychosocial component. In Burgess, Ann W., ed. *Psychiatric Nursing in the Hospital and the Community,* 3rd ed. Englewood Cliffs, NJ: Prentice-Hall, 1981, pp. 637–647.

Koldjeski, Dixie. The mental health role of primary care nurses. *Journal of Clinical Child Psychology* 7(1):37–39, Spring, 1978.

Kramer, Marlene. Field notes on the head nurse. In Davis, Marcella Z., Kramer, Marlene, and Strauss, Anselm L., eds. *Nurses in Practice: A Perspective on Work Environments.* St. Louis: C. V. Mosby Co., 1975, p. 9.

Lego, Suzanne. Nurse psychotherapists: How are we different? *Perspectives in Psychiatric Care* 11:144–147, October–December, 1973.

Leininger, Madeleine. Caring: A central focus of nursing and health care services. *Nursing and Health Care* 1(3):135–143 and 176, October, 1980.

Leininger, Madeleine. The phenomenon of caring. Part V. Caring: the essence and central focus of nursing, *American Nurses' Foundation Nursing Research Report* 12(1):2,14, February, 1977.

Mellow, June. Nursing therapy. *American Journal of Nursing* 68:2365–2369, November, 1968.

Orlando, Ida Jean. *The Dynamic Nurse–Patient Relationship.* New York: G. P. Putnam's Sons, 1961, pp. 31–60.

Paterson, Josephine G., and Zderad, Loretta T. *Humanistic Nursing.* New York: John Wiley & Sons, 1976.

Peplau, Hildegarde. *The Interpersonal Relations in Nursing.* New York: G. P. Putnam's Sons, 1952, pp. 3–43.

President's Commission on Mental Health. *Report to the President from the President's Commission on Mental Health,* Vol. 1. Washington, D.C.: Government Printing Office, May, 1978.

Sarosi, G. M. A critical theory: The nurse as a fully human person. *Nursing Forum* 7:349, 1968.

Smoyak, Shirley A. Family therapy. In Huey, Florence L., Compiler. *Psychiatric Nursing 1946 to 1974: A Report on the State of the Art.* New York: The American Journal of Nursing Company, 1975, pp. 36–49.

Stokes, Gertrude A., Williams, F. S., Davidities, R. M., Ballulyan, A., and Ullman, M. *The Role of Psychiatric Nurses in Community Mental Health Practice: A Giant Step.* New York: Faculty Press, 1969.

Ujhely, Gertrud B. The nurse as psychotherapist: What are the issues? *Perspectives in Psychiatric Care* 11:155–160, October–December, 1973.

Watson, Jean. *Nursing: The Philosophy and Science of Caring*. Boston: Little, Brown and Company, 1979.

Zahourek, Rothlyn, and Tower, Margene. Community mental health nurses question "care, cure, and coordination." In Goldman, Elaine, ed. *Community Mental Health Nursing*. New York: Appleton-Century-Crofts, 1972, pp. 6–19.

3 | COMMUNITY MENTAL HEALTH NURSING: A SOCIAL PSYCHOLOGICAL MODEL OF MENTAL HEALTH AND MENTAL ILLNESS

INTRODUCTION

Concepts of mental health and mental illness are important in community mental health nursing because they have a major organizing effect on the clinical frameworks that guide nursing practice. Traditionally, the conceptual frameworks developed by other mental health disciplines have served to organize a considerable amount of clinical practice in this subspecialty of nursing. Today, there are different views about the definitions and meanings of mental health and mental illness in light of new theories of human functioning and research. Because of this ferment, community mental health nursing is in a good position to examine its current clinical practice frameworks and develop new ones or modify existing ones and encourage the development of new roles and functions. Such development would intensify the examination and identification of relationships between nursing and community mental health nursing as well as those between community mental health nursing and clinical practice roles in regard to both mental health and mental illness.

Traditionally, concepts of mental health and mental illness have focused on the mental status of the individual personality. This approach is based on a medical model of mental illness. This model assumes that a disease process exists within the personality structure of an individual in much the same way that a disease process exists within the body of a person to produce physical illness. The medical model of mental illness does not explicitly consider the fact that human behavior is caused in part by the interactions of people as these occur in social settings and is influenced by cultural values, social norms, and role expectations.

For centuries, bizarre and aberrant behavior has been known as insanity. Such behavior is probably as old as mankind, however the causes were a mystery until this century. Historically, the explanations of insanity reflected the beliefs of the time and had their roots in demonology, mysticism, and religion. Successive redefinition of insanity over time has resulted in behaviors once labeled as insanity being routinely diagnosed today as mental illness.

The process of redefining insanity to mean mental illness has been facilitated by the development of the science of human behavior in both its scientific and humanistic aspects. Advancements in understanding some of the general principles of normal and abnormal behavior have had the effect of bringing the study and treatment of mental health and emotional problems into the mainstream of modern scientific health care. Through research and clinical innovations, new and different approaches to assessment and therapeutic interventions have been developed. Furthermore, the right of the mentally ill to receive humane care and medical treatment is well established as a criterion of modern psychiatric care.

New concepts of mental health and mental illness continue to evolve as theorists, scientists, and clinicians use new knowledge and clinical experiences to test research findings. Social and psychological concepts of mental health and mental illness integrate several dimensions of the human experience that are known to contribute to both normal and deviant behavioral development and maintenance. Of major importance are the primary group settings in which child and adult socialization occur throughout the life cycle. Such group experiences contribute to the development of the self in mentally healthy ways and facilitate individual self-actualization.

An emphasis on social psychological concepts in clinical frameworks for community mental health nursing orients the nurse to consider mental health and mental illness in various ways. For example, the mental health of family systems must be considered in assessing the mental health of family members. Furthermore, the mental health of communities relates to the mental health of families and their members and influences how and whether positive mental health can be promoted and maintained.

Some years ago, nursing began to move away from an overreliance on disease models as the primary basis for orienting clinical practice. Today, social, psychological, humanistic, and personal dimensions of health and illness have been incorporated in nursing theories and in the frameworks for clinical nursing practice. However, nursing practice in the field of mental health continues to be oriented in large part by psychiatric problems and illnesses and the related theories that provide causative explanations. This orientation is reflected in the kinds of therapeutic activities that are taught to nurse clinicians and in the services provided to people who experience emotional stress and mental disorder.

The model of mental health and mental illness presented in this chapter tries to make more explicit a conceptual base for community mental health nursing that includes theory and research from the social, psychological, and nursing sciences; humanism; and systems concepts. It builds on the traditional emphasis in nursing that health and illness have many dimensions that must be addressed in professional nursing practice.

The model of community mental health nursing unifies a number of more limited theoretical approaches about particular aspects of mental health and mental illness and related clinical nursing practice. There comes a time in the development of the science of a profession's practice base when it is possible to consolidate into a more unified whole some of the smaller theories and research to formulate a slightly different clinical practice framework. Such unification efforts, although incomplete and imperfect, present new ideas and models that may be used by others to advance further.

In this chapter, the social psychological model of mental health and mental illness is presented by first examining some of the changing concepts about mental health and mental illness over the past several decades. Following this discussion, basic assumptions are identified. Mental health and mental illness are defined. The social psychological model of mental health and mental illness is then presented with schematic representation. Implications for community mental health nursing are discussed.

CHANGES IN CONCEPTS ABOUT MENTAL HEALTH AND MENTAL ILLNESS

Concepts of mental health and mental illness have proven very difficult to define with any precision and have meant different things at various times. One reason for this difficulty is that these labels have always been used to cover a variety of conditions, disorders, and factors associated with social and psychological functioning.

The evolutionary process of redefining insanity to mean mental illness has generated controversy about what mental health and mental illness actually mean in terms of behavior. Different perspectives of behavior have led to definitions for both conditions. Once-accepted concepts of mental health and definitions of mental illness have changed as new theories and research have provided some answers and raised new and different kinds of questions. Four well-known concepts about mental health and mental illness are discussed. The discussions establish a basis for the model of mental health and mental illness that is presented.

Concept: Mental Illness Is Like Any Other Illness—Or Is It?

The concept that mental illness is like any other illness has been promoted over the past three decades. The most influential theory of mental functioning to support this concept is the psychodynamic theory of behavior (Freud, 1933). Freud postulated that psychic energy generated within the structure of the personality is analogous to physical energy generated by biological processes in the body.

Although Freud never elaborated the concept that mental illness is like any other illness, his theory of mental functioning has served as the basis for this latter-day slogan, which was popularized in the 1950s. The Freudian theory of mental functioning conceives of mental and emotional problems as conflict between the three parts of the personality structure: the id, ego, and superego. The *id* represents the unconscious part of the personality. In the *id*, psychic energy is generated from basic primitive needs, desires, and impulses, including socially forbidden ones that cannot be directly expressed. Conflicts no longer in conscious awareness are repressed in the *id* and continue to generate psychic energy. The *superego* is the conscience part of the personality. It is the last part to develop, usually by 7 years of age. It acts as a force to give meaning to our desires, wishes, and behaviors, and to enable us to judge them. Superego values may be narrow and rigid and become punitive in monitoring our actions. The *ego* is the reality-testing, or conscious, part of the personality. It mediates between the impulses coming from the id and the controlling messages coming from the superego. The three parts of the personality compete with and influence one another and in this process generate conflict. The ego, superego, and id must be integrated to permit charactistic and adaptive patterns of responses to develop in order to interrelate thoughts, feelings, and actions.

Theories based on the Freudian theory of mental functioning have come to be known as psychodynamic theories. The relative emphasis accorded the different parts of the personality structure varies from theory to theory. Freud, for example, placed great emphasis on the influence of id functions, whereas Neo-Freudians place greater emphasis on ego functions.

Psychodynamic theories of mental functioning have oriented psychotherapeutic interventions on the feelings and emotions of people to effect changes in these. More specifically, psychotherapeutic interventions are designed to uncover psychological conflicts within the self and between the self and others and to encourage the client to recognize the related feelings attached to such relationships. Once recognition occurs, the client can work through such feelings with a therapist. Overall, the goal of psychotherapy is to help clients develop insight about the hidden and obscure reasons why they feel and act as they do.

The concept that mental illness is like any other illness has led to the use of interventions other than psychological ones in the treatment of mental and emotional problems. In general, these interventions have focused on applying various kinds of treatments to the human body in order to change thoughts, emotions, and behavior. Among these are psychopharmacological products that have the ability to control behavior, regulate one's mood up and down, and alter thought patterns. Electroconvulsive therapy continues to be used as a somatic treatment. Psychosurgical procedures such as lobotomy are undergoing a resurgence in use.

The idea that mental illness has a biochemical basis like physical illnesses is becoming more credible each passing year. There is evidence, particularly from the neurosciences, that a number of "mental illnesses" have some biochemical bases, but the well-known psychiatrist Torrey (1974) pointed out that this does not make them *mental diseases* in the medical sense because all activities of the brain have chemical and neurological components. Depression is an example of a mental condition that has been found to entail a definite chemical malfunction, and it responds to drug therapy. At the same time, social and psychological interventions used in conjunction with chemical therapies bring about a greater change in behavior than when drug treatment alone is used. This indicates that depression has social and psychological components as well as chemical ones, so the kind of "illness" depression represents is an open question.

Torrey (1974), was also very critical of the concept that mental illness is a disease. He pointed out that our language shapes our thoughts and that the thought of "mental diseases" creates a strange category of diseases without known causes. Torrey stated that a disease is something you *have*, behavior is something you *do*.

The various kinds of mental, emotional, and behavioral conditions that are today called mental illness may all turn out someday to have causes of a psychophysiological chemical nature, but until such causes are known, the concept that mental illness is like any other illness is more of a slogan than a basis for clinical practice. To consider mental illness processes analogous to physical illness processes ignores the personal and social consequences of being mentally ill. The idea that mental and emotional problems are an "illness" has been challenged by social and behavioral scientists and some psychiatrists on the grounds that much of the behavior that is labeled mental illness is actually violations of social norms and personal rules of behavior.

The concept that mental illness is like any other illness will continue to be challenged because the theoretical underpinnings for this assertion have little or no basis in science. Alternative ways of conceptualizing normal and abnormal behavior will more accurately describe a considerable amount of the behavior that is currently classified as mental illness.

Concept: Mental Health and Mental Illness Have Social and Cultural Components as Well as Psychological Ones

In recent years, theories of mental health and mental illness that have not explicitly considered the social and cultural components of behavior have increasingly come under question as to their completeness. In mental health, the causes of behavior have proven to be quite elusive and multidimensional in nature. Furthermore, research and clinical experiences have raised serious questions about the validity of psychodynamic principles of mental functioning. A major contribution to this dialogue has been the work of social and behavioral scientists who looked at different factors and situations that they believed were involved in mental health and mental illness. For example, social scientists were among the first to point out that strange and unusual behavior, such as hallucinations in public places, can lead to a person's being labeled mentally ill some of the time but not all of the time. Furthermore, in some cultures, such behavior is considered holy and endows the person who has it with special powers. The recognition that both mental health and mental illness have social, cultural, and situational components has altered to some extent the ways in which these aspects of health are considered today.

Another influence that has changed concepts of mental health and mental illness has been the use of behavioral theories of learning. A major principle of these is that all behavior is learned and can be unlearned. The structure of mental functioning is not the concern in behavior modification theory and strategies; rather, the conditions under which behavior can be changed are the emphasis. Applications of principles of behavioral theory have demonstrated that both normal and abnormal behavior are indeed learned. Learning such behaviors occurs as a result of reinforcements from other persons and the social conditions under which the behavior evolves. Research using behavior modification has demonstrated that the bases of behavior are not necessarily psychological in nature. Rather, there is a complex interplay between the events and situations causing behavior to emerge and the reinforcements provided to a person to use such behavior.

Concept: Multiple Theories on the Motivation of Behavior Are Now an Accepted Part of Mental Health Theories

The emergence and acceptance of theories of personality, behavior, and mental functioning based on different sources of motivation other than that proposed in psychodynamic theory have had a significant influence on ideas about mental health and mental illness. One that has had a major impact is self-actualization theory. Self-actualization theories emphasize humanistic and phenomenological principles of living and being. People are assumed to act in rational, socially organized, and constructive ways. Self-actualization is achieved when perceptions of one's self and perceptions of the world are congruent.

Self-actualization theories identify anxious and disturbed people as maladjusted when they are threatened by the incongruity between concept of self and perceptions of experiences. This incongruity causes a distortion and denial of experiences; these then become inconsistent with the concept one holds about oneself (Rogers, 1951).

This theory of personality has quite different assumptions about causes of behavior as compared to psychodynamic and behavioral theories. Psychodynamic theories all assume that expressed feelings and behavior are closely related to the content, fantasies, feelings, and urges repressed in the unconscious part of the personality. This means that people are primarily motivated by irrational, destructive, and unsocialized forces of which they are not aware. On the other hand, behavioral theories locate the impetus for man's actions in the rewards and punishments provided by others or those rewards and punishments that are present in the situation in which behavior emerges. Self-actualization theories hold that a person can know and liberate herself or himself to achieve aspirations and goals.

Social psychological theories of behavior having an interactionist perspective hold that a person is motivated to act on the meanings attributed to the intention of present and future actions of others. In addition, definitions of situations, appraisals of threat to self, problem solving, and feedback from emergent social interactions are also used. Such theories lead to the conceptualization of people as rational, optimistic, and caring persons whose mental health is influenced by factors in social settings and contexts and cultural values and beliefs. Further, people use their distinctly human qualities and abilities to reflect on themselves and on their thoughts, actions, and feelings and to use the results of these reflections as a basis for further actions.

Concept: The Unity of Mind and Body as a Mental Health Concept Needs to be Reflected in Services Provided in Mental Health Care

The traditional focus in the fields of mental health and physical health has been to consider each of these areas as separate entities. This has had the unintended consequence of creating a division in the wholeness of a person's experience. The schism between mental and general health care systems is evident today by separate care systems.

A number of changes are occurring in systems of health care that will improve the unity of direct care services and preserve the wholeness of people's experiences. One is the increased use of liaison nursing between different systems to establish better referral and coordinating activities between health care providers. Another is the reorganization of health services to include both mental and general components making mental health care more accessible and less stigmatic.

Efforts to bring together services in ways permitting clinicians to implement the concept of unity of mind and body are a step forward. For community mental health nursing, it will make it easier to use a holistic perspective of nursing care as a guiding principle for clinical practice.

ASSUMPTIONS ABOUT MENTAL HEALTH AND MENTAL ILLNESS

All models of mental health and mental illness have certain assumptions that underlie basic concepts and principles. The social psychological model presented is no exception. Eight assumptions are identified and discussed.

> *Assumption 1: Mental health and mental illness are two mutually exclusive categories of life experiences that are used to organize selected aspects of behavior.*

This assumption underlies a model of mental health and mental illness that conceives of each category as having distinct and qualitatively different experiences. The behavior of people considered in the context of role expectations, cultural values, and social settings plays an important role in the placement of a person in one category or the other. This discrete, or two-category, model of mental health and mental illness assumes that different patterns of coping responses may be used by people as they function in daily living experiences and in the special experiences designed to help people correct emotional and mental health problems in institutional settings. These patterns vary in terms of their effectiveness for handling stress for promoting the development and maintenance of mental health, and for restoring mental health to people who are mentally ill.

The model is based on the realities of what it means to experience being mentally ill and being mentally healthy. When a person is medically and legally diagnosed as mentally ill, the kind and quality of life experiences undergo abrupt changes. The two-category model of mental health and mental illness differs from ones that place mental health and mental illness at endpoints on a continuum.

The continuum model assumes that one or more common mental processes govern the development and maturation of emotional and mental behavior and underlie both mental illness and mental health. Although biological, developmental, maturational, and physical growth do have principles of development that are common to humans, the assumption that similar principles operate in the development of mental and emotional health is questioned. The reason this is questioned is that the development of emotions, feelings, and cognitions are primarily social and cultural in nature—not biogenetically determined—thus there is great variation in what is learned, the rate of learning, and the meanings attributed to emotional, and cognitive experiences.

It is true that in the early years of life, certain physical, social, and psychological tasks and skills need to be learned at appropriate times, and on these the learning of more complex ones are based. The acquisition of essential social and interpersonal competencies is related to some extent to neuromuscular development of various systems of the body. Although there are some relationships between social psychological development and phases of physical development, there is also considerable independence between these two particularly in adulthood.

Social and cultural aspects of the human experience have great variability not only in terms of their uniqueness for people but also in terms of differences in experiences from subculture to subculture, from culture to culture. Thus, the principles of anatomy and physiology, of biophysical growth and development, of biochemical and neural development cannot be assumed to operate in like manner where the social, cultural, and psychological aspects of growth and development are concerned. If a poor self-concept develops, is distorted or warped, the principles that govern this maladaptive response cannot be assumed to be similar to those that underlie biophysical illness. It is the generalization of the biophysical and genetic model of health and illness with an underlying principle of continuity for human development to social, emotional, and mental development that is questioned. It is in this framework that mental health and mental illness are conceived of as two distinct kinds of social and personal experiences rather than being on a continuum.

Continuum models of mental health and mental illness further assume that the difference between the two conditions is one of degree. In actual practice, the endpoints of the continuum—mental health and mental illness—are usually used as categories to designate mental status in a general sense. It is very difficult to assign someone a place on a mental health–mental illness continuum when the distinctions or diagnoses in mental health are made on categories of behavior rather than on a degree of mental health or mental illness.

Table 3.1
A Two-Category Model of Mental Health and Mental Illness Experiences

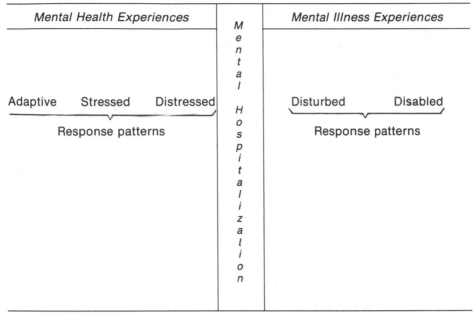

A social psychological model of mental health and mental illness addresses a different set of considerations about life experiences. Socialization of adults and children is important over the life span and is a major force in fostering and maintaining the mental and emotional health of people. The experience of being labeled mentally ill is believed to have consequences for people so labeled and their significant others that are far beyond the immediate situation that caused such a label to be applied.

A two-category model of mental health and mental illness is shown in Table 3.1. Behaviors that place people in one category or the other are different in kind. Data obtained from assessment and from history provide the information to category responses. In each of the categories, responses are a matter of both kind and degree. In a general sense, individual mental health is equated with a general sense of wholeness of mind, body, spirit, and group membership. It is characterized by an ability to cope and adapt without too much stress and getting some satisfaction and enjoyment out of living.

Mental health, in the model in Table 3.1, is characterized by three patterns of responses: (1) adaptive, indicating that life is being handled without undue difficulties; (2) stressed, indicating that there are recurring problems and tensions in coping in daily living experiences, roles, and relationships; and (3) distressed, indicating major systems and role problems in coping and handling relationships.

It is recognized that, theoretically, a number of gradations could be identified to indicate mentally healthy responses; however, in clinical practice, the difficulties of using precise measurements for placement on such a scale are impractical since such measures are not available. Within the mental health experience category, the continuum of responses is on the basis of effectiveness in coping. Experiences in the mental health category differ in kind and quality from those that patients experience in the mental illness category.

The mental health experience category is open-ended and indicates ongoing growth potential for new patterns of coping and adaptive responses to develop. At the individual level, coping and adaptation are related to the outcome of self-actualization and realization of personal autonomy and life goals. These goals are akin to high-level wellness identified by Dunn (1977) and are characterized by maximization of a person's potential within the environments in which she or he functions. Mental health is oriented toward learning and using less stressful ways of coping in order to achieve the fullest measure of satisfaction possible from living and preventing the development of emotional problems and mental illness. Mental health is more than the lack of mental illness. The opportunities for having mentally healthy experiences are infinite, and healthy functioning families and primary socialization groups have a responsibility to see that a variety of these are made available to their members, depending on their age, interests, and stage of development.

Mental illness, in the model in Table 3.1, is characterized by behavior indicating disturbed and disabled coping response patterns to living. This means that communication processes are disturbed or disordered to such an extent that the person cannot effectively communicate with others. Communication and relationship difficulties seriously impair the ability of a person to fulfill roles and functions in family, friendship, and work groups and situations.

In the mental illness category, two patterns of responses are identified and signify coping and adaptation problems: (1) disturbed, indicating diminished ability to perform expected roles, functions, and responsibilities in family, friend, and work systems; and (2) disabled, indicating disability and failure to perform social work and familial roles and expectations and a marked inability to integrate social, cognitive, and psychological aspects of self and the experiences that are happening to the person. The disabled response pattern refers to a person who is severely mentally disabled and requires other people to assist in control of behavior, testing of reality, and establishment of relationships. Professional care and treatment for people using both of these types of behavioral responses are usually provided in protective environments such as hospital psychiatric units, mental hospitals, and psychiatric units in penal institutions.

The major event placing a person in the mental illness category is that of mental hospitalization. This event signifies that a medical and/or legal label of mental illness has been assigned. The acquisition of such a label has serious consequences for the person so labeled, for the family, for significant others, and for some career choices. The stigma and stereotypes associated with mental illness continue to be a problem in our society. This is especially true when a person who has been a mental patient reenters social, familial, friend, and work roles and relationships. Hospitalization for mental and emotional illnesses is a medical and psychiatric decision and is often made without adequate consideration of the long-range consequences for other areas of the person's life. The decision to hospitalize a person needs to be weighed in terms of immediate benefits against future social costs and consequences.

Mental illness experiences are bounded; that is, they are limited in scope and variety. They differ in both kind and quality from mentally healthy experiences not only in their limited and repetetive aspects but also in their interpersonal, familial, social, and psychological ones. Mental hospitalization changes the nature of these experiences as much as and perhaps even more than the effects of emotional and mental problems themselves.

> *Assumption 2:* Mental health and mental illness are related to the experiences that people have in primary groups where socialization takes place.

This assumption specifically relates to the linkages between mental and emotional health and the environments in which people are socialized. Primary group settings of various kinds in which people spend a large portion of their time are major environments for learning a range of behaviors and experiencing different kinds of relationships, all of which are necessary for the development and maintenance of positive mental health.

Social settings may be ranked in terms of their probability for being able to provide children and adults with a milieu conducive to the development of positive mental health. The ranking of settings is based on small-group, organizational, and family theories and research, individual development, and decades of clinical experiences. In Table 3.2, settings are ranked in terms of their potential for providing a milieu for the promotion, maintenance, and enhancement of positive mental health; rankings range from excellent to poor.

A setting in which the potential is *excellent* for development of positive mental health is the *natural* family system in which important socialization processes occur. Socialization starts at birth, thus the family of birth has an optimal potential for providing a healthy growth-promoting environment over the life span. When this potential is realized, the young receive the nurturing care, emotional and social development opportunities, and adult guidance they need to become ready for adulthood. Adults receive emotional and social support and are encouraged to continue personal growth and development. Families who adopt children are also ranked as having an excellent potential, since they in fact try to become natural family systems in the fullest sense. The potential of these systems to provide milieus that support the development of positive mental health of members is related to community and social networks that interrelate family life to cultural values, social norms, and sources of community support. In assessing the mental health of individuals, an understanding of the stability, interrelationships,

Table 3.2
Ranking of Potential of Settings for Development of Positive Mental Health

Ranking of Socialization Potential	Socialization Settings
Excellent	Natural families
	Adoptive families
Good	Surrogate families
	Primary socialization groups in small residential settings
	Primary groups in school, work, and recreational settings
Fair	Family-like groups in residential treatment homes
	Psychiatric units in general hospitals
	Residential treatment centers
Poor	Mental hospitals
	Psychiatric units in penal institutions

and values of the family is necessary because of their interactional influences on the personal and emotional growth and self-actualization of family members.

Surrogate families such as foster families have a *good* potential for providing milieus for promotion, development, and maintenance of the mental health of their members. Such families are substitutes for natural family systems. Surrogate families may provide a home for children and adults and supply the requisite nurturing and social relationships needed for love, growth, and safety. However, these family systems are ranked lower than natural and adoptive families because the potential for social, cognitive, and psychological growth and self-actualization for their members is more uncertain for several reasons. First, foster parents or companions must genuinely like children or adults who need foster care and not view such care as just a means of making a living. Such parents must be mature adults who are comfortable about their own self-identities and achievements in life. They must also be able to experience personal satisfaction in contributing to the development of and in meeting the emotional and physical needs of human beings who require positive family experiences. Foster parents must be able to support each other in their own continued personal growth and actualization. Furthermore, foster families must have adequate resources to provide both the necessities of life as well as creative and educational opportunities for growth. Finally, foster parents must be able to welcome each new member to the family as a person in his or her own right; thus, they must be able to accept considerable diversity in behavior and relationships in the family system.

The socialization of young children and adults may not always occur in natural adoptive, or surrogate family settings. It may take place in settings such as orphanages or halfway houses or in other kinds of special residential settings organized for this purpose. Such settings are ranked as having *good* potential for providing milieus that promote positive mental health. They are characteristically organized in small groups and foster the development of intergroup relationships that are caring, provide direct feedback and communication, and foster the development of a group identity. At best, these settings cannot replicate the roots and relationships that develop in natural families that have, rely on, or can have help from kith and kin networks. Group socialization settings of the kinds described may be organized and managed primarily for pecuniary purposes. In such cases, the potential of such settings to foster and promote the mental health of members may be compromised if resources are so scarce as to jeopardize profit making.

Special residential socialization settings that establish primary groups in which a child or adult can be a member and develop a sense of belonging may provide many of the necessary warm and caring relationships and experiences that are essential for the development of positive mental health. These settings, as a general rule, are limited in the extent to which they can meet individual needs. Therefore, such settings do not have as high a potential as natural and adoptive families for the kind of socialization that promotes and fosters mental health. Such social groups usually interrelate with each other and with other kinds of groups in the community and may be able to provide considerable variation in the number and kinds of situations that people face and are challenged to learn to cope with and adapt to.

In social organizational settings where the potential for the development and maintenance of mental health of people is good or excellent, health promotion and primary prevention activities are the focus of applications in community mental health nursing. Where families and other primary groups experience stress and relationship problems as interacting systems, it is assumed that persons living and working in these settings also experience difficulties in coping. In such situations, interventions are appropriate.

Primary groups in school, work, and recreational settings have a *good* potential for continued socialization in ways that promote positive mental health because of the opportunities for continued learning of essential social, cognitive, and interpersonal competencies. Settings such as these are usually organized for special purposes, however socialization and learning do occur and influence the mental and emotional health of people in many ways. One reason why such settings are ranked good in potential is because of the ability of people to shape them in ways to meet their own needs. There are some settings such as schools that pay particular attention to the socialization of their students; thus, these settings are especially important in promoting and maintaining mental health.

The majority of people in the population are mentally healthy. They do not experience prolonged symptoms of mental and emotional stress to the point of illness. People tend to find effective and satisfying ways of coping before emotional and mental problems become so severe that they need medical and psychiatric attention.

When a person does have mental and emotional problems severe and extensive enough to be diagnosed as mental disorder, mental hospitalization is usually necessary. Hospitalization for a mental disorder is a major personal and social event for the patient. It has a number of implications for the patient both during hospitalization and after a return to family and community roles and functions. Many of these implications are related to the stigma and stereotypes that continue to be associated with mental illness and being a mental patient. In the perceptions of a large number of people, mental illness is simply different from physical illness in many important ways: There is fear about what a mental patient may do, fear of violence, fear of "catching" the illness, and uncertainty in knowing how to act and talk with former patients.

Social settings organized for hospitalization of patients who experience emotional and mental disorders may be ranked in terms of their potential for providing the kind of socialization and relationship experience necessary for recovery of a person's mental health.

Special kinds of socialization are provided in settings designed to provide corrective experiences for maladaptive or deviant behavior. Such settings may be in the form of residential treatment homes, psychiatric units in general hospitals, and residential treatment centers attached to some larger institution. All of these kinds of settings are ranked *fair* in their potential for being able to provide the kinds of milieu that promote and maintain positive mental health. Activities in such settings are sometimes organized to provide social experiences designed to address the personal and emotional needs of residents, inmates, or patients; however, programs are most often organized to accommodate deficits of one kind or another experienced by residents rather than on growth-promoting experiences. This need to accommodate social, emotional, and mental deficits in cognitions, behavior, and relationships makes it extremely difficult to organize a milieu that is conducive to the development of positive mental health. In special socialization settings, residents show the effects of accumulated lags in learning effective coping strategies and ways of relating to others. Furthermore, the provision of creative learning opportunities may not be possible to any extent, and where such opportunities exist, the social and emotional status of residents may hinder their effective use. While residential settings have only a fair potential for the development and maintenance of positive mental health in people, they are more supportive to this effort than total institutions.

Mental hospitals and prison hospitals are total institutions. They have a *poor* potential for providing the kinds of essential individual and group relationships and role experimentation needed for new patterns of coping to be tested and for the self-concept to be enhanced as knowledge and understanding about how one relates to others is experienced and examined.

Mental hospitals and psychiatric units in penal institutions are not organized for promoting the development of social and emotional health behaviors that characterize positive mental health. This is true for settings where both children and adults are institutionalized, although settings for children seem to have more flexible organization and diversity of learning opportunities.

Total institutions are characterized by the following:

1. Basic daily living plans of residents or inmates are drastically altered in that working, playing, and sleeping activities, which under ordinary circumstances are conducted in entirely different arenas of living and with different groups of people in each arena, are broken down, and all these aspects of living occur in the same place under the same single authority.

2. Each day, every day, residents or inmates must conduct all of their activities of daily living in a group; rules and regulations are set up for group management and not for individual concerns.

3. Events of daily living tend consistently to be scheduled by the system of authority deciding in effect who, when, where, and how such activities occur.

4. The daily plan, rules, regulations, and expectations for the group of residents or inmates "fit" a rationale that is supposed to allow the institution to reach its official aims. (Goffman, 1961)

Institutions, such as total institutions, are organized primarily to control and manage deviant behavior. They cannot by their aims and organization provide the kinds of experiences that people need to develop positive mental health. Basically, efforts are made to provide corrective experiences for behavior that is not tolerated socially in order to help patients, residents, or inmates change selective aspects of such behavior that are noxious to others. In this process, it is hoped that some understanding will occur of why any one individual uses certain kinds of behavior or thinks about herself or himself in ways that are not conducive to development of independence, autonomy, and self-actualization. Total institutions are not settings in which mental health is developed or even maintained; they are settings in which deviant behavior is controlled and socially accepted ways of relating are learned so that deinstitutionalization can occur.

Secondary and rehabilitative activities are needed to assist patients in mental hospital settings to learn new behaviors and ways of coping and to achieve some understanding of how usual response patterns are perceived by self and others. Fortunately, only a small minority of persons in our society need mental hospitalization, but this minority has special interpersonal, social, and communication needs. Psychiatric nursing, the care of the hospitalized mentally ill, is the branch of nursing that accepts a major responsibility for providing such care. The complexity of psychiatric nursing is recognized when one examines the competencies relating to therapeutic care of the mentally ill that are needed to fulfill this role: in psychotherapy, sociotherapy, humanistic caring, behavior modification, health education, socialization, therapy, and milieu management (McDonagh, 1980).

The social psychological model of mental health and mental illness interrelates personal, interpersonal, and group experiences that contribute to the development and stabilization of emotional and mental health of adults and children. Social organizational theories relating to primary groups and total institutions are important to the model because they play an important part in learning and structuring the behaviors characteristic of both mental health and mental illness. The organizational structures of different social and institutional settings have different potentials for providing the kind of socialization experiences needed for mental health development. Such structures also have different potentials for assisting people to regain mental health after experiencing a problem.

Socialization is continuous and dynamic over the life span and occurs in whatever settings living activities take place. Not all settings have the same potential for providing the socialization activities and opportunities needed for positive mental health. Settings may be organized for different purposes, have different rules and regulations, and be concerned to different degrees about the development of warm and caring relationships. Major socialization settings have been ranked in terms of their potential for promotion of mental health on the basis of organization, purposes, and ability to create warm and caring milieus in which learning and emotional development can occur. Because of the great influence that milieus have on emotional development and learning, it is recognized that behaviors indicative of both mental health and mental illness can be promoted and maintained in any of the settings but that mental health has a potentially higher probability of developing in some settings than in others. The social psychology of relationships between individuals and organizations suggests that settings will socialize people to learn the behaviors necessary to get along. But such behaviors may be considered deviant outside a particular setting. The ranking of the socialization potential of a number of settings provides a framework that community mental health nurses can use to systematically relate social settings, socialization, and potential for development of positive mental health so that these can be assessed and incorporated as part of a comprehensive data base for providing community mental health nursing.

Assumption 3: Characteristic patterns of interaction, coping, and relationships within families and the behavior of individual members usually indicate whether a person will be placed in the mental health or mental illness category.

Characteristic patterns of responses such as interactions, coping strategies, and communications usually provide some indication of the kind and quality of relationships in the family system. Family members also use characteristic patterns of behavior in their efforts to cope with and adapt to the stresses, joys, and problems of daily living. Certain kinds of behaviors help to place a person in either the mental health or mental illness category of experience. Some of the major behavioral areas are identified in Table 3.3. In general, the behaviors are ones that are observable by other people. Significant changes in a person's level of functioning will be noticed by others. Such changes may be an early indication that a person is having difficulty fulfilling social, personal, work, and familial roles.

The behaviors identified in the categories indicating mental health and mental illness are primarily behavioral and social in nature. People experiencing difficulties such as those described in the mental illness category may also have a number of psychological and familial problems. Even so, it is usually when such problems become intense enough to cause disruptions or significant changes in roles, relationships, and functions that mental illness is considered.

Ten areas of behavior are identified about which judgments are made in determinations of adaptive or maladaptive functioning. In order to be placed in the mental illness category, a person has to use behaviors that indicate difficulties or an inability to function in most of the areas to some extent and in several key areas to a considerable

Table 3.3
Behaviors That Characterize Placement in Either the Mental Health or Mental Illness Experience Category

Mental Health	Mental Illness
Role expectations	
Role expectations and performances are effectively met in family, social, and employment situations; usual and unusual situations with both known and unknown outcomes and familiar and unfamiliar relationships are handled without undue difficulties.	Role expectations and performances are not effectively met in family, social and employment situations; coping efforts show difficulties in handling familiar situations with known outcomes and old relationships.
Role expectations associated with new experiences are used to develop role expansions and relationships that lead to novel solutions to daily living situations and problems.	New role expectations are met with usual response patterns, although they may be ineffective; new experiences are not sought and if they occur, are not used to expand roles; problem solving is not used to address problems that arise as the result of ineffective role performances.
Communication	
Communications are coherent in content, process, and patterns; they link social, cultural, and psychological aspects of group and individual experiences in meaningful ways.	Communications are disturbed and altered in content, process, and patterns; they show an impaired ability to develop and maintain satisfying experiences that promote the development and maintenance of self, group identity, and a sense of community.
Reality testing	
Reality is tested through use of response patterns that, on balance, are effective for coping with both the stressful and unstressful aspects of life experiences and situations encountered in daily living.	Reality is tested through use of response patterns that distort relationships, events, and situations to the degree that subjective perceptions of reality are incongruent with objective reality; the inner meanings of experiences cannot be validated in whole or in part with the perceptions of others.
Interactions with significant others	
Social and interpersonal interactions with significant others are developed in ways that optimize the ability of people to engage in mutually satisfying close relationships.	Social and interpersonal interactions with significant others are altered in their quality and number; there is a decrease in intimacy, closeness, and clarification of mutually understood meanings about relationships.

Self-organization Self is organized by group and individual experiences that facilitate intergration of inner psychological needs, social expectations, situational demands, and meaningful relationships.	Self experiences some disorganization by the diminished ability of person to use and integrate social and interpersonal experiences, inner psychological needs, meet situational demands, and participate in meaningful relationships.
Coping Strategies characteristically used for coping and problem solving are, on balance, effective and go beyond known solutions to discover new ones.	Coping strategies tend to be stereotypical and repetitive; information about their effectiveness is not used to the fullest extent to try out new or modified coping strategies.
Learning Learning takes place with a degree of personal anxiety that enables a realistic evaluation of what happens in the learning process in respect to group, interpersonal, and social relationships; contributes to the continued development of the personal self and behaviors indicative of mental health.	Learning characteristically takes place under a high level of personal anxiety that create distortions in the learning process; only selected aspects of personal and group experiences are examined in terms of their satisfactions and potential for personal growth of self and learning of competencies essential for mental health.
Self-identity The person labels herself or himself as being mentally healthy and uses in a positive way the feedback from others to enhance self-identity, relationships, and social role performances.	The person is labeled by others as having "a mental illness," uses feedback from others on the basis of this label to reinforce a deviant self-identity, exhibits an inability to perform effectively social role performances.
Socialization Socialization experiences in natural and primary group settings are used for continued development and maintenance of self and achievement of self-actualization.	Socialization experiences in mental hospital settings orient and socialize the person to accept a mental patient role, adopt institutional expectations about behavior, and accept that medical treatment and mental hospitalization will restore emotional and mental health.
Role development Roles of different kinds are developed and tried out in social, familial, and work settings and situations and used to maintain and foster development of self and mental health behaviors.	Sick role and attendant behaviors are adopted; an identity of self incorporates identity of a mental patient; there is limited use of different and novel roles that would provide experiences congruent with those needed for functioning outside of mental hospital settings.

extent. Key areas of difficulty are role expectations and performances, communications, reality testing, and the ability to develop and sustain interactions with significant others. Difficulties in these areas are often experienced first by family members and close friends and, if they continue, become noticeable in work, school, and outside-of-family relationships.

The behaviors in both the mental health and mental illness categories may be used in the comprehensive community mental health nursing assessment. The mental health behaviors are those associated with positive mental health. Diminished ability in the performance or learning of such behaviors is reflected in social, psychological, communication, and learning deficits. Continued diminished functioning has a high probability of being assessed and labeled as some form of emotional problem or mental illness.

Behavioral indicators of emotional and mental problems are now widely used in mental health. For example, in many states, selected kinds of behavior are used as indicators of mental illness or emotional problems, especially for emergency commitments to mental hospitals or psychiatric services. Three kinds of behavior are widely used for this purpose: danger to other persons, danger to self, and inability of a person to care for herself or himself because of confusion or disorientation. In respect to dangerous behavior toward others, some research has found that knowledge of the home setting, sociocultural background, and prevalence of stress events that the person has had to cope with are important predictors (Levinson & Ramsay, 1979).

The social and psychological behaviors identified as characteristic of the mental health and mental illness categories are different from those usually of concern in psychiatric assessments. Such examinations usually assess selected aspects of the personality presenting problems, family background, and personal history. They focus on the affect or mood; thought processes, content, fantasies, and aspirations; associations between ideas or lack of same; perceptions, memory, and judgments; and level of maturity. The mental status examination is appropriate to the concept of mental illness as a psychological disease. Unless it is expanded to include roles, relationships, communication, and patterns of coping, a great many aspects of daily living may not be considered. In such cases, a determination of the mental status of a person may be based on a fairly limited cluster of behavior.

The model of mental health and mental illness emphasized as a basis for the clinical practice of community mental health nursing is much broader than traditional ones of mental illness as faulty mental functioning. The behaviors that place a person in a mental health or mental illness category are consistent with the overall emphasis that mental health and mental illness both have social and cultural components and these have to be included in the clinical frameworks of community mental health nursing.

Mental Health and Mental Illness Considered as Two Different Life Experiences

Early in the community mental health movement in the 1950s, a number of social and behavioral scientists and mental health professionals noted that mental health and mental illness are two different life experiences. Unfortunately, this view of mental health and mental illness was not pursued primarily because of the prevailing view in psychiatry that considered mental illness analogous to a physical illness. The idea that two distinct kinds of experiences for mental health and mental illness existed was not supportive of the medical model of mental illness—and this model was then and continues to be the dominant one in American mental health.

Smith (1950) noted 30 years ago that a positive concept of mental health spoke to an experience that is entirely different from an experience with a mental disease or abnormality. He proposed three different indicators of mental health: adjustment, integration, and cognitive adequacy, with individual circumstances and sociocharacteristics considered. A couple of years later, Conrad (1952) suggested the need for mental health clinicians to think beyond psychopathy to a positive concept of mental health. She proposed two major categories: health and pathology. Mental health was conceived of as different in many respects from mental illness and more than the lack of mental illness. Kroner (1958) later proposed that mental health and mental illness be considered as two distinct continua rather than one continuum. On the mental health continuum endpoints would be mental health and mental injury; on the mental illness continuum, susceptibility and mental illness.

In a classic analysis of concepts of mental health, Jahoda (1958) proposed that mental health and mental illness be considered as entities of health potential and not as endpoints on a continuum. Each entity would address two qualitatively different kinds of phenomena. These discussions about the nature of mental health and mental illness occurred early in the community mental health movement but gained little support at that time because most mental health professionals conceived of mental health and mental illness as a continuous health–illness process.

The continuum model of mental health and mental illness assumes that differences between the two conditions are a matter of degree, not a difference in kinds of behavior that characterize each condition. This model further assumes that the behavior of a person can be placed with some precision and confidence on the scale on the basis of assessment data at any particular time. Even if this model had validity, precise criteria are still not available for using it. This problem was recognized many years ago by Menninger (1963), who identified the need for distinctive criteria that would allow such placement.

Manning and Zucker (1976) are among a number of scientists who stated that normality in relation to mental health and abnormality in relation to mental illness are mutually exclusive conditions. They noted that although these conditions are often treated as if they were continuous and overlapping, a person cannot have both conditions or be in both categories at the same time. Osborne (1970) also questioned the notion of a mental health–mental illness continuum and described a two-continua model of mental health and psychiatric nursing. This model in effect conceives of mental health and mental illness as mutually exclusive categories.

Several years ago, Clausen (1968) rejected the notion of a mental health–mental illness continuum because it could not accommodate the numerous facets of behavior that relate to the two different kinds of life experiences. He conceptualized mental health as multidimensional in scope and included factors that do not necessarily evolve on the basis of an underlying characteristic. He identified such factors as: (1) the ability to relate to others in mutually satisfying and enduring relationships; (2) the ability to mobilize one's personal resources to meet the demands of unexpected or difficult circumstances; (3) the substantial degree of autonomy or ability needed to regulate one's life; and (4) a perception of oneself and others that is reasonably accurate or realistic and free from distortions arising from one's own psychological needs.

Political and professional considerations, rather than research, have to a large extent shaped the concepts of mental health in this country as well as the directions for establishing service. When the community mental health movement was seeking support from many groups and the public, a major effort from the outset was to blur and minimize distinctions between mental health and mental illness. The reason for this strategy was to diminish the stigma and stereotypes attached to mental illness in order to increase the acceptability of community-based mental health services and the community residence of former mental patients.

Differences between mental health and mental illness were minimized to change the attitudes and beliefs people attached to insanity and mental illness. If mental health is a desirable condition that everyone has to some extent but not in all extents, then mental illness is an exaggeration of those aspects of mental health in which one is not quite up to par! Thus, mental illness is not alien to an individual's health experience. Over a decade ago, Grinker (1966) pointed out some of the values associated with such shifts in terminology in the field of mental health. He observed that the term "mental health," which has a sweet sound and hopeful connotation, has rapidly replaced the feared words "mental illness." Furthermore, he noted that clinics are no longer called psychiatric but "mental health centers" even though their stench remains.

The continuum model of mental health and mental illness helped to stimulate the development of the community-based mental health services and care. However, at the direct patient care level where theory is used to guide assessment of mental health and related problems and to orient clinicians toward particular kinds of interventions, the use of a continuum concept has limitations. Although the strategy of blurring the meanings between mental health and mental illness may have been useful in the early years of the community mental health movement, it is time to examine critically whether this model of mental health and mental illness is one that advances clinical management of emotional problems, promotion of mental health, and generation of research in community mental health nursing.

> *Assumption 4: There are differences in the quality of the life experiences of poeple who are labeled mentally ill and those considered to be mentally healthy.*

This assumption holds that people who are medically and legally labeled mentally ill have quite different kinds of life experiences than people who have never been so labeled. Rüemke (1955) made a strong plea for understanding these differences by emphasizing that understanding the mentally ill person does not contribute to understanding the mentally healthy normal person. Psychiatry has been criticized for trying to understand mental illness without prior knowledge of mental health.

Qualitative differences occur in a person's experiences when mentally ill that involve a number of basic human processes. Changes occur in the feelings a person holds about herself or himself and toward others. Thoughts and actions may not occur as intended.

Irrespective of what may be the cause of behavior, the actual behavior that a person uses is what sets into motion changes in personal, interpersonal, and group relationships. These changes are experienced and given meaning by significant others with whom interactions occur and they have an immediate impact on further relationships.

The Qualitative Changes in Interpersonal and Group Relationships

When a person is having difficulty coping and the coping responses are not appropriate, qualitative changes in interpersonal and group relationships occur. These changes follow a developmental process. The labeling of odd and unusual behavior as a mental and emotional problem usually does not occur abruptly unless behavior is so bizarre or dangerous that it constitutes a psychiatric or medical emergency. The person who is experiencing stress and a feeling of loss of control of behavior and situations also experiences difficulty trying to maintain close relationships, performing usual roles and functions, and using appropriate and adaptive behavior in daily living situations. Family members, close friends, and colleagues in work situations notice the difficulties and changes in behavior and soon begin to experience unease about the stressed person. Slowly and surely, family, personal, and work relationships undergo qualitative changes. Changes occur in the intensity, spontaneity, and frequency of relationships and communications. Patterns of interactions undergo changes in order to decrease emotional and physical closeness. Role expectations and responsibilities undergo redefinitions in order to accommodate the decreased ability of the stressed person to function as effectively as she or he once did. The perceptions held by significant others about the person who is experiencing difficulties undergo a change, and the social labeling of the individual as a person who has a mental or emotional problem occurs.

Once labeling occurs, the perceptions that significant others hold about the distressed person lead to the reinforcement of perceptions that the person is developing about herself or himself. These perceptions become the basis for further interactions and have a continuing effect on the quality of interpersonal and group relationships. By this time, it is difficult for both the distressed person and significant others to achieve and experience satisfying relationships. When this happens, mutual withdrawal occurs. At this point in the developmental process, the distressed person is deprived of many opportunities to test reality with friends and associates and to find acceptance for the best behavior that can be mustered. There will now be a further reallocation of roles and responsibilities that reduces the need for face-to-face relationships between the person who is experiencing difficulties and significant others. Potential conflicts will be avoided by minimizing opportunities for the distressed individual to try out new behaviors or modify old ones that have been used to handle situations in the past. The subjective changes and perceptions that are part of the inner world of the distressed are played out in social settings and reflected in changes in key relationships.

Interactions generated under these circumstances set into motion a cyclical process that becomes mutually reinforcing between the person experiencing difficulties and significant others. If hospitalization in a mental hospital becomes necessary, all key interpersonal and group relationships undergo drastic changes.

Becoming a Mental Patient in a Mental Hospital

When a person becomes a mental patient in a mental hospital, there is an abrupt transition in role and status for the person. There is the adoption of the sick role entailing the adoption of social constraints and expectations associated with the label "mental patient." When hospitalization in a mental hospital setting takes place, segregation occurs for people who have a similar label and mental illnes problems. For patients, there is a loss or curtailment of freedom and control over their personal actions and daily living activities. There is constant monitoring or surveillance by caretakers day and night. Expectations of these caretakers about appropriate behavior in the hospital setting and the information that they provide to patients for getting along in the mental hospital milieu may have little or no relevance for application for roles outside of the hospital that the patient hopes to reenter as soon as possible.

Changes occur in the relationships that the sick person has with family members, friends, and co-workers. In trying to relate to and communicate with a mental patient, everyone involved often experiences anxiety, guilt, and fear. The patient's relatives and friends often do not know what to say or how to say it. These uncertain aspects of interpersonal relationships alter the flow and ease of interactions. This unease is transmitted by both verbal and nonverbal communication. It is not long before all of these changes come to have an effect on the self-concept of the patient as well as on significant others who are trying to maintain a meaningful relationship.

Another change for the mental patient concerns her or his ability to cope and adapt to situations. The sick person may recognize that something does not seem quite right with her or his response to a situation. Behavior often has meaning for the patient but there is difficulty in communicating these meanings to others. If the patient acts on inner-world fantasies and feelings, the gulf between the patient and those around her or him becomes even greater. Significant others experience even greater difficulties trying to communicate and maintaining loving and caring relationships. Changes in the quality of these personal and interpersonal relationships are reflected in patterns of interactions by avoidance of contact, guarded communications, cautious selection of topics, and careful maintenance of physical space and emotional distance.

The world of the mental patient differs in several respects from a mentally healthy person's world. A major difference is the loss or serious impairment of communality, that is, the ability to experience group unity, group cohesion, and group purpose. Not being able to fully experience being a member of a community deprives the patient of needed experiences in group membership, sharing of group interests, and providing and receiving support from others. Group experiences are essential for patients in mental hospitals because they attest to and support the patients' humanity. Such experiences also provide opportunities to learn essential social and relationship competencies and a milieu in which such competencies can be tried with others without fear of failure.

There are also qualitative differences in the consequences of hospitalization for a mental illness and those of hospitalization for other kinds of illness. The consequences of mental hospitalization operate in social relationships, job opportunities, and family and marital relationships after such hospitalization. These consequences may be experienced keenly when the former mental patient tries to establis relationships with associates in personal, social, group, and work situations. Negative stereotypes about mental illness and insanity are remembered, whereas other illnesses tend to be associated with more socially accepted beliefs. Negative beliefs are reflected in the ways in which close associates structure and control their relationships and expectations.

When so many changes occur in the basic processes of the human experience as a result of being mentally ill, the experience is quite different in kind and quality from that with other kinds of illnesses. Such changes cumulate to make being mentally ill an unique experience. No other illness in our society creates the special combination of circumstances that is set into motion when a person is hospitalized for a mental illness.

Mental health professionals are wont to say that mental illness is like any other illness. People who have been mentally ill, their families, friends, and co-workers do not experience mental illness and its personal, familial, and social consequences in the same way that other kinds of illnesses are experienced.

> *Assumption 5: Both mental health and mental illness are multidimensional experiences and there is a need for mental health professionals to consider a broad array of data in providing mental health services.*

The assumption holds that both mental health and mental illness are far more than psychological experiences. Both include multidimensional factors involving social, cultural, behavioral, situational, and psychological aspects of living. Many of the difficulties that are involved in trying to define mental health and mental illness are due to differences in concepts about the role such factors have in the development and organization of the self. A further problem is that mental health and mental illness tend to be defined as conditions inherent within *individuals*, thus, definitions that include social, cultural, and community aspects as part of these conditions are difficult to reconcile.

Pasewark and Rardin (1971) classified theoretical models of community mental health in two broad categories to make more explicit some of the dimensions involved as person-focused and population-focused. The person-focused model is concerned primarily with the individual and emphasizes the treatment of already existing emotional and mental health problems. This category includes the medical, ego, actualization, behavioral, and social models of behavior. The population-focused model focuses on broader environmental, cultural, and social factors that are involved in the mental health and mental illness of populations. This category includes public health and social models of health and illness.

The social psychological model of mental health and mental illness is multidimensional and uses concepts from both the person-focused and population-focused models. Concepts have been consolidated and added to develop a focus on the primary group settings in which child and adult socialization takes place from birth to death and where the major dramas of life occur. This focus is important because family settings are important, especially in the early years of person's life, when nurturing and growth needs are high, and in later years in the stabilization of adult personalities and the realization of interpersonal satisfactions. Other kinds of primary groups are also important in mental health because it is in these settings that much of communal living in a complex society occurs. The model explicitly addresses the interrelationships that exist between individuals primary groups in which they are members, and the social and cultural contexts in which these relationships occur.

Jahoda (1958) cited the need for mental health professionals to consider more fully the conditions under which mental health is acquired and maintained. She noted that behavior needs to be considered not only on the basis of individual personalities but also on the basis of primary and reference group memberships, all of which influence the mental health of individuals. This observation was based on evidence that individuals adjust their behavior not only in interactions with other people but also in response to situations and institutional expectations. All of these factors are more or less independent of the particular personality a person may have. Jahoda also commented on environmental considerations that take into account the people with whom a person interacts at different phases of development. By this she meant that as the world of a person expands, the impact of environment on mental health occurs through a variety of channels such as schools and community experiences.

Mental illness and mental health are two different kinds of experiences that occur in the total context of living. Models that consider mutlidimensional factors that influence the development of mental health need to conceive of a framework that assists the clinician in making distinctions between being mentally ill and being mentally healthy.

> *Assumption 6: Mental wellness and mental illness are integral aspects of general wellness and illness.*

Traditionally, concepts of mental wellness and mental illness have been conceptualized as if they had little relationship to general health and general illness. Many personality and psychopathology theories assume that fragments of the human experience—the emotional and cognitive aspects—can satisfactorily explain the complexities of behavior associated with mental functioning. This assumption creates an artificial dichotomy between body and mind. Mental illness continues to be regarded as a special illness that requires mental health specialists to administer care and treatment in special kinds of psychiatric services. This division of health into mental and physical aspects carries over to the organization of services and to education and training programs for mental health professionals.

A concept of health needs to be broad enough to encompass the essential unity of mind and body. More important, it should lead the mental health clinician to raise questions about the health status of a person that look to connections between the mental and physical aspects of health. Neal (1975) pointed out that health is a crucial concept in medical systems because it informs theory, directs activities, and generally shapes the contours of clinical practice. Moreover, concepts of health and illness have consequences for theories that are used for clinical application. An example of this principle is the definition of health by Illich (1976): a process of adaptation during which one can actively change one's life situation. Such a definition directs the clinician's attention to a particular range of data and a particular way of conceptualizing the data.

Mental Health Related to the General Health of a Person

The health of the psychological structure of the personality that makes up the personal organization of the self is related to a person's general health status. General health in turn is interrelated to the social, cultural, and work settings in which the person spends most of her or his time. To consider the organization of the self in isolation from the general health of the person is to ignore the unity of mind and body as they function in concert. Health in its broadest context takes into account physical, mental, and social functioning of a person and the environments in which the person copes in order to try to achieve a measure of satisfaction in life.

Besson (1967) portrayed health as a health–illness spectrum. In this model, health is defined as a state of interaction between self and environment and not a condition of the individual. It is a ceaseless struggle between a basically hostile environment and a series of defenses that people are endowed with and add to when necessary. Environmental hazards are physical, biological, social, and cultural in nature. In another view, Murray and Zentner (1975) distinguished between health and illness by defining health as purposeful adaptive physical, emotional, and social responses to internal and external stimuli in order to maintain stability and comfort. Illness is described as disturbed adaptive responses to internal and external stimuli resulting in disequilibrium and inability to use health promotion resources.

Dunn (1977) proposed that health be viewed as high-level wellness. Good health is a relatively passive state of freedom from illness, whereas wellness is thought of as dynamic—a condition of change in which a person moves forward, climbing toward a higher potential of functioning. High-level wellness is defined as an integrated method of functioning that is oriented toward maximizing the potential of which an individual is capable within the environment in which she or he is functioning.

A more contemporary approach to defining health and illness is to identify health and illness behaviors. Douglass (1971) defined health behaviors as actions taken to avoid becoming ill or to detect disease in the presymptomatic stage. Illness behaviors are actions taken when a person believes herself or himself to be ill and seeks a diagnosis or treatment regimen. Factors associated with health behaviors that integrate the unity of mind, body, and sociocultural factors are concept of self, psychophysiological expression of stress, coping strategies, and role. It is being increasingly recognized that a majority of the emotional problems being encountered in community mental health are related to stress, anxiety, depression, and ineffective ways of coping. All of these problems are social, physical, and multidimensional in nature.

Primary Prevention of Mental Illness in Well Populations

Integral to a concept of health is the primary prevention of mental illness in well populations. The public health model of primary prevention, based on biophysiological processes, has not been especially useful for planning programs that prevent illnesses and conditions that have unknown or have multiple causes.

Primary prevention in mental health has received maximal verbal and minimal financial support in this country. A major reason for this situation is that clinicians in mental health are oriented by education and practice to provide care and treatment to the people with emotional problems and mental illnesses. Thus, decisions about services, budgets, and program directions are usually made by mental health professionals who do not hold strong public health orientations about primary prevention.

A 30-year debate over how to define and implement primary prevention programs to prevent mental and emotional illnesses has had the unintended consequences of slowing down the development and test of different approaches. The ethical and philosophical issues involved in changing social and cultural patterns and beliefs that have a relation to mental health are difficult to resolve in a democratic society that places great value on diversity and freedom of choice. More recently, at the national level, health care policy is emphasizing primary prevention. In respect to this emphasis in mental health, Goldston (1977) suggested four different frameworks by which primary prevention in mental health might be categorized: (1) mental illnesses with known etiology; (2) mental illness with unknown etiology; (3) emotional stress, maladaptation, maladjustment, needless psychopathology, and human misery; and (4) promotion of mental health.

The social, psychological, and somatic linkages that unify physical, mental, and social health are not well understood but they do exist. Maps of these linkages will evolve through further discoveries in neurophysiology, biochemistry, and social psychology. However, a person's health status at any given time is a holistic response to internal and external demands and stimuli. Thus, a comprehensive approach to health is necessary in community mental health nursing.

> *Assumption 7: Placement of a person in the mental illness category depends on changes in social relationships, situational demands, and cultural contexts in which odd and unusual behavior occurs.*

The behavior of a person in and of itself does not necessarily indicate who is mentally ill. A considerable amount of unusual and abnormal behavior is not defined as mental illness because of a number of mediating circumstances. These circumstances are varied and involve such things as the tolerance of a person's family to odd and unusual behavior, the degree to which such behavior disrupts relationships in work and other primary group settings, the context in which the behavior occurs, and the cultural values and beliefs that are attributed to the behavior by observers. In recent years, legal definitions of mental illness have become increasingly more limited and specify particular kinds of behaviors for which a person may be hospitalized involuntarily in a psychiatric facility. However, a person may use behaviors such as those specified in legal codes and not be hospitalized in a mental institution or setting because of the number of mediating factors that may deflect such an action.

In some of the classic studies of paths to the mental hospital, a number of social and familial factors were identified that prevented diagnosis and mental hospitalization. For example, Yarrow and Clausen (1955) found considerable variation in the kinds of behaviors that families, the individuals themselves, and significant others considered "crazy." Odd and even bizarre behavior was not recognized as such, or it was ignored or rationalized as having a cause not associated with mental illness. Variations such as these continue to operate when decisions have to be made about people who have behaviors suggestive of mental illness.

Scheff (1966) found that five major conditions operate to determine whether a person will be labeled mentally ill for odd and unusual behavior: (1) the degree, amount, and visibility of the odd and unusual behavior; (2) the power of the person who engages in the behavior; (3) the social distance between this person and the individual(s) who would exert means to secure control over the person's behavior; (4) the tolerance level of the community in which the behavior occurs; and (5) the availability in the community of alternative roles for the person to adopt. Koldjeski (1974) found that the most important factor that caused labeling of odd and unusual behavior to be mental illness was for it to occur in crisis situations. Research suggests that the labeling of odd and unusual behavior—the kind of behavior that has a high probability of being labeled as "sick" behavior—is dependent on many factors other than the behavior itself.

Placement of a person in the mental illness category may also be done on an informal basis by social labeling. This process involves the labeling of a person as "sick" for nonconforming behavior. The unfortunate thing about this practice is that the label is picked up and transmitted to others who may not know the person personally and therefore not have data either to support or to refute the use of it. Other people then begin to act toward the individual who has been labeled as if the label was real and valid. At some point, it no longer matters whether the label has any basis in fact. It becomes associated with the person as if it were in fact true. Unfortunately, once labeling occurs and begins to be used by others, changes then occur in ongoing relationships and in employment potential for the person so labeled.

Placement of an individual in the mental illness category may be done more formally by application of a psychiatric diagnosis (a medical–legal label) of mental illness by a physician. The type of diagnosis and the decision of whether to hospitalize in a psychiatric facility are related more to social and situational factors than to distinctive behaviors that indicate a particular kind of mental illness. For example, beginning with Hollingshead and Redlich (1958), a considerable body of literature has established a relationship between the kind of diagnosis a person receives and social class. Certain kinds of behaviors are diagnosed as mental illness when the person is in a low social class; the same behavior is called a personal idiosyncrasy when the person comes from the upper class (Hollingshead & Redlich, 1958). Other social factors that have been identified as influencing the diagnosis and kind of treatment a person receives in psychiatric services are race, sex, and role in family.

The assumption that placement in the mental illness category depends on behavior that has many social and cultural factors as well as on odd and unusual behavior that is often situation specific is related to difficulties of establishing differential diagnoses on the basis of a mental illness concept. The community mental health nurse who relies on a selected group of personal behaviors being used by patients or clients and considered apart from social and cultural contexts must be sensitive to the limitations of such an assessment.

> *Assumption 8:* The "mental health" of a community is essential for the mental health of people who live and work there because of the need for supportive personal, familial, and social relationships.

The concept of "mental health" of a community relates to the interrelationships between social and community networks and the mental health of families and individuals who live in that community. The community must provide many of the resources essential for its members to experience satisfying and growth-promoting personal, interpersonal, and group relationships. The degree to which this goal is met is one measure of the mental health of a community.

More specifically, the mental health of a community can be measured by the extent to which it provides for life experiences for children and adults that contribute to the development of positive mental health over the life span. Mental illness and emotional stress are positively correlated with poverty, social status, family structure, race, and sex. For example, a black woman who is separated from her husband, has children, and earns the minimum wage in house-cleaning jobs has quite different community service and resource needs than does a white man with a spouse and children who earns an income that places the family in a high-income bracket and a high social status. In this case, the kinds of services and resources that the community provides to help the black mother organize socialization experiences conducive to her children's mental health and the maintenance and uplifting of her own are indicative of the mental health of a community.

The community is a major social setting that influences on the kinds of behavior that people and groups use in public places. This influence is felt through community networks and the interrelationships between networks, families, and other kinds of primary groups. This transmission of influence through system networks is facilitated by the sense of identity that people develop about their community. This sense of community is reflected in community values, norms, and the kinds of social networks that are developed and supported. In turn, all of these are linked to some extent to religious institutions, schools, employment settings, and leisure organizations through interrelationships and participation.

The Mental Health of a Community

A community's mental health may also be evaluated by conceiving of it as having three major dimensions: emotional, structural, and functional (Archer & Fleshman, 1979). The *emotional community* is the place where one has feelings of belonging. It is often the place where one was born and grew up and has family and kin roots. The emotional community is important because it has a relationship to the personal identity people hold about themselves. The longing to know where one belongs and comes from can be gauged to some extent by the unparalleled interest in genealogy that occurred after the publication of *Roots* (Haley, 1976), the psychohistory of a black family across time, space, generations, and human experiences.

Urbanization and industrialization continue to be important factors in creating a need for mobility of individuals and families. Mobility involves relocation across states, regions, and continents. The enrichment of human interactions and support that comes from stable family and friend relationships and the putting down of roots can be diminished or lost with mobility. Career advancement, economic improvements in one's standard of living, and personal freedom in terms of increased autonomy and privacy may be gained by moving away from one's emotional community. However, these gains have concomitant losses. A major one is the loss of caring and supportive relationships of families and friends. Another is the change in the intimacy and feeling of belonging in one's emotional community to a sense of social and personal isolation in a new geographic community.

The *structural community* relates to time and space relationships among people. Of the several aspects of the structural community Archer and Fleshman (1979) described, three have been found to be particularly useful in community mental health nursing: the primary community, the community of solutions, and the ecological community. The *primary community* represents the primary social groups within the community that relate and interrelate on a continuing basis. In these groups, members know one another, communication networks tend to be short and direct, and the concerns of the community are known to the members. The *community of solutions* defines a community as an entity around which boundaries may be set in order to look at concerns and arrive at solutions. This way of looking at the community cross-cuts other ways of organizing the community and leads the community mental health nurse to examine a mosaic of resources that people in the community have access to outside the community. The political jurisdictions that get involved in community affairs, and the different kinds of people who come together to work on a common mission. The *ecological community* addresses the distribution patterns of health and illness as well as environmental, social, and technological conditions that contribute to health and illness patterns.

The ecological community concept is congenial with the concept of a catchment area, the geographical area in which a particular community mental health center has the responsibility for providing mental health services. Catchment areas are organized on the basis of population density, hence the geographical area may be quite small in urban areas and very large in sparsely settled ones. Each federally funded community mental health center in the country has a designated catchment area. Population of the area may range from 35,000 to 75,000 people. In practice, the assignment of a geographical service area on the basis of population density has caused communities, primary groups, and neighborhoods to be fragmented and separated, often adversely affecting the "mental health" of the community that community mental health centers are designed to serve.

The *functional community* is based on the identification of groups of people who have common interests about the community and work on its everyday problems and concerns. These groups can be drawn together to address things that the community needs in order to improve the quality of life and provide essential services to its citizens.

Each of these facets of the community may be used to obtain data from families, groups, and individuals in order to establish some of the interrelationships between them and the community. It is important in the comprehensive community mental health nursing assessment to obtain a picture of participation and the use of resources in the community by the family or individual being assessed.

MENTAL HEALTH DEFINED

Mental health is an integral component of the total health experience. It is defined as the outcome of interactions that individuals and families use in the process of coping, adapting and achieving satisfactions in loving relationships, in daily activities and in work and community activities and relationships. This definition is enhanced by the inclusion of one proposed by Williams (1972): Mental health is a particular human endeavor in which people do things in describable and relatively organized ways. Both of these definitions assume that people in primary group settings are able to integrate personality and social and cultural factors to perform roles and meet situational demands, and in this process, experience both satisfaction and challenge. Conflicting forces and demands are handled in ways that, on balance, make it possible for people to achieve satisfying and enduring relationships, enjoy creative expression, experience personal autonomy, and achieve rewards in social and work situations. These outcomes are made possible by the development of problem-solving skills and adaptive coping responses and the expression of feelings and emotional responses in ways that facilitate the management of expected and unexpected relationships and situations.

MENTAL ILLNESS DEFINED

Mental illness is defined as a special life experience involving individuals, their families and the primary groups in which their daily living and working relationships and activities occur. It is characterized by the use of disturbed and disabling interactions by people under stress who are trying to cope with the realities of role performances, maintain key interrelationships in their lives, and fulfill familial, social, and work responsibilities. The inner turmoil and conflict a person may experience in mental illness may be acted out in different ways in the social settings and situational contexts encountered in daily living. Disturbed and disabling interactions interfere with a person's ability to perform institutionalized roles and related tasks; to function in interpersonal, family, group, and employment relationships; to test the reliability of these experiences; to communicate meaningfully with others; and to manage aspects of her or his environment. In mental illness, these impairments are severe enough that a person is unable to function in most or all of these areas in a consistent and effective manner and to achieve satisfactions in relationships and achievements.

Mental illness is multidimensional in that it has social, psychological, biophysical, and cultural aspects of behavior. Furthermore, situational experiences, with their rules and norms for conduct, tend to act as triggers for certain kinds of actions and interractions. For people under great stress and experiencing considerable inner turmoil, such triggers may evoke the emergence of odd, unusual, inappropriate, and even bizarre behavioral responses.

An inability or greatly reduced ability to handle personal and social stress for any length of time has a high probability of resulting in mental hospitalization. Hospitalization legitimates acceptance of the sick role and assumes that four kinds of conditions exist: (1) the individual cannot overcome the incapacity by decision making or actions on her or his accord; (2) the sick person is exempted from normal role and task obligations; (3) the role is legitimated by medical authority (inherent in this legitimation is the assumption that the individual will follow the regimen and use her or his energies to get well); and (4) the individual seeks competent medical assistance and cooperates in getting well (Parsons, 1958).

On reentry to the community, individuals discharged from a mental hospital or psychiatric service are assumed to have learned more adaptive patterns of responses for handling the stresses and problems in their lives. Therefore, posthospitalization mental patients are assumed to have regained a measure of mental health. The goal of community mental health nursing is to assist these persons to structure life experiences, not as former mental patients, but as mentally healthy people who are able to function to some degree in the community, in their families, and in work roles. It is assumed that people who have undergone the special experience of being mentally ill will have some stress as they reintegrate into family, work, social groups, and community life. Therefore, it is important that this normal kind of response not be interpreted in ways to justify setting up *"patient–nurse"* relationships. Rather, the goal is to establish relationships with these citizens on the basis of their being responsible individuals who have had a unique experience learning to more effectively handle the stresses and problems in their lives and achieve greater satisfaction from life.

SOCIAL PSYCHOLOGICAL MODEL OF MENTAL HEALTH AND MENTAL ILLNESS

The model of mental and mental illness that has been developed to this point includes multidimensional aspects and conceives of mental health and mental illness as two distinct categories of life experiences. A more complete model is now presented to show some of the interrelationships between the different dimensions. The model is shown in Table 3.4.

Earlier in this chapter, in Table 3.1, a two-category model of mental health and mental illness experiences was presented in which three kinds of response patterns are associated with mental health: adaptive, stressed, and distressed. Characteristic response patterns associated with mental illness experiences are identified as disturbed and disabling. Mental health responses are open-ended and have the potential for growth and use of innovative and creative experiences. Mental illness experiences tend to be selective and are limited in range, scope, and innovativeness.

Building on the two-category model of mental health and mental illness experiences, the social psychological model incorporates additional dimensions of these experiences. Major ones are the potential of different kinds of socialization systems for promoting and maintaining the positive mental health of members, expected kinds of response patterns that characterize such systems, the potential for opportunities to develop autonomous and independent behaviors, and participation in community activities and networks.

Given the potential of socialization systems to provide milieus conducive for the development of the positive mental health of their members, each system can be assessed to determine the level of actual functioning and to identify characteristic response patterns of behavior. Once characteristic response patterns of behavior have been validated with sufficient evidence, the nurse can estimate the extent to which the potential is not being realized. For example, the nurse assesses a natural family system to identify characteristic patterns of interactions and communication patterns to determine whether the milieu is one in which there are loving and caring relationships, whether opportunities are provided for adults and children to learn essential social competencies, and whether the structure and relationship network provides stability and helps the family to achieve its goals. If the potential of the family is being realized, then the nurse would expect to find on balance adaptive patterns of responses. However, it is possible that potential is good even though there is stress in characteristic response patterns. Or the family may have response patterns that clearly indicate distress. On the coping response continuum, it has already been noted that a number of additional gradations could be added; however, for use in clinical situations, small incremental gradations are not practical.

Some distinctions are made in the model about the kinds of therapeutic activities that the community mental health nurse may find appropriate for socialization systems experiencing different degrees of stress. Preventions are recommended for healthy and adaptive functioning systems. Counseling and interventions are provided to systems that are stressed, while specialized interventions may be needed to help distressed family and other kinds of primary socialization systems.

In mental illness experiences, the potential of specialized settings to provide healthy and growth-promoting experiences in some small group situations is fair, while in larger total institutional-type settings it is poor. Because of various institutional expectations about management of people's behavior when they are hospitalized with mental illness, the experiences that promote mental health are usually not readily available on a consistent basis.

Once mental hospitalization occurs, treatment tends to be both psychiatric and medical in nature and involves specialized psychological modalities and medical interventions. In this setting, psychiatric nursing plays an important role in the establishment of milieus that provide specialized learning opportunities, making available a group of professionals who care and provide assistance and support, and coordinating the many facets of daily living activities.

The social psychological model of mental health and mental illness is a picture of interrelationships that may exist between selected dimensions of these experiences and the potential for such experiences to occur. It also relates response patterns to systems of socialization and therapeutic activities in community mental health nursing. In clinical practice, the responsibility of the community mental health nurse is to determine how closely actual situations fit those described in the model so that clinical judgments may be made about particular situations. The model is an integral part of the clinical organizing framework that guides nursing practice.

IMPLICATIONS FOR COMMUNITY MENTAL HEALTH NURSING

There are always implications for community mental health nursing in whatever model of mental health and mental illness is used. The assumptions of the social psychological model shape clinical practice and orient the kinds of client outcomes the nurse hopes to help clients achieve. The dimensions of mental health and mental illness orient the nurse to ask certain kinds of questions in the assessment process, and they serve as the basis for interpretation of data and evaluation.

Prevention and promotion of mental health are derived from mental health models rather than from mental illness ones. The community mental health nurse must develop some sensitivity about the inappropriateness of using mental illness frameworks with mentally healthy families and individuals and when working with socialization groups of any kind.

Another kind of awareness that must be heightened is that the official classification of mental disorders used in mental health services exerts a pervasive influence on clinical concepts of both mental health and mental illness. This influence also affects the clinical judgments that nurses make about the emotional and mental health of clients and families. The official classification system orients clinicians to consider certain kinds of data to the exclusion of others. It provides criteria for putting data together in ways to arrive at certain kinds of conclusions. This shaping process was described by Wilson and Kneisl (1983) (*see* page 90).

Table 3.4
A Social and Psychological Model of Mental Health and Mental Illness Experiences

Interrelationships Among Social Settings, Characteristic Responses, and Potential for Mental Health

Mental Health Experiences

Dimension	Potential/Responses		
Potential for mental health promotion and maintenance in primary socialization systems by rank	Excellent for Natural families Adoptive families	Good for Surrogate families Family-like groups Primary groups in schools and work settings	
Characteristic response patterns in primary socialization milieu; open-ended experiences	Adaptive	Stressed	Distressed
	Actual patterns determined by assessment		
Participation in community/social activities and networks	Excellent	Good	Fair

Interrelationships Among Specialized Social Settings, Characteristic Responses, and Potential for Mental Health

Mental Illness Experiences

Dimension	Potential/Responses	
Potential for mental health experiences in specialized socialization systems by rank	Fair for Small residential settings Psychiatric units in general hospitals Residential treatment centers	Poor for Mental hospitals Psychiatric units in penal settings
Unusual response patterns in socialization systems; experiences limited in scope, kind, and intensity	Disturbed	Disabled
	Actual patterns determined by assessment	
Participation by patients/inmates in community/social activities and networks	Fair	Poor

88

Potential to learn roles, relationships, coping patterns, autonomy, independence, and other kinds of *mental health* behaviors	Excellent	Good	Fair		z a t i o n		Potential to learn new roles, relationships, coping patterns, autonomy independence, and other kinds of *mental health* behaviors	Fair	Poor

Therapeutic nursing experiences	Preventions
	Mental health promotions
	Primary preventions
	Mental health education
	General health promotion
	Self-care
		Interventions
		Counseling
		Secondary preventions
		Mental health education
		General health promotion
		Self-care
			Interventions
			Therapy
			Secondary preventions
			Mental health education
			Family therapy
			General health promotion
			Self-care
							Therapeutic nursing experiences	Interventions
								Special therapies
								  Social
								  Psychological
								  Milieu
								Nurse-patient relationships
								Psychopharmacologic treatments
								Somatic treatments
								Group experiences
								General health monitoring
								Education
								Socialization
								Tertiary preventions
									Interventions
									Special activities
									Rehabilitation
									Supportive
									Psychopharmacology
									Milieu
									Psychopharmacologic treatments
									Somatic treatments
									Custodial and humane care
									General health monitored
									Tertiary preventions

Estimate of population in each category	Majority						Estimate of population in each category	Minority	

89

Minor distortions of reality, such as excessive fantasizing, inability to cope, and worrying, supposedly all lead the diagnostician to consider a broad category of disorders that were called neurotic disorders or neuroses before DSM-III. Major alterations in perceptions of reality (such as hallucinations and delusions), massive withdrawal, and major disturbances of affect (feelings) lead to the consideration of psychotic disorders or psychoses. The basic difference between neuroses and psychoses presumably depends on how clients perceive the world and how they behave in light of these perceptions.

A new classification system of mental and behavioral disorders has recently come into use. Five different axes of behavior are identified around which relevant information can be organized: I and II—all of the mental disorders; III—physical disorders and conditions; IV—severity of psychosocial stressors; and V—highest level of functioning in past year (American Psychiatric Association, 1980). This classification system expands the data base on which diagnostic decisions are made about mental illness. It is too early to know how this new system will shape decisions and judgments about the mental health of individuals and families.

In the clinical practice of community mental health nursing, the clinician at times may need to focus on the mental and emotional problems of an individual in crisis and other unusual situations. The social psychological model allows for this kind of focus; however, the clinician should recognize the limitations of this approach. The unique feature of community mental health nursing is the use of a comprehensive data base that relates specifically to the multidimensional aspects of positive mental health and how it can be promoted and maintained in adaptive and healthy functioning families and other kinds of primary socialization groups. This focus is realized when community mental health nursing focuses on preventions.

The concept that mental health is more than and different from mental illness directs the community mental health nurse to think in a different way about what constitutes mental health and the kinds of behavior that characterize it. It encourages the use of different kinds of strategies and preventions.

The assumption that mental illness and mental health are two mutually exclusive categories relating to two different kinds of life experiences has considerable use for community mental health nursing. Such a view helps the nurse to organize a specific clinical practice framework and to use this to sort out the complex phenomena that is collected from clinical assessments and counseling interactions. In this respect, the model is an example of how new concepts or modifications of old ones help to advance both the practice and research bases of this special area of nursing practice. Last, it helps community mental health nurses to explicate more clearly their roles and functions in community mental health and special psychiatric settings.

SUMMARY

Conceptions of mental health and mental illness over the past three decades have changed. These changes have occurred as a result of the development of different theories about mental functioning; basic research from the neurological, social, biochemical, and behavioral sciences; and community mental health nursing theory. Theories have been tested in clinical practice and have resulted in many innovative and effective ways of changing behavior and attitudes of people.

The different theories of explaining mental functioning have helped mental health professionals realize the importance of psychological, social, cultural, and situational factors in mental health. Such formulations have also provided information about the linkages between the mental health of communities and the mental health of their citizens.

A social psychological model of mental health and mental illness experiences focuses on the interrelationships between social settings, social and psychological responses of groups in such settings and their members, and the potential of such settings for promoting and maintaining the mental health of members. In primary socialization groups, such as families and surrogate families, characteristic response patterns may be adaptive or healthy, stressed, or distressed. Mental health experiences are open-ended, with opportunities for families and members to fulfill their potential for self-actualization.

Mental illness experiences are considered quite different from mental health ones. Mental illness experiences are bounded, or limited, in scope and kind. Response patterns may be assessed as disturbed or disabled. The placement of a person in this category has major social and personal consequences for the individual so labeled.

The use of the proposed model in community mental health nursing practice is a way of emphasizing mental health in its family aspects and recognizing the relationship between these and individual mental health. It can serve as the basis for organizing preventions as well as interventions in clinical practice and helps to make distinctions between community mental health nursing, mental health nursing, and psychiatric nursing.

REFERENCES

American Psychiatric Association. *Diagnostic and Statistical Manual of Mental Disorders*, 3rd ed. Washington, DC: Division of Public Affairs, American Psychiatric Association, 1980.

Archer, Sarah, and Fleshman, Ruth. eds. *Community Health Nursing: Patterns and Practices*, 2nd ed. Scituate, MA: Duxbury Press, 1979, pp. 23–29.

Besson, Gerald. The health–illness spectrum. *American Journal of Public Health* 57:1101–1104, 1967.

Clausen, John A. Values and norms, and the health called "mental": Purposes and feasibility of assessment. in Sells, S. B., ed. *Definition and Measurement of Mental Health. Washington, D.C.: HEW, 1968, pp. 117–130.*

Conrad, Dorothy C. Toward a more productive concept of mental health. Mental Hygiene 36:456–466, 1952.

Douglass, Chester W. A social psychological view of health for health science research. *Health Services Research*, 6:6–14, Spring, 1971.

Dunn, Helbert L. What high-level wellness means. *Health Values* 1:9–17, January–February, 1977.

Freud, Sigmund. *New Introductory Lectures on Psychoanalysis*. London: Hogarth Press, 1964.

Goffman, Erving. *Asylums: Essays on the Social Situations of Mental Patients and Other Inmates.* Garden City, NY: Anchor Books, Doubleday, 1961, pp. xiii and 5–6.

Goldston, Stephen E. An overview of primary prevention programming. in *Primary Prevention: An Idea Whose Time Has Come*, HEW Publication No. (ADM) 77-447. Washington, DC: National Institute of Mental Health, HEW, 1977, pp. 24–26.

Grinker, Roy. Foreword. In Offer, Daniel, and Sabshin, Melvin, *Normality*. New York: Basic Books, 1966, pp. vi–viii.

Haley, Alex. *Roots*. New York: Random House, 1976.

Hollingshead, August, and Redlich, Frederich. *Social Class and Mental Illness: A Community Study*. New York: John Wiley & Sons, 1958, pp. 172–176.

Illich, Ivan. *Medical Nemesis*. New York: Pantheon Books, 1976.

Jahoda, Marie. *Current Concepts of Mental Health*. New York: Basic Books, 1958, pp. 106–108.

Koldjeski, Dixie. Social factors influencing processing of mental illness. In *Proceedings of Eastern Region Research Conference*, Williamsburg, VA. Richmond, VA: Virginia Commonwealth University, 1974, pp. 91–107. Also in *Dissertation Abstracts International* 34:10:6760A, 1974.

Kroner, Ija N. Mental health vs mental illness. *Mental Hygiene* 2:315–320, 1958.

Levinson, Richard M., and Ramsay, Georgean. Dangerousness, stress, and mental health evaluations. *Journal of Health and Social Behavior* 20:178–187, 1979.

Manning, Peter K., and Zucker, Martine. *The Sociology of Mental Health and Mental Illness*. Indianapolis: Bobbs-Merrill, 1976, pp. 98–104.

McDonagh, Mary, Tribles, Virginia, and Crum, Ann. Nurse-therapists in a state psychiatric hospital. *American Journal of Nursing* 80:103–104, 1980.

Menninger, Karl. *The Vital Balance*. New York: Viking Press, 1963, pp. 134–138.

Murray, Ruth, and Zenter, Judith. *Nursing Concepts for Health Promotion*. New York: Prentice-Hall, 1975, pp. 6–7.

Neal, Ann. An analysis of health. In *The Joseph and Rose Kennedy Institute for the Study of Human Reproduction and Bioethics Quarterly Report*, Georgetown University, Washington, DC, Autumn, 1975.

Osborne, Oliver. A theoretical basis for the education of the psychiatric-mental health nurse. *Nursing Clinics of North America* 5:699–712, 1970.

Pasewark, Richard, and Rardin, Max. Theoretical models in community mental health. *Mental Hygiene* 55:358–364, 1971.

Parsons, Talcott. Definitions of health and illness in the light of American values and social structure. In Garth, Jaco, ed. *Patients, Physicians, and Illness* New York: Free Press, 1958, p. 176.

Rogers, Carl R. *Client-centered Therapy*. Boston: Houghton-Mifflin, 1951.

Rüemke, H. C. Solved and unsolved problems in mental health. *Mental Hygiene* 39:178–195, 1955.

Scheff, Thomas. *Being Mentally Ill*. Chicago: Aldine Press, 1966, pp. 96–97.

Smith, M. Brewster. Optima of mental health. *Psychiatry* 13:503–509, 1950.

Torrey, E. Fuller. *The Death of Psychiatry*. Radnor, PA: Chilton Book Company, 1974, pp. 36–42.

Williams, Richard H. *Perspective in the Field of Mental Health*. Rockville, MD: National Institute of Mental Health, 1972, p. 3.

Wilson, Holly, and Kneisl, Carol. *Psychiatric Nursing*. Menlo Park, CA: Addison-Wesley, 1983, p. 19.

Yarrow, M., and Clausen, J. The psychological meaning of mental illness in the family. *Journal of Social Issues* 11:12–24, 1955.

CHAPTER | TRADITIONAL AND
4 | CONTEMPORARY
FACTORS
INFLUENCING
MENTAL
HEALTH

INTRODUCTION

Community mental health nursing is based in large part on the conceptual and ideological bases of community mental health. As community mental health was developed, the directions of clinical services, organization of systems of care, and roles of mental health professionals were all profoundly affected. The recent changes in mental health legislation and implementation of these changes through various policy decisions continue to influence the development of community mental health nursing and has implications for future role development and the contribution of the field to the implementation of some of the new initiatives that have been recommended in mental health care.

The implementation of a concept of community mental health is of fairly recent origin. Selected mental health services have been available to people in this country for a long time. In 1909, the first child guidance clinics were put in operation. Rossi (1962) reported that by 1925, over 400 clinics in the country were providing various kinds of services for mental problems.

The more contemporary concept of community mental health goes considerably beyond earlier ideas of mental health care in clinics in community settings. Bloom (1977) defined community mental health as all the activities undertaken in a community in the name of mental health. He suggested that community mental health is also distinguished from the more traditional mental health–related activities by its emphasis on practice in the community as opposed to practice in institutional settings.

Community mental health is legally defined to cover a variety of activities. It includes primary prevention activities that focus on the prevention of mental and emotional disorders, secondary prevention activities that try to reduce the likelihood of mental and emotional illness from developing in persons at risk, and tertiary activities that address the care and management of people who experience serious and long-term psychiatric problems and who may need episodic or continuous hospitalization in a mental institution or psychiatric unit.

Traditionally, mental health had been defined as the mental and emotional status of a person. Community mental health is defined in terms of the location of services, the system through which services are provided, and an array of direct and indirect services to clients. Its conceptual underpinnings are held together by principles and concepts from a variety of theories relating to mental health of individuals, groups, and families, and the interrelationship of their mental health to the life of their communities.

The emergence of community mental health in this country has been an evolutionary process. A major breakthrough came when an urgent need arose to develop a new approach for handling an ever-increasing number of people who were being institutionalized for various kinds of mental illnesses. The Second World War was instrumental in focusing attention on this enormous problem as it related to men and women in the armed services. In the catastrophic experiences encountered under the pressure of combat stress, the emotional and mental health problems of men and women became starkly revealed. During the Second World War, innovative approaches for handling combat stress were developed quite literally in the field, applied, and found to be successful for handling many of the problems. Out of these experiences came new theories, ideas, and approaches about the treatment and management of mental illness.

After the Second World War ended, influential psychiatrists such as the Menninger brothers began to sound the cry for the need to improve the mental health care of citizens and returning veterans in this country. Exposés of various kinds showed appalling conditions in mental institutions and the lack of a sufficient number of adequately trained mental health professionals to provide the leadership and expertise for professional mental health care and therapy. The efforts of concerned professionals, former patients, and laypersons to inform the people in the United States about the condition of mental hospitals and the state of psychiatric care were successful and resulted in major reforms. This impetus for change was accelerated and became focused through a national commission that was charged to present new approaches to mental health care.

The establishment of community-based mental health care was conceived as more than a change in the location of services. This concept embodied ideas that mental and emotional problems could be prevented; that the earlier problems were treated, the more optimistic the outcome; and that different therapeutic approaches could be used and effectively applied by other than medical mental health professionals. Attempts were made to lessen the stigma associated with mental illness, of "being crazy." Mental health education programs on a national scale were launched to try to change the attitudes and ideas that many Americans held about mental illness.

The directions in which community mental health has developed for the last quarter century have attracted both praise and criticism. As a concept around which considerable ideology has developed and been operationalized, the praise has been deserved. There is no doubt that emotional and mental health problems have become somewhat less stigmatic and more accepted as an integral aspect of living in modern contemporary society. With this change in attitudes, people have become more willing to seek assistance before serious problems develop. Furthermore, the necessity of providing therapeutic services to people with considerable cultural diversity and various kinds of stresses related to problems of living has generated many new approaches and theories.

At the same time, criticisms have also been leveled and are equally deserved. A major one is that the centers have not adequately served the mental health needs of underserved and traditionally unserved populations. Moreover, the traditional therapies that mental health professionals have become proficient using have not been effective with population groups who have different social and educational backgrounds. Rather than develop new theories and approaches to handle the emotional and mental health problems of these clients and families, therapists have declared these people "unsuitable for therapy." Recent evaluation of persons served by community-based mental health services shows that a limited population is served, namely, white, middle-class, and articulate clients who are not experiencing serious emotional or mental health problems.

Another criticism of contemporary community mental health involves the cost of providing specialist care in first visits for mental health problems. Usually, specialist services are made available to people on a need basis through referral, with a professional health generalist making an initial assessment or tentative diagnosis. In community mental health, this approach was reversed: Specialist care was to be provided on first contact with clients. Over time, this policy has been expensive and has had the effect of trying to make generalists out of mental health specialists. Mental health professionals have been expected to provide a core of generic therapeutic activities and treatment modalities. This has come to be the model of mental health services in most community mental health centers and services. This approach has had the unanticipated consequence of deprofessionalizing the mental health work force. Special knowledge, competencies, and unique contributions of mental health specialists from the core professional disciplines have not always been used to best advantage.

The practices of the core mental health disciplines—community mental health nursing, psychiatry, psychology, and psychiatric social work—have been greatly influenced by community mental health. Some of the warping of roles, functions, and responsibilities in community mental health nursing have already been identified. The directions that clinical practice will take in these respective disciplines in community mental health is open. There are challenges for all of the mental health disciplines to use the respective talents and expertise of their members to develop new practice models and roles in community mental health.

In order to appreciate what some future directions might be for community mental health nursing and selected factors that may influence these, some traditional and contemporary aspects of community mental health are examined. These factors cover a number of social, political, and professional concerns.

COMMUNITY MENTAL HEALTH AS
SOCIAL POLICY

Community mental health has developed to its present form as the result of several converging forces, one of which was an evolving social policy to improve the care and treatment of the mentally ill in the United States. The efforts of reformers and concerned professionals to improve the care and treatment of the mentally ill in the United States reached levels in the government where policy is changed and made. One overriding belief in this effort was that the pattern of mental hospitalization in large state hospitals was not the answer to the psychiatric needs of citizens. However, it was not until this and other concerns were translated into social and national health policy through federal legislation that initiative and direction were given to community mental health as an alternative.

Mechanic (1969) linked mental health and social policy by calling attention to the fact that a coherent mental health policy had to make decisions among various alternatives, recognize issues in mental health that are relevant to such policy decisions, and consider probable advantages and disadvantages of each alternative. Bloom (1977) identified the social policies inherent in the Community Mental Health Centers Act of 1963. These policies include a complex set of interdependent roles involving community, state, and federal responsibilities and rights, with each jurisdiction given limited rights and responsibilities. At the federal level, the administration ensures that the state meets certain requirements. The state ensures that a local community meets certain requirements. The local community ensures that the program of mental health services meets the needs of the people in the community, are provided by appropriate professionals, and are cost effective. The right of local communities to plan and control their own human services was ensured. The right of the state was preserved for monitoring, coordinating, and funding programs that its citizens needed. The right of the federal government was stated as that of providing national leadership and initiative in programs that addressed the national mental health needs of the country, for controlling, planning, and maintaining the regulations and guidelines for use of federal funds.

Another social policy that Bloom (1977) identified is one that implements a concern for poor states that cannot support community mental health services as envisioned in the Community Mental Health Centers Act (1963). Funds allocated for support of the community mental health centers and certain mandated services were allocated on a formula that took into account the population in the state, the need for services, and the financial condition of the state and communities to be served. In general, a policy was established that the poorer the state, the larger the allotment of federal funds and the less the proportion that such a state was expected to contribute for its share of support.

A third social policy was the requirement that a "catchment area" be defined for each community mental health center. Geopolitical and geocommunity boundaries had to be established so that each mental health center had the responsibility for providing a range of comprehensive community-based services. This idea was based on a policy of providing services in the communities in which people live so that they would be accessible and community relationships and control could be maintained. In reality, the concept of a catchment area has been difficult to apply, particularly in urban and sparsely populated rural areas. Nevertheless, the idea has had a lasting impact as a model by which other kinds of community-based health and human services might be organized.

A fourth social policy inherent in the Community Mental Health Centers Act of 1965 dealt with the consolidation of mental and general health services in each of the community settings, a policy not supported by many medical and mental health professionals. Generally, this policy of consolidation was achieved by a compromise: Psychiatrists were to be directors of the community mental health centers and responsible for psychiatric clinical programs with medical doctors responsible for other aspects of health care. This model, designed to decrease the fragmentation between mental and general health care and services, did not decrease this fragmentation. Needless to say, it has not been implemented in the way in which it was envisioned. This compromise ignored the fact that many of the emotional and mental problems experienced by people in contemporary society are social, cultural, and behavioral in nature and require different kinds of treatment and management, thus decreasing the need for both traditional therapies and medical care. Instead of integrating the experiences of clients and patients to form a wholeness in which connections between parts of experiences could be understood, the model served further to fragment care and treatments relating to mind and body and allocated each of these to physicians with quite different kinds of specialized knowledge and medical expertise. It also failed to take into account other models of mental illness and mental health in which professionals from nonmedical disciplines are more than competent to provide a range of services for a broad array of mental and emotional problems.

A fifth social policy, identified by Bloom (1977) in the Community Mental Health Centers Act, concerns the accessibility of community groups to mental health services. This access was not to be denied to anyone for any reason. Traditionally, quality psychiatric care and treatment have been the province of people who could pay. For people who could not afford to pay for private psychiatric care and treatment, mental hospitalization in a state facility was the usual pathway for getting mental health care. The policy established access to services for community mental health care and removed major barriers for obtaining mental health care.

There can be no doubt that linking the concept of community-based mental health care to social policy goals at a national level provided the impetus for revolutionary change. Consensus was created that provided the support for interested professional groups to get legislation passed and funded. A process of rapid change was set into motion and the enthusiasm and momentum generated were major factors in the acceptance of the federal role in mental health. This role was radically different from any that had ever been assumed before at the national level.

Mental health services in community-based settings were mandated in the Community Mental Health Centers Act (1963), which identified the essential services to be provided. A three-way partnership between federal and state governments and local communities was established to implement the law. These changes contributed to the redefinition of professional roles and functions of mental health professionals, and the development of some new strategies of clinical management. They established a framework in which professionals could use creativity and ingenuity to develop new service models that would have the potential of reaching populations not generally reached in traditionally oriented mental health care.

MENTAL HYGIENE MOVEMENT

No account of traditional factors that have influenced the development of community mental health would be complete without noting the contributions of the mental hygiene movement in the United States. In the early part of this century, this movement developed and focused on the concerns of people who had mental and emotional problems and on the lack of services to provide proper care and treatment. In 1909, the movement was formalized by the establishment of a National Committee for Mental Hygiene. The committee had supporters in high places, among them William James, a psychologist; William Welch, a pathologist; Adolph Meyer, a psychiatrist; and Clifford Beers, an articulate and influential ex-mental patient who wrote a book about his experiences in an asylum that shocked the nation. The use of the term *mental hygiene* was important. The intent was that it would place emotional and mental illness problems in a new framework rather than the traditional one of insanity. Meyer, a visionary, oriented the movement toward prevention of mental illness. This effort failed to arouse enough public interest to generate broad government and professional support. The movement was the forerunner of the community mental health movement that reemerged in the 1960s and that was to revolutionize the organization and concept of mental health care in the United States.

MAGNITUDE OF THE PROBLEM OF MENTAL ILLNESS

The enormity of psychiatric problems in the military during World War II has already been mentioned. It was brought home to many families who had a son or daughter in the services and made the treatment of psychiatric illness a personal and family concern. There was good reason. Levenson (1974) reported that approximately 40% of the 5,000,000 men rejected for military services for medical reasons had neuropsychiatric problems. Added to this number were the thousands of servicemen who became temporarily disabled from psychiatric problems while serving in combat.

On the home front, by the end of World War II, state mental hospitals were full to overflowing with patients. Many of these large institutions had populations of from 12,000 to 15,000 and were known as "cities of the sick." However, these institutions had in fact become warehouses for very disturbed and mentally sick people. By 1945, there were approximately 450,000 patients in state hospitals in the United States, and by 1955, this number had increased to 550,000 (Levenson, 1974).

The enormous financial, personal, social, and human costs of maintaining a system of care that constantly admitted patients with few discharged to return to productive lives became recognized. At this time, the care and treatment of mentally ill people were primarily state responsibilities because families could not pay the enormous costs of care required for what was essentially lifetime treatment in a mental institution. It was in this climate of approaching financial and institutional crisis that Congress enacted a Mental Health Studies Act in 1955. As part of this legislation, a Joint Commission on Mental Health and Mental Illness was appointed to study the needs and resources of the mentally ill in the United States and charged to make recommendations for a national mental health program (Joint Commission on Mental Health and Mental Illness, 1961).

REPORT OF THE JOINT COMMISSION (1961)

The report of the Joint Commission, called *Action for Mental Health*, had five major recommendations that were designed to address the problems in mental health and provide directions for a national mental health policy. Summarized, they recommended the following:

1. Take action to support research and development of research centers.
2. Use existing knowledge and experience more broadly by adopting a liberal philosophy of what constitutes treatment and who can provide it; nonmedical mental health workers with competencies should be permitted to do short-term therapy.
3. Increase the number of mental health professionals through federal support of education in the mental health professions.
4. Increase community mental health services and psychiatric units in general hospitals.
5. Increase federal funding for mental health care and improvement of mental health services. (*Action for Mental Health*, 1961, pp. vii–xxiii)

In developing its report, the Joint Commission contracted for a number of studies to be conducted that related to different important aspects of mental health care. These reports in the form of monographs served as the support base for the mental program that the Joint Commission recommended. One of the monographs explored different concepts of mental health and was published as *Current Concepts of Positive Mental Health*, by Jahoda (1958). This publication has had an enormous influence on conceptualizations of mental health. A social psychological rather than medical model of mental health was elaborated. It presented a framework that nonmedical mental health professionals could use to expand their roles and functions and provide the mental health services needed by so many people in the United States. Other monographs covered such things as the cost of mental illness, manpower needs, and national surveys about attitudes held by the nation about mental illness.

The recommendations of the Joint Commission were received favorably by the government and professional and interested lay groups. In 1963, President John Kennedy used the work of the Joint Commission as the basis for his address to the nation on the crisis in mental health care. (See Appendix I.) In response, Congress passed the first Community Mental Health Centers Act. (See Appendix II.) This unprecedented legislation established the principle of comprehensive community mental health care and put forward the set of relationships already discussed that were to be established between the federal government, states, local communities, and citizens. The act changed traditional roles about states' rights and responsibilities and federal obligations for national mental health problems. By 1965, the first community mental health centers were in operation.

In the Community Mental Health Centers Act of 1963, community mental health centers were expected to provide five essential services: inpatient care, outpatient care, emergency services, partial hospitalization, and consultation. Later, additional legislation mandated five additional services: diagnostic services, rehabilitation services, precare and aftercare, training, research and evaluation.

TRADITIONAL AND CONTEMPORARY FACTORS INFLUENCING MENTAL HEALTH

It is sometimes difficult to appreciate today how revolutionary the concept of community-based mental health care was in 1963. In offering an alternative to hospitalization in a mental institution, beliefs and traditions of the centuries were challenged. This was especially true in relation to the perceived need to protect the public from dangerous lunatics (who, by the 1960s and in consideration of a more humanistic label, were being called "mentally ill"). On the basis of this long-held stereotype, most state mental hospitals were built well away from town and communities; this has been and continues to be a factor in virtually isolating staff and patients from the community with little or no social exchange.

For the majority of people experiencing mental or emotional illnesses, hospitalization meant commitment to a state mental institution unless a person could afford private psychiatric care. The quality of psychiatric care in mental hospitals varied from state to state, from hospital to hospital, and ranged from excellent to disgraceful. The history of psychiatric care in the United States, particularly that provided in large state mental hospitals, has been characterized by a cyclical process of exposé of inadequate, inhumane, and often brutal treatment of patients; followed by investigations of various sorts that resulted in resignation of administrators or physicians and recommendations for change; followed by an increase of monetary resources to secure personnel and upgrade facilities; followed by a period of official and professional complacency; followed by a gradual deterioration of the quality of mental health care as resources are cut and priorities given to other social needs; followed by another exposé, at which time another cycle is underway. In truth, the idea that there might be another and better way of providing care to people outside of mental hospital settings was a startling notion.

Another factor that had to be considered in implementing community-based mental health care involved changing the negative attitudes about mental illness that had been found prevalent in the United States. Success in this effort was imperative if people labeled as mental patients were to be tolerated in social and community settings.

Other more practical matters had to be addressed on a national scale. The professional mental health work force had to be increased rapidly. A broader array of services had to be developed. Educational institutions had to develop specialized programs to teach mental health professionals. It was recognized—but not fully appreciated until some years later—that the provision of mental health care in community-based settings would be quite different because of the conditions under which services would be provided, the differences in patients and clients who would use the services, and the fact that the protective environment of mental hospitals could no longer be used as a major mode of treatment and management.

Ideology of Mental Health

An ideology of community mental health was developed to organize the beliefs and ideas about community mental health care and organization of services. Underlying this ideology was an assumption that traditional concepts of mental illness and the need for mental hospitalization were antithetical to new alternatives for providing mental health care. The new set of ideas and beliefs about mental health, or the ideology of mental health, raised many questions about old views and stereotypes about mental illness and mental health, as did the proposed new directions for addressing the *mental health needs* of populations in communities.

The ideology of community mental health embodies at least 10 beliefs that continue to be used. These beliefs have been summarized from Bloom's (1977) discussion of the meaning of community mental health. Community mental health will

1. Provide mental health care in the community as opposed to institutional settings.
2. Focus services on a total community or population rather than on individual patients; catchment areas will define the population of concern for a particular community mental health center.
3. Focus on prevention services as distinguished from therapeutic ones.
4. Provide continuity and comprehensiveness of services rather than care based on illness episodes.
5. Provide indirect services such as consultation and mental health education rather than direct services to patients and clients.
6. Innovate clinical strategies designed to meet more promptly the needs of larger numbers of people.
7. Plan realistically by using demographic data and community involvement to establish priorities for needed mental health services.
8. Develop and train new mental health workers who bring dimensions of mental health care not generally provided by the core mental health disciplines.
9. Identify sources of stress within communities on the assumption that individual pathologies do not always arise as a result of intrapsychic conflict and tensions.
10. Obtain commitment of community involvement for mental health planning and programming. (Bloom, 1977)

It is by this ideology that the effectiveness of community mental health is evaluated and, in many cases, found wanting. Although imperfectly implemented up to the present time, this ideology has exerted a profound influence on changing attitudes about mental illness and the organization and financial support of services for the emotionally and mentally ill. The ideology of community mental health serves as a baseline by which the four core mental disciplines may evaluate their contributions and determine services that need fuller development.

Discovery of Psychotropic Drugs

The discovery of psychotherapeutic drugs has been a major factor in the development of community mental health. Until the early 1950s, major conceptions of mental illness focused on models of psychological and intrapsychological disorders. These models orient psychiatric care and treatment toward psychological and somatic therapies that are intended to influence emotions and cognitions through applications to mind and body. Electroshock and insulin therapies have been commonly used for somatic treatments, whereas psychotherapy has been the major application for emotions and the mind. Custodial and protective management made up the third emphasis of psychiatric treatment.

In 1953, new drugs were discovered that could be used to alter feelings, cognitions, and behaviors of persons suffering from both mild and severe mental and emotional disorders. Such discoveries opened up a new era of clinical management for mental and emotional illness by use of biochemical treatment. In time, such medical management of mental and emotional illness was instrumental in calling into question the adequacy of psychological and intrapsychic models of emotional problems and mental illness.

The first of the drug discoveries was almost an accident. A laboratory worker was working with a chemical product and consumed some of the product and discovered that he had a marvelous sense of well-being for some time after the incident. Once the connection was made between the effects of the chemical product, which was named chlorpromazine, and the feelings and behavior of the laboratory worker, a new era of treatment for the emotional and mental illnesses began. The role and use of mind-altering and emotion-altering drugs in the practice of psychiatry are enormous. Ideally, psychopharmacological therapy is based on a comprehensive assessment of the mental, behavioral, and medical status of a person with careful delineation of symptoms. There is then a matching of the proper drug to clinical symptomology.

The field of psychopharmacology has advanced so rapidly and produced so many different kinds of drugs, the use of appropriate ones can be a clinical problem. Efforts to simplify the array of possible drugs has been facilitated by various classification schemes. A simple one that provides an orientation to major kinds of drugs is that proposed by Hollister (1973). He related groups of drugs to clinical symptoms such as psychoses, psychotics, depressants, mania, and anxiety. This simple yet useful classification provides a schema showing there are drugs to elevate, calm, or depress a range of human emotions and behavior.

The effectiveness of psychopharmacological products in the medical management of mental and emotional problems has been instrumental in helping to make the goals of community mental health become a reality. Without such drugs, many patients and potential patients would have required continued mental hospitalization because of poor control of thoughts, feelings, and behaviors. The general effect of such therapy began to be evident in 1955. In that year, a reduction of populations in mental hospitals occurred, the first such change in memory. This reduction in the number of mental hospital patients was underway before community mental health centers were in operation. The use of pharmacological therapy and community management of people with mental health problems began to potentiate each other to further reduce the number of people hospitalized for mental and emotional problems.

The use of drugs that produced such profound changes on the emotions and behaviors of people with mental and emotiional problems also produced changes in the clinical practice, roles, and functions of the core mental health professions. These aspects of clinical practice underwent restructuring and expansion. Inherent in such changes, are role conflicts, which became evident as one discipline vied for new and expanded roles vis-à-vis other disciplines with similar claims. In general, community mental health nurses were not able to be as successful in negotiating expanded roles and functions as some of the specialists from the other professions. Too often, roles and functions in community mental health nursing were shaped and defined by other professionals rather than by nurses and nursing. Some of this legacy remains today and is illustrated by perceptions that community mental health nursing has one major and distinct function in this area of practice: the administration of medications.

The medical use of psychopharmacological drugs in mental health and mental illness is expected to increase as more and more discoveries are made. It is already possible to prescribe a drug regimen to fit the mood and behavior that an individual wishes to experience, although in mental health, one would expect that such drugs would be used on the basis of medical needs. In community mental health, nurses need to be specially aware of the importance of drug therapy in the practice of psychiatry and the expectation that nurses will administer these drugs and monitor their outcomes on patients. However, if care is not taken to structure a more comprehensive role of clinical practice, this function can take on such proportions in community mental health center programs that the nurse will find little time left for the implementation of therapeutic nursing activities.

Legalization of Mental Illness

The increased use of the legal process to make decisions about commitment and treatment of mental illness is another factor influencing community mental health. This phenomenon has gradually occurred over the past three decades. The *legalization* of mental illness means that people who experience mental and emotional problems severe enough to require mental hospitalization must have a due process that protects their civil and personal rights in the courts. Legal definitions of mental illness have to be met before a person can be committed to a mental hospital. These definitions include criteria that relate to (1) the legal behaviors that constitute mental illness; (2) the length of stay; (3) the rights of a patient if she or he is committed, such as access to a lawyer and minister, the right to receive and send out mail, the right to have a periodic review of the treatment program to judge its effectiveness, and the right to outside communication; and (4) the right to have an individualized treatment program designed to help the mental and emotional problem for which commitment was granted. Today, patients may decline to take medications that alter their mind and emotions and make them less than effective in daily living activities and situations.

The legalization of the treatment and management of mental illness in mental hospital settings will no doubt increase; these same rights of patients must be respected in the clinical management of illness provided in community-based mental health settings.

Establishment of due process and the rights of patients committed to mental institutions have altered many policies and practices in mental hospitals and services. The domination and control of the commitment process and medical management of treatment regimens by psychiatrists alarmed civil libertarians, social and behavioral scientists, legal scholars, some psychiatrists, and patients and their families. This domination included almost complete control over patients' lives once institutionalization occurred. In the name of psychiatric treatment and hospitalization, psychiatrists and physicians in mental hospitals were the sole authority on the kind and length of treatments, evaluation of progress or lack of progress, and discharge decisions—all of which raised conflict-of-interest questions from a legal standpoint in terms of who represented the patient on civil rights.

Social scientists were leaders in conducting research about ways in which clinical and legal decisions were made about commitment (Kutner, 1962; Scheff, 1964; Dinitz et al., 1961). They found that psychiatrists often made recommendations for commitment on the basis of cursory mental examinations and inadequate information and used a number of social and familial factors. Psychiatric recommendations actually turned to be legal decisions, as judges tended not to question psychiatric opnions, even where the evidence did not support previously determined criteria as a basis for commitment. Such research generated a powerful effort to examine the mental health laws in the United States. Today, all states have laws governing the processing, commitment, and treatment of mentally and emotionally ill persons. Due process is required for all commitments and there are usually provisions requiring release of patients in certain periods of time if no unusual or bizarre behavior occurs. An important outcome of this process has been the placement of important legal controls in the decision-making process about commitments to mental hospitals and the treatment process rather than having these depend on the professional judgments of psychiatrists.

Current Issues and Concerns

Changes in social and political priorities have had and will continue to have a major influence on community mental health. In 1977, another Presidential Commission was established by President Jimmy Carter to examine the present state of mental health in the United States and to establish an agenda for mental health for the next decade (President's Commission on Mental Health, 1978).

This Presidential Commission, under the honorary chairpersonship of the President's wife, Mrs. Rosalyn Carter, held hearings around the United States to obtain grassroots information about the advantages and shortfalls in mental health services. Commission members also wanted to get a sense of direction about establishing the new agenda for mental health. The Presidential Commission established a number of task forces to study particular concerns and problems and to develop a data base for support of recommendations. These task forces recommended changes in service mandates and pointed out the need for new initiatives. Important ones are a focus on prevention of mental illness; provision of services for the elderly, minorities, children, adolescents, and people suffering from chronic mental illness problems; preparation of a sufficient and qualified number of mental health professionals in the core mental health disciplines each year; and removal of financial barriers to mental health services. In response to these broad and general needs, the Presidential Commission made the following recommendations:

1. Support community mental health systems and expand these as the basic mental health system in the United States.
2. Provide mental health services in the least restrictive settings to help clients and patients maintain and achieve independence.
3. Phase out the large state mental hospitals; in the meantime, improve and upgrade services.
4. Protect the civil rights of people needing mental health services and mental hospitalization.
5. Provide clinical mental health services under the supervision of professionals from one of the core mental health professions.

6. Strengthen and promote the development of natural support systems and networks in communities.

7. Make primary prevention a strong emphasis in program implementation.

8. Coordinate and integrate mental and general health services.

9. Step up mental health education.

10. Increase monetary support for research and expand the capacity for such research.

11. Change laws that govern third-party payments to permit clients to have more options for selection of mental health providers. (President's Commission on Mental Health, 1978, pp. 12–57)

By 1980, these recommendations were enacted into law and are now part of the laws and regulations that govern community mental health administration and financial management.

The Presidential Commission was established by the President because mental health as a national concern had declined and political support diminished. The cause of mental health had lost a considerable amount of support from the various groups that traditionally supported changes in the national agenda and obtained federal support for such changes. Federal funding for mental health began to decline in 1970. Each succeeding year saw further erosion of political support and a decrease in monetary support, which, in turn, placed a great responsibility and strain on state and local levels of government to support already established and legally mandated services.

Dissatisfaction had increased about the way in which community mental health services had developed clinical services. The ideology of community mental health that emphasized prevention and focused on populations at risk rather than on providing treatment and rehabilitative services to individuals had somehow been shifted in the years since the first legislation was enacted and community mental health services established. Instead of the services identified as central to community mental health, the Presidential Commission found that services provided in most community mental health centers were the traditional ones and emphasized individual adjustment and assistance. Services were provided to individuals representing population groups who had the cultural, social, and educational backgrounds to participate in such therapeutic endeavors, thus excluding populations that could not participate to the satisfaction of therapists.

By 1980, the enthusiasm and optimism felt in the United States in 1963 about the new concept of community mental health had greatly diminished. Mental health as social policy and as a "political disease," that is, one that generates political interest in Congress and enjoys the support of large constituencies, had been replaced by other social and legislative agendas. Community mental health increasingly had to justify and compete with myriad programs that met other kinds of health and human service needs.

Community mental health has been an innovative force for 30 years in providing the leadership for more humane and effective mental health care and treatment for the nation's citizens who need such services. It has now become an established institution and has developed a cadre of professionals, paraprofessionals, technicians, and lay supporters who have vested interests in existing arrangements and resist major changes in program directions. However, if the recommendations developed by the Presidential Commission are to be implemented in ways that effectively meet the mental health needs of the nation, then strong leadership has to be forthcoming to help create a national consensus that will regenerate interest in mental health. These needs are of critical importance because the cycle of exposé of brutal and inhumane care and treatment in various kinds of mental hospitalization facilities has begun anew. Both mental hospital care and community mental health care face challenges in support and will have to respond to various issues and charges raised about each of these systems of mental health care. Borus (1978) noted that the community health movement is in a "state of crisis."

Professional, interested laypersons and people who have benefited from mental health care have to become more articulate spokespersons for mental health at state and national forums in which program and policy decisions are made and financed.

Future Concerns About Community Mental Health

There are a number of concerns that will affect the future direction of community mental health in both positive and negative ways. One of these is the overstatement of unrealistic expectations about community mental health care that mental health professionals have made to the public. Claims about the efficiency of community mental health services in handling an array of mental and emotional health and human service problems have been tempered by some harsh realities. One of these has been the release of mental patients into community settings without adequate social, personal, and community support services being in place to assist them at such an important time of transition. A second reality has been that some mental illness and behavioral problems need to be handled by mental hospitalization in order to protect the community as well as persons suffering from the problems. It is now recognized that there are mental and behavioral problems about which there is insufficient knowledge, thus making community treatment and care exceedingly difficult. In such cases, mental hospitalization may be the best treatment option even though it is a highly restrictive environment.

A concern stated in the recent Presidential Commission report and reflected in one of the recommendations is the emphasis in community mental health on a small range of services. The development of services in community mental health centers has focused on the development of direct services primarily to individuals. Family and group services have been less available. This focus has minimized the development of a direction that addressed a major emphasis that was articulated when the community mental health ideology was expressed in the middle of the 1960s, namely, the provision of indirect services such as consultation to other human and health service providers, the setting up of programs of mental health education, and the provision of primary prevention programs for the public. Based on past experiences, it seems that although both kinds of services have to be provided, direct services should not occupy most of the budgetary and staff resources. It seems clear that in order to implement the recommendations in the Presidential Commission report (1978) that the community mental health system be the basic one in the United States and that primary prevention as well as treatment modalities be provided, the community mental health system has to provide services that are both different in kind and more expansive than what has previously been possible. For example, if state mental hospitals are to be phased out as much as possible, there is a need to provide mental health services to help people that these institutions have traditionally served. Furthermore, if community mental health is to focus on prevention activities and mental health education programs, budget allocations must reflect this increase in responsibilities more realistically in the future than they have in the past.

A concern for the future is becoming increasingly real each year as the level of financial support necessary to provide the existing services decreases. Budget limitations make it difficult to provide the new services required to make the community mental health system the primary system of mental health care in the United States. Traditionally, when mental health budgets have been placed in competition with those of other health and human services, they have not fared well and tended to take disproportionate cuts. It is unfortunate that community mental health systems have to compete with state hospital systems for mental health monies. It has proven to be very difficult to phase out mental hospitals even where there are ample reasons and alternative services available. Until it is decided whether community-based mental health care or mental hospital–based psychiatric care is the basic system, community mental health will continue to experience chronic underfunding and conflict about its role in mental health. This will minimize the introduction of more diverse services to currently underserved populations groups and slow down the development of innovative prevention projects designed to decrease the incidence and prevalance of mental and emotional illness.

Another area of concern is the planned withdrawal of support for mental health training and education by the federal government. This action raises fear among mental health professionals that the already existing shortage of mental health professionals will increase yearly until a point is reached when the provision of professional services will be severely hampered because of insufficient number of qualified professionals. Pardes (1982) noted that the present administration plans to phase out support for clinical training by the end of fiscal year 1982. If this occurs, a national shortage of mental health professionals in all of the core disciplines can be anticipated in the future.

There are positive aspects for the continued support of community mental health. Although research may not be available to support the contention that community-based mental health care is more humane and effective than state mental hospital care, clients receiving services know this to be so, professionals recognize this reality, and the public accepts it as a welcome change. Community mental health will continue to develop in the direction of being the primary mental health system of care. This development will probably be slower than over the past two decades, but it is a change that needs to be made.

Community mental health ideology helped to guide the establishment of programs to change the attitudes of people about mental illness and modified stereotypes that were held about the personal characteristics of people who suffered from mental and emotional illnesses. The availability of services in community settings seems to have been a factor in lessening these factors, in part, because the stereotypes were challenged as family members, friends, and neighbors used them. Services in community settings can be less costly in both human and financial terms. The idea that prevention of mental health problems is possible still has to be more widely accepted by professionals and the public alike because they hold the key for promoting and maintaining positive mental and emotional health.

One positive outcome from the report of the Presidential Commission (1978) has been the increase in mental health research. Pardes (1982) reported the new emphases are in neuroscience, new technologies for studying brain functioning, and therapeutic management of mental and emotional problems with a broad spectrum of new and improved psychopharmacological agents. Unfortunately, the social and psychological aspects of mental and emotional illness and health are being deemphasized in favor of biochemical and neuropsychiatric research.

FROM COMMUNITY MENTAL HEALTH CENTERS TO COMMUNITY MENTAL HEALTH SYSTEMS

The advances, concerns, criticisms, and pressures of community mental health over the past two decades are helping to focus attention on community mental health systems and away from community mental health centers as entities. Over the past few years, it has become fashionable to refer to the mental health system as a nonsystem. This label has been used because of the traditional emphasis of mental hospitals, community mental health centers, and psychiatric units in general hospitals to be "different and apart" from other kinds of health services and systems and to function independently of each other.

The Presidential Commission (1978) recommended the integration and coordination of mental health and general health service systems because of the need for closer collaboration and referral mechanisms. One effort to achieve these has been to appoint "linkers," that is, people responsible for providing liaison activities between patients and clients entering one system and needing services in other systems.

At health system levels, several models have been identified that integrate and coordinate mental health and general health services in different ways. From research about the organization and service implementation systems in 19 neighborhood health centers, four patterns of integration and coordination of services have been identified.

1. Joint Endeavor Model—where the mental health program is provided at the health center site by a combined health and mental health staff
2. Autonomous Neighborhood Health Center Model—where centers operate and fund a mental health service as one of many health services
3. Community Mental Health Center Outpost Model—where a component of mental health services is funded and provided by a community mental health center
4. Consultative Model—where a neighborhood health center is contracted to provide consultation and mental health service (Borus et al., 1978)

With increased budget and policy pressures being brought to bear on costs of health care, efforts to develop more cost-effective services in community mental health are going to increase. Koldjeski (1979) pointed out that community health and mental health systems have evolved from different perspectives. Community health centers were established in the 1960s as part of the War on Poverty to make general health care more accessible to underserved and unserved populations. Community mental health centers evolved as an alternative to the large mental hospital system in this country and the need to provide a wider variety of therapeutic services and management alternatives.

For the most part, community mental health and community health systems have tended to be discrete operations although both have a common goal—that is, to provide community-based health care. In this respect, the recent Presidential Commission report (1978) noted

> General health care settings represent an important resource for mental care in the community. There is ample evidence that emotional stress is often related to physical illness and that many physical disorders coexist with psychological disorders. While general health care settings frequently serve as an entry point to the mental health care system, many millions of persons are never referred to mental health specialists. . . .

While the interdependence of the mental health and general health care system is evident, cooperative working arrangements between health care settings and community mental health service programs are rare. If we are to develop a truly comprehensive system of mental health services at the community level, greater attention must be paid to the relationship between health and mental health. (p. 20)

The challenge for both community mental health and community health systems seems clear. The issue is whether the interrelationships between mental health systems and health systems will be defined by the professionals who are familiar with advantages and disadvantages of various arrangements or will this task be decided by political decisions as a result of pressures by special interest groups.

IMPLICATIONS OF TRADITIONAL AND CONTEMPORARY FACTORS FOR COMMUNITY MENTAL HEALTH NURSING

Community mental health nursing has been influenced by the same factors that helped to shape and regulate community mental health. As one of the four core mental health disciplines, community mental health nursing has experienced changes in roles, functions, and clinical practice in somewhat different ways than other disciplines in this field. A number of these changes have been discussed in previous chapters. In this section, some present and future concerns are discussed.

The Medicalization of Health and Mental Health

The medicalization of health, mental health, and mental illness seems to be in an accelerated period in both professional and policy-making bodies. Fischer (1979) called attention to a series of articles in the newsletter of the Michigan Psychiatric Society that cited a need for psychiatrists to identify with their medical colleagues and cease support of mental health programs that emphasize the "autonomy" of nonmedical mental health professionals. The current emphasis on biochemical, neuropsychiatric and psychopharmacological research is at the expense of social and psychological research. Each of these major research areas will no doubt yield knowledge that will be useful to many mental health clinicians. It is unfortunate, however, that a policy has been set into motion that minimizes research in the area of social, psychological, and cultural aspects of mental health and mental illness. Social, psychological, and behavioral aspects of mental health and mental illness are also needed to apply new knowledge and develop innovative approaches to management. People do have to learn new behaviors and change older ones that have not been particularly productive in helping them relate to others and get along with any kind of satisfaction in living and work. The ever increasing use of drugs in psychiatry to manage basic problems in relationships and to decrease the awareness of the need to learn basic social and interpersonal competencies necessary for living is developing into a national concern. This medicalization process is being applied to other areas of health and health care. Increasingly, health care is being defined as medical care and under the control of physicians.

The move to define mental and emotional problems as medical in nature has several implications for community mental health nursing. In recent years, this specialty of nursing began to define a role and related functions for working with healthy people, families, and groups. If this emphasis in mental health becomes defined as an arena of medical practice, it limits one of the most fruitful areas of clinical practice in which community mental health nursing can make a major contribution. A second implication is that when emotional problems are defined as medical disorders, the social cultural, psychological, and behavioral aspects of mental and emotional problems become secondary to medical treatments that can be provided only by a physician and psychiatrists. This minimizes the role of the community mental health nurses in the very aspects of clinical practice in which they excel.

The Joint Commission Report (1961) called for use of nonmedical mental health professionals to provide social and psychological therapies to persons suffering from emotional and mental illness. The intervening years have more than amply demonstrated that mental health professionals can provide effective and quality therapeutic care to people suffering from a variety of disorders of stress experiences. In spite of this record, there is an ever increasing domination of medical treatment in psychiatry through pharmacological, biochemical, and somatic therapies. This suggests that the management of mental illness is becoming increasingly medical rather than psychological and behavioral in nature. Social and behavioral sciences that have contributed to the development of various kinds of therapeutic experiences over the past two decades are now being minimized in favor of sciences that rely on development of outside agents rather than inner strengths to cope and deal with mental and emotional disorders. As mental health professionals, community mental health nurses must become more aware of the implications of these changes on clinical nursing practice.

With the increased medicalization of mental illness and mental health, community mental health nursing will no doubt experience great pressure to define the clinical nursing process in terms of technical support for physicians and psychiatrists. Roles in community mental health nursing that focus primarily on therapeutic functions of a social and psychological nature may become more difficult to establish and maintain. Nursing will be especially vulnerable as the medicalization of mental illness increases because of the traditional interdependencies between it and medicine.

Today, the majority of registered nurses employed in community mental health centers are prepared at the technical level of nursing education. This group of nurses for the most part fit a model of mental health care and treatment that sees nurses in technical roles and functions. Technically prepared nurses are willing to accept salaries lower than nurse generalists and clinical nurse specialists, thus are deemed to more cost effective. Because professional nursing roles compete with those claimed by other mental health professionals, the control of clinical nursing practice in community mental health centers has been managed indirectly by low salaries, limited functions, and role allocations that are not consistent with professional nursing education.

One of the challenges today in community mental health nursing is to more clearly define the role of the professional nurse generalist. Furthermore, there is a need to identify the unique competencies and knowledge of general nursing that can be best used to advance the cause of providing more effective prevention activities and therapeutic care to persons experiencing mental and emotional problems. Such a distinction would assist clinical nurse specialists, whose role has been more clearly defined in mental health, to assert that they bring competencies and expertise to community mental health that would improve the overall quality of care.

Need for Clearer Conceptual Models

There is a need to refine and develop models of community mental health, mental health, and psychiatric nursing that clearly distinguish these from each other and from the practice models of other professions. On the whole, nursing models in this subspecialty of nursing practice have not been too innovative; rather, they have tended to modify roles developed by other disciplines. This approach has minimized the use of the distinct aspects of nursing practice and accentuated therapist roles modeled on those from other disciplines.

Role modeling from other mental health professionals is also evident in the emphasis that has been placed on securing the right for clinical nurse specialists to secure third-party payment for services. This emphasis promotes the individual practice model and delivery of traditional therapeutic services. Fee-for-payment should be accorded all nurses who provide professional community mental health nursing services. Unfortunately, the effort to secure third-party reimbursements has obscured some major clinical problems in this area of practice involving many issues and nurses working in other than small independent practices.

Conceptual models of community mental health nursing that identify innovative approaches through which role and functions could be upgraded and expanded are needed. A part of this effort must be centered on the personnel classification systems that most states use, which place nurses in this area of practice at levels of responsibility and functions that are inconsistent with professional nursing education and practice. The job descriptions of nursing positions support a role of technical and support functions to physicians and other mental health professionals. Salaries of nurses in many state classification systems in community mental health are too low in relation to the responsibilities, roles, and functions of the professional nurse. Advanced prepared clinical specialists in many mental health systems occupy positions with generic titles, such as coordinator of services. However, until due regard is given to the *clinical roles* in community mental health nursing, a self-fulfilling prophecy operates in staffing community mental health centers and services: Nurses who apply and are willing to work for the salaries offered are usually technically prepared; therefore, there is no need to provide clinical positions for more qualified nurses in community mental health nursing because salaries are not high enough to attract and hold them.

Like psychiatrists, both nurse generalists and nurse specialists have abandoned a share of their responsibility for the psychiatric care of patients in mental hospitals. In 1979, a special program was initiated at the federal level to develop programs that would provide education and training with people needing mental hospitalization. This was an effort to attract mental health professionals who would work in these settings. This action indicated the serious maldistribution of mental health professionals; that is, they do not necessarily choose to work where the need for their expertise is great. This is indeed ironic when one considers that today, the patients in mental institutions constitute very sick populations who cannot be managed in community-based mental health services. These patients are also likely to have mental and emotional disorders that have failed to respond to conventional treatment modalities. Such patients in public mental hospitals are increasingly being cared for and treated by a work force that has less education and few professional skills. This work force, like that in community mental health centers, continues to undergo deprofessionalization as changes in mental health management focus on enough people to "cover" services, rather than qualified professionals who provide therapeutic care and treatment.

Nursing, in the subspecialty areas of community mental health and psychiatric nursing, has traditionally been involved in providing mental health and psychiatric care to patients and clients in both major mental health systems: community-based services and mental hospitals. A renewal of the commitment to mental hospital service requires the development of more contemporary roles and functions of nursing in this area. Such efforts need to more clearly elaborate the interdependence of technical, generalist, and specialist roles.

Primary Mental Health Care Role

The primary mental health care role of the nurse will increasingly become important over this decade. As general health and mental health systems of care are pressured or mandated to integrate and coordinate services, the nurse in community mental health will need to have broader and more comprehensive practice bases that encompass the physical basis of health as well as the social psychological, cultural, and behavioral ones. The move toward primary mental health care will speed up the definition of roles in this area so that holistic health care can actually be provided to persons in both health and mental health services.

The primary mental health nurse role for the advanced prepared nurse generalist that has been discussed by Koldjeski (1978, 1981) has not attracted much attention to date. It is, however, a promising new direction that may have more relevance as service systems change the emphasis of mental health and general health services to provide these in integrated systems of care. This and other such roles deserve more attention from educators and clinicians.

It is already recognized that the professional nurse generalist in primary health care makes a substantial contribution to mental health care. This role can be expanded by teaching these nurse providers to conduct more comprehensive and complete health assessments that identify emotional and mental health problems. Skillful applications of generic intervention strategies such as crisis intervention techniques, therapeutic listening, and supportive counseling would enhance the nurse's abilities to provide first-line nursing care and management of health and mental health problems.

The professional nurse generalist in community mental health can assume leadership in providing services in primary prevention, particularly working with family systems and individuals that have a "normal" amount of stress. With family systems that experience stress or with individual clients, the professional nurse generalist can provide interventions that involve personal, social, situational developmental, and maturational experiences. Nurse generalists are situated in all types of health care systems and can help people recognize and handle anxiety. They can work with families to identify strengths and promote potential to achieve emotional and mental health of their members.

New Roles

New role development for nurses in mental health for both the generalist and specialist levels is needed. Nursing has a central role in the implementation of the recommendations of the Presidential Commission (1978). To do so means that there is a necessity for identifying more clearly what such roles may be and how to implement them. There may be merit in asking whether community mental health nursing is focusing too much on efforts to maintain existing roles and the status quo in clinical practice. Although there is always a need to consolidate and improve past gains and current practices, there is also a need to look to the future, to advance this area of nursing practice.

Koldjeski conducted a survey of the literature over the past four decades from 1940 to 1981 to determine whether a consistent pattern of role development could be identified in psychiatric and community mental health nursing. She found that from 1940 to 1950, the role of the psychiatric nurse, particularly in mental hospitals, was the focus in the literature. This role centered on the provision of custodial, technical, and protective functions by the psychiatric nurse. Such functions included administration of medications, physical care to patients, assisting physicians in the application of a variety of somatic therapies, and administration of ward units as the "home away from home" for mental patients. The idea of the psychiatric nurse as a clinician who would provide various kinds of therapeutic activities to patients was an idea whose time had not yet come or that had at least not been published.*

In the early 1950s, the social and psychotherapeutic role of the nurse in psychiatric nursing and in nursing in general began to evolve and be discussed in the literature. By the end of this decade, this role was coming to be widely accepted by nurses and other mental health professionals. This acceptance meant that nurses in general hospitals and on psychiatric wards were having to participate in a considerable amount of new learning, undergo clinical training, and learn how to function in new kinds of relationships that included the therapeutic use of self. By 1970, a sociopsychotherapeutic role in nursing had been incorporated as a core aspect of nursing in most generalist nursing programs in the country.

Out of the psychotherapeutic role of the nurse generalist, the role of the clinical nurse specialist in psychiatric nursing was also evolving. By the mid-1950s, a few programs were in place to prepare nurses in this new role at the master's level of study. By the end of this decade, the clinical nurse specialist had come to be accepted as an advanced practice role for both psychiatric nursing and community mental health nursing.

During the 1960s and in the 1970s several roles evolved in conjunction with the clinical nurse specialist role, namely, those of consultant and liaison nurse. During these decades, the therapist role was used in a host of health care settings with clients and patients have a wide variety of medical, social, and mental health problems. Consultation was provided to nurses and other health care providers in mental and general hospital settings and with various community groups. The liaison role has never been used as extensively as the therapist and consultant roles, but it has the potential for being very important as general health and mental health services are coordinated or integrated. Nurses who serve as linkers between general and mental hospital settings and services have already found this role to be useful.

The only other role written about in the literature by the end of the 1970s was the primary mental health care role. However, this role may have difficulty in being advanced because it has an orientation and involves functions that differ from specialized therapist roles. This role and its related practice model need some different conceptual bases from the ones underlying many of the therapeutic modalities that clinical nurse specialists routinely provide.

At the same time that new roles need to be developed, there is also the need to define them in ways that they can more adequately be explained to employers, to nurses themselves, to other mental health professionals, and to policy-making and law-making bodies. The professional nurse generalist in community mental health may be an endangered species and the assistance of all clinicians in the field is needed to define practice models more clearly so they can be learned and applied. The emphasis that is placed on specialist care in community mental health services makes the definition of roles for the professional nurse generalist difficult.

One way of discerning more clearly some of the distinctions between specialist, generalist, and technical nursing care in community mental health is to use the conceptual

---

* Dixie Koldjeski. *Psychiatric and Mental Health Nursing: State of the Art*. Paper presented at the Third National Symposium on Psychiatric/Mental Health Nursing, Atlanta, May 6, 1981.

model that has been tested by Benner (1982). Using a modified Dreyfus model, she identified five stages of nursing practice: the *novice*, who as the beginner has no experience with the situations in which tasks are to be performed; next, the *beginner* who demonstrates marginally accepted performances; then, the *competent practitioner* who has experiences in different situations, uses long-range goals to plan actions, and uses conscious, abstract, and analytic contemplation of nursing problems; then, the *proficient nurse* who perceives situations as wholes and whose performance is guided by maxims; and last, the *expert nurse* who uses experience and an intuitive grasp of situations to assess these to arrive at solutions without waste of time and effort. This, or some other schema, would be useful to begin to make some distinctions in the clinical practice of community mental health nursing.

Recruitment of Nurses

The recruitment of nurses to community mental health nursing continues to be a problem. Community mental health, mental health, and psychiatric nursing have never been subspecialties favored as a career by large numbers of nurses. Miller (1982) reported that this clinical preference pattern continues. In a recent survey, she found that nursing students are not especially attracted to this special area of nursing practice. Negative undergraduate experiences in mental health appear to be related to a lack of interest in this clinical area as a career option.

There are no doubt many reasons why nurses do not choose this subspecialty as a career. One is the expected salary the nurse can get in return for study and advanced educational practice. The relatively low—even ridiculous—salary levels that are characteristic of state personnel systems do absolutely nothing to attract new recruits to the field. These systems are very resistant to changes in personnel classifications and the salaries assigned to positions. Therefore, it should be expected that nurses who do elect this subspecialty will seek alternative systems in which to practice rather than community-based and mental hospital ones in spite of the need for their services and leadership. In many cases, there are no positions as a clinician for the advanced prepared nurse. As already noted, advanced prepared nurses may have to accept administrative positions in order to secure salaries at a level commensurate with their qualifications. This, however, lessens the amount of direct services these skilled clinicians provide to clients. Until positions, functions, and roles are brought in line with professional qualifications, expectations, and salaries, it is reasonable to assume that the shortage of nurses in mental health will increase, the recruitment of young nurses to this career choice is not very promising.

With federal support for education and training costs, nursing in mental health has been able to attract motivated and bright students; however, never enough to meet the demands of established services and to staff the new services that have evolved over the past two decades. As federal funding decreases or stops altogether, this action will no doubt hasten the decline of recruits to the field.Chamberlain and Marshall (1982) presented data showing that since 1968, full-time enrollments in psychiatric and mental health nursing have declined more than in other clinical areas in advanced study. From 1976 to 1982, the number of programs funded by the National Institute of Mental Health dropped from 122 to 78.

In recent years, nurse practitioner programs of various types have proven to be very attractive to large numbers of nurses. These programs are viewed by many nurses as the route to independent practice roles and third-party payment. Both of these reasons may be quite illusionary in many states. Nursing practice of expanded functions is often controlled by a joint commission of physicians and nurses. In several states, the use of the expanded role and related functions of nurse practitioners is being legally challenged on the grounds that such functions are in fact medical practice and must be under direct medical supervision.

It may well be that the role of primary mental health nurse will combine aspects of both community mental health and nurse practitioner functions. Such a role would provide enlightened mental care to the large group of aftercare patients that now reside in most communities by the nurse being the primary mental health care provider. This role would be useful in mental hospitals where nurses could assume the responsibility for providing health care to patients and be the provider who ensures continuity and care over time.

SUMMARY

Traditional and contemporary factors have influenced mental health and community mental health nursing. Two major Presidential Commissions have made recommendations about how to improve mental health services in the United States. Recommendations from the first Presidential Commission (1961) made a significant impact, particularly the recommendation that nonmedical mental health professionals be used to provide therapeutic care and services. A second recommendation that has been of enormous importance was that funding at the federal level should be provided to develop and support education and training of mental health professionals, a practice now being phased out. The most important recommendation was that the nation should move toward community-based mental health care.

The second Presidential Commission (1978) made some judgments about the effectiveness of the community-based mental health care established over the past two decades. Gaps in services were found for unserved and underserved populations. It was recommended that mental health care be provided in the least restrictive environment necessary to the mental and emotional health of clients. One of the most important recommendations was that primary prevention programs be more fully developed.

At a time when new challenges face the professions that provide the bulk of mental health care in this country, the policy to curtail or cease support for training and education will adversely affect the number of qualified professionals available to implement recommendations. Community mental health nursing has been particularly affected by this action.

There is a need for professional specialists and generalists in community mental health, mental health, and psychiatric nursing to define more clearly the roles of the technician, generalist, and specialist in community mental health. Concerted action by the profession to address both practice and economic problems is needed to promote the recruitment and retention of nurses in mental health.

REFERENCES

Benner, Patricia. From novice to expert. *American Journal of Nursing* 82:402–407, March, 1982.

Bloom, Bernard L. *Community Mental Health: A General Introduction.* Monterey, CA: Brooks/Cole Publishing Co., 1977, chapters 1 and 4.

Borus, Jonathan. Issues critical to the survival of community mental health. *American Journal of Psychiatry* 135(9):1025–1035, 1978.

Borus, Jonathan F., Burns, Barbara, Jacobsen, Alan M., Macht, Lee B., Morrill, Richard G., and Wilson, Elaine M. *Neighborhood Health Centers as Providers of Coordinated Mental Health Care.* Paper prepared for the President's Commission on Mental Health. Washington, DC: Institute of Medicine, Academy of Sciences, 1978.

Chamberlain, Jeanette, and Marshall, Shallie. Recruitment problems from the Psychiatric Nursing Education Branch Perspective. In *Proceedings: Psychiatric Mental Health Nursing Recruitment to the Specialty.* Washington, DC: National Institute of Mental Health, 1982, pp. 8–15.

Dinitz, Simon, Lefton, Mark, Angrist, Shirley, and Pasamanick, Benjamine. Psychiatric and social attributes as predictors of case outcomes in mental hospitalization. *Social Problems* 8(1):322–328, Spring, 1961.

Fischer, Lorene. Problems, conflicts, and issues facing psychiatric and mental health nursing today. In *Proceedings: Fourth National Conference on Graduate Education in Psychiatric and Mental Health Nursing.* Kansas City, MO: American Nurses' Association, 1979, pp. 3–6.

Hollister, L. *Clinical Use of Psychotherapeutic Drugs.* Springfield, IL: Charles C. Thomas, 1973.

Jahoda, Marie, *Current Concepts of Positive Mental Health.* New York: Basic Books, 1958.

Joint Commission on Mental Health and Mental Illness, *Action for Mental Health.* New York: Basic Books, 1961.

Koldjeski, Dixie. The mental health role of primary health care nurses. *Journal of Clinical Child Psychology* 7(1):37–39, Spring, 1978.

Koldjeski, Dixie. Mental health and psychiatric nursing and primary care: Issues and prospects. In *Proceedings: Fourth National Conference on Graduate Education in Psychiatric and Mental Health Nursing.* Kansas City, MO: American Nurses' Association, 1979, pp. 30–34.

Koldjeski, Dixie. Primary health nursing: The psychosocial component. In Burgess, Ann W., ed. *Psychiatric Nursing in Hospital and Community.* Englewood Cliffs, NJ: Prentice-Hall, 1981, pp. 636–647.

Kutner, Luis. The illusion of due process in commitment proceedings. *Northwestern University Law Review* 57:383–389, September–October, 1962.

Levenson, Alan I. A review of the Federal Community Mental Health Centers Program. In Arieti, Silvano, ed. *American Handbook of Psychiatry*, vol. II. New York: Basic Books, 1974, pp. 593–604.

Mechanic, David. *Mental Health and Social Policy.* Englewood Cliffs, NJ: Prentice-Hall, 1969, p. viii.

Mental Retardation Facilities and Community Mental Health Center's Construction Act of 1963, Public Law 88-164, Title II and Title IV, U.S. Congress, Washington DC, 1963.

Message from the President of the United States Relative to Mental Illness and Mental Retardation, The White House, February 5, 1963. Address by President John F. Kennedy.

Miller, Jeanne. BSN/MSN preliminary data report. In *Proceedings: Psychiatric Mental Health Nursing Recruitment to the Specialty.* Washington, DC: National Institute of Mental Health, 1982, pp. 45–61.

Pardes, Herbert. Overview of national mental health issues. In *Proceedings: Psychiatric Mental Health Recruitment to the Specialty.* Washington, DC: National Institute of Mental Health, 1982, pp. 1–7.

President's Commission on Mental Health. *Report to the President of the President's Commission on Mental Health.* Washington, DC: Government Printing Office, 1978, pp. 12–57.

Rossi, A. M. Some pre–World War II antecedents of community mental health theory and practice. *Mental Hygiene* 46:78–94, 1962.

Scheff, Thomas. Social conditions for rationality: How urban and rural courts deal with the mentally ill. *American Behavioral Scientist* 7:21–27, March, 1964.

THEORY AND RESEARCH BASES FROM MENTAL HEALTH AND RELATED SCIENCES

OVERVIEW

In Part Two, the social and psychological bases of community mental health nursing are explored. Theory and research from nursing, social, psychological, and mental health sciences are brought together to formulate a base for community mental health nursing.

First, basic concepts and principles of a social psychological perspective of human behavior and functioning are discussed. Then, several social psychological theories about the development and organization of the self and of the individual as a person are described. Last, indicators of positive mental health for families, communities, and individuals are identified. Profiles of adaptive, stressed, and distressed family systems have been developed from theory and research.

In Chapter 5, six concepts basic to a social psychological perspective of human behavior are discussed. Socialization is a very important one and serves as an organizing concept. Adaptation and coping have received special attention because they relate and interface with clinical nursing practice in that they represent patterns of responses that people as individuals and groups use in getting along in personal, work, and social relationships.

Social psychological principles of behavior are set out. These principles tie together some of the social, psychological, and situational aspects of human behavior and the levels or organizations that have to be considered when implementing a holistic concept of nursing practice.

In Chapter 6, several social psychological theories for the development and organization of the self and selfhood are presented. The interactionist perspective is emphasized because of its usefulness in conceptualization of community mental health nursing practice. Interpersonal and psychodynamic theories of behavior offer different ways to conceive of the organization and development of a self.

117

For each of these, assumptions, motivational sources, and the relationship of self, mind, and society are discussed.

Some adult perspectives about the continued development of self in late and late late adulthood in the social psychological tradition are presented. Each view addresses developmental tasks, life restructuring, and changes in roles and relationships. Differences in developmental phases for men and women in middle adulthood show a need to rethink the kind of opportunities that are needed for continued growth across the life span.

In Chapter 7, indicators of mental health for families, communities, and individuals have been developed from a broad array of theory and research. Relationships and linkages between family systems, daily living groups in school and work settings, and other kinds of social organizations are related to positive mental health. Models and profiles of healthy or adaptive, stressed, and distressed family systems are presented. Each shows some distinctive characteristics in terms or organization, function, relationship between spouses, and world view.

The indicators of mental health and profiles of family functioning provide the nurse with specific referents of behavior. These may be easily used in making assessments and clinical decisions and judgments and deciding on appropriate clinical strategies.

5 | SOCIAL PSYCHOLOGICAL CONCEPTS AND PRINCIPLES OF BEHAVIOR

INTRODUCTION

A social psychological concept of behavior is an important part of the theoretical base underlying the theory and practice of community mental health nursing. Although this concept serves as the major orientation, concepts from other theories are also used to develop a comprehensive conceptual framework on which to base community mental health nursing. In social psychology, the overall approach focuses not so much on the individual per se as on the interactions and interrelationships among people (Lindesmith et al., 1975).

Social psychological theories of behavior that incorporate principles from different perspectives have specific meanings associated with various concepts and relationships. Of particular interest are principles from an interactionist perspective. Concepts from this view postulate the development and organization of a self in a way that differs from other social psychological theories. Major emphases are on the self as social in nature and the relationship of man and society. In general, sociologically oriented theories emphasize social and personal organization and development of self, whereas more psychologically oriented ones emphasize interpersonal and intrapsychic development of personality.

Social psychology as a basic scientific discipline addresses the incomplete aspects of sociology and psychology. Lindesmith and Strauss (1956, 1968) observed that traditionally psychology has stressed the individual and slighted the situation by focusing on the study of individual personalities and the processes of learning. Sociology, on the other hand, has focused on the study of the social systems, structures, organizations, groups, roles, and communication and has slighted the individual. In seeking to balance these orientations, social psychology tries to link the sociocultural, psychological, and situational aspects of human experiences by broadening the conceptual frameworks through which behavior is organized, observed, and synthesized.

Levinson and colleagues (1978) described social psychology as a boundary discipline. That is, it creates a structure of theory and knowledge linking disciplines that deal primarily with the individual and those that deal with society, culture, and collective life. In this view, a social psychology of human growth and development must consider both the nature of the person and the nature of society because there is an interpenetration of self and world so that each is inside the other with no divisions between self and society. To put it another way, the self is the world and the world is the self.

Many concepts derived from social psychological theories are abstract and imprecise in meaning when compared with concepts derived from laboratory-tested and clinically derived theories of behavior. This is true because by definition the social sciences are concerned with phenomena that often have indirect referents. Commonly used concepts

119

that fall in this category are role, status, and social structure. Over a decade ago, Blumer (1969) called attention to the difficulty of working with concepts that are hard to define and do not attach readily to concrete data. But he also noted that turning away from such concepts because of these difficulties means a loss of their use in guiding observations and opening up new perspectives of human behavior.

Theories from the social sciences differ in another way from clinically oriented theories of health and illness. Although some disciplines have been able to develop a large part of their knowledge base from research conducted in controlled laboratory settings, the social sciences for the most part have conducted research in the social milieus in which people live, work, and play. Because of the variability of factors that operate in such settings, the principles of behavior that evolve out of such research may not have the degree of certainty that principles in the natural and behavioral sciences have. However, principles that are developed under natural social conditions may have more relevance to the clinical practice of community mental health nursing than principles derived from research conducted in artificial milieus.

The interactions generated when people come together to relate and communicate and the contexts in which these occur are assumed to have major influence on the kinds of behaviors that people learn and use in their efforts to adapt and cope. How and under what conditions family, group, and interpersonal relationships develop, grow, and change are important in this learning process. Socialization experiences involve learning, adaptation and coping, and development of the self, all of which relate directly and indirectly to the mental health of individuals, their families, and other kinds of primary groups in which they are members.

Cardwell (1971) noted that most behavior is cultural in nature because it is in response to valued symbols. This linkage between behavior and cultural symbols is important in community mental health nursing because the values and beliefs held about mental health and mental illness are primarily social and cultural in nature. An integral part of ongoing socialization in social, employment, and community groups is the transmission and inculcation of values and beliefs. These are then used to appraise one's own behavior. Such appraisals become a part of the organization of the self and the view one holds about oneself. Within these contexts medical definitions of health and illness are shaped into meanings in terms of symptoms or lack thereof, causes of illness, methods of management, and prognosis. These social definitions are particularly important in relation to the social and emotional ills that are associated with daily living and working stresses as well as for more severe psychiatric problems.

If there were comprehensive theories of social psychology that could be modified to include the basic concepts of nursing theory and practice and concepts of mental health and mental illness, then the development of nursing frameworks using this approach would be greatly simplified. But such is not the case. Until more unified theories of human growth and development of health and illness are developed, it continues to be necessary to develop nursing frameworks that include a synthesis of research and theory from a number of sources in order to establish a comprehensive theory base for the practice of community mental health nursing. The difficulty of this task has been expressed by Pasquali and co-workers (1981) who noted that professional nursing acknowledges the complexities of human nature and promotes a holistic view of man. To implement this view requires knowledge and understanding of the complex interactions and interrelationships between the biological, psychological, and cultural dimensions of behavior as each individual continually adapts to his or her internal and external environments.

The social psychological concepts and principles identified in this chapter have been important in elaborating a conceptual framework for community mental health nursing.

They are used to identify sets of interrelationships for basic groups in which people live. Using this perspective, the concept of mental health is given specific referents as it applies to family functioning and individual and community mental health.

Use of a community mental health nursing framework has the potential for bringing about different outcomes of behavior for patients, clients, and families. This is true because different aspects of life experiences may be addressed by other than use of traditional nursing strategies. The framework permits a focus on changes in the systems in which people have to function in their private lives and jobs as well as on individual changes in behavior.

The development of individuals as fully functioning, autonomous, and self-actualizing persons is a major goal of families. Interrelationships between the personal growth of family members for adulthood and positive mental health and socialization experiences in the family are considered.

BASIC CONCEPTS

Six basic concepts from a social psychological perspective are considered as to their meanings. These concepts are used in the social psychological principles of behavior that follow this section.

Socialization

From a social psychological perspective, socialization is the process through which an individual acquires social norms and roles and cultural values and symbols. These become an integral part of the organization and concept of self. In this process people learn to be human and experience the joy, anxiety, and grief of human relationships.

During socialization, society and culture acquire individuals just as individuals acquire culture and society. Society and culture acquire individuals by making them representatives who use and transmit valued norms, roles, beliefs, and symbols. Socialization also concerns the ways in which children and adults become members of different kinds of groups and how they are able to inculcate their norms, perspectives, and values in individual members (Lindesmith et al., 1975).

Consistent with a social psychological approach, Grace and Camilleri (1981) defined socialization as the means by which people acquire the behaviors, competencies, and attributes they need in order to "fit" adequately into groups to which they belong. Two aspects of the socialization process are: (1) learning performance behaviors, that is, discovering and acquiring the kind of behavior that is approved by the social group and shaping it accordingly; and (2) learning to play a variety of roles and developing a view and evaluation of self that is consistent with the view held by a person's significant others.

Society recognizes that a child is not social at birth but he or she is immediately exposed to interactional experiences on a face-to-face basis. This is the beginning of the socialization process. Once these interactions begin, they continue throughout life and are necessary for continued growth and development. In this process, people learn to be human from their contacts and relationships with other humans. Feldman and Orford (1980) reviewed research on social and psychological functioning that has used a variety of conceptual approaches and found repeatedly that conclusions point to the fact that "people need people" to grow, develop, and become humanized.

In the socialization process, relationships are formed by people that use culturally shared symbols and beliefs in their personal, social, community, and organizational experiences. These symbols and beliefs help them structure their daily living and working relationships. The cultural symbols and beliefs involved in this process are pervasive and include both general and specific ones that have come to be valued over time and often have continuity over generations. They help shape perceptions of reality, influence definitions of situations, and mold expectations that people hold about themselves and others in terms of participation in significant roles and relationships.

Social values and cultural symbols and beliefs vary from culture to culture. The social settings in which particular values, beliefs, and standards are emphasized may also differ. For example, there are some unique characteristics associated with the behaviors, values, and standards taught and expected in interactions and relationships in families that have distinct ethnic, racial, and social class traditions. At the same time, the family holds and teaches to its members values, standards, and behaviors common to the culture.

Families, communities, and individuals may hold culture-bound perspectives. Such perspectives lead people to believe that their beliefs and standards of conduct are the best and perhaps the only way of believing and doing. Such ethnocentric views can be persistent and enduring because socialization experiences may set limits on the adoption of world views as well as reward behavior, expressions, and expectations that support a particular view.

Adult socialization is a continuous process throughout life. This process is closely associated with the social and personal experiences that occur in many kinds of groups. Such experiences make available diverse views, relationships, and opportunities for learning. Group experiences for adults provide quite different kinds of challenges to learning than those provided in infancy and childhood. Understanding and appreciation of the importance of adult socialization has increased over the past decade as research has focused on mid and later phases of the life cycle.

The social psychological theory of adult socialization proposed by Levinson and colleagues (1978) developed the concept of a succession of life structures, that is, the need to restructure the underlying patterns or designs of a person's life at given periods throughout adulthood. Life structures address three important things: (1) the sociocultural world of the individual as it impinges on her or him and the meanings and consequences that accrue; (2) the aspects of self that are lived out; and (3) the participation of the person in the world.

Several other theories of adult socialization have been developed in recent years from different perspectives. Such theories note that as the population in this country gradually becomes older in terms of average age, opportunities for learning and establishing meaningful relationships need to be widely available.

Cultural and Social Systems

Cultural and social systems are intertwined; however, the cultural system is considered to be the master. Cultural systems are preeminent because once man evolved a culture with enduring symbols, beliefs, norms of conduct, and language, culture has "been there" in some form or another. People are born in whatever culture is present and the family is the major social system for transmission of its values and beliefs.

Culture may be defined as an ordered system of shared and socially transmitted symbols and meanings that structure a person's world view and guide behavior (Geertz, 1957). Culture systems refer to the concepts and symbols that men live by: a complex whole that includes knowledge, beliefs, art, morals, law, customs, and other habits and behaviors an individual acquires as a member of society (Kluckhohn, 1967).

The impact of culture is general in one sense and specific in another. General beliefs and values are reflected in specific standards of conduct. These standards guide behavior and development of the attitudes that are used in daily living situations. They take into account the particular needs of people, situations, and contexts. Thus, the interrelationships between social and cultural systems are always present and influence and guide the behavior of people as individuals and members of groups. Such influences may be overt and easily identified or they may be subtle, pervasive, and not easily recognized.

Social systems are the patterns of social organization that people develop and use in order to live together. In coming together for common purposes, social interactions and relationships are generated and provide order by which life in groups and organizations can be satisfying and productive. Mutual influences flow back and forth through interactions and are reflected in communications, reactions, and actions. The quality of interactions and relationships, especially in relation to emotional involvement and commitment to others, is important particularly in primary socialization systems where rearing the young and stabilizing adult personalities are major responsibilities.

The concept of social systems calls attention to the diversity of interchange and interdependence of thoughts, feelings, and behavior that people experience as they adapt and cope in different social contexts. This means there are relationships and linkages between a number of systems. In the case of family systems, such linkages influence the definitions of family structure and functions, shape the relationships between family members and of the family as an interacting unit, provide direction to the socialization of children and adults, and orient relationships with the community.

Social systems have different levels of organization. These may be organized in a number of ways. One was presented earlier that used the size of systems and scope of influence as a way of providing structure. The size of systems influences the development of certain kinds of human interactions and relationships, the kinds of decisions that may be made, the scope of influence such decisions have on people in systems at other levels, and the kinds of social organizations found at different system levels (Mullen & Dumpson, 1972).

Social systems may be organized in other ways. One that has been used in mental health and group work for a long time is as follows: (1) interpersonal relations, (2) group relations, and (3) social order. At the interpersonal level, only two people may be involved in a relationship. This relationship need not necessarily be intimate, as *interpersonal* literally means that two people are relating. The group level is concerned with the interactions of groups and group process as well as the way in which they organize, carry out functions, change, and dissolve. The social order level focuses on the distinctive and interwoven patterns of social organization of a community or, on a broader scale, a society (Baron & Byrne, 1981). This organization of systems, as Lakin (1972) pointed out, leads to group experiences and individual experiences in groups being treated as if they correspond with each other rather than as interrelated phenomena. This view of group experiences minimizes interrelationships outside the group.

The concept of social system has also been used to describe the network of roles that operate in social organizations. Such networks have to be considered in relation to specific systems as these are the pathways by which relationships occur.

The behaviors used by individuals in social settings may deviate from culturally shared patterns and have stigmatic labels applied to them. For example, much of the behavior that gets labeled as mental illness is deviation from social norms. The community mental health nurse needs to obtain data about perceptions and tolerance of peer and community groups to behavioral deviations that by consensus are highly likely to be labeled as mental illness. At stake is whether an individual using such behavior can be maintained in the family and community with a resumption of personal, social, and work roles and responsibilities.

Sensitivity to an understanding of social and cultural systems are essential in community mental health nursing because these systems relate directly and indirectly to how individuals, families, and groups behave as they do. Cultural values and social norms have been consensually accepted in a community and subculture when individuals, families, and groups participate in their application.

Social Interactions and Social Relationships

Social interactions refer to the reciprocal behaviors expressed and the influences people have with one another in face-to-face presence (Goffman, 1959). These influences come from all persons involved in the social interactional process. A common aspect of social interactions is the sequence of behaviors that evolves as actions and reactions occur. Social interactions are the adjustive responses that one person makes to another in face-to-face encounters.

When a pattern of specific and recurrent interactions are established between people, social relationships evolve and are related to individual and group needs and goals (Miller, 1963). Relationships are more stable than interactions and occur with enough frequency over a period of time to develop patterns and emotional involvement.

In the health professions, the provision of helping relationships is the major social psychological approach through which personal and familial assistance is provided. Traditionally, it has been assumed that helping relationships extend over a span of time long enough for a patterned sequence to occur (Sundeen et al., 1981). Increasingly, however, professional nurses have to provide preventions and interventions in brief encounters with people. In a relatively short time, these activities have to make an impact in some way on the thoughts, feelings, and behavior of people. This means there is a need to develop and try out a variety of strategies and approaches in nursing practice that take into account such changes in nurse-patient relationships.

Social relationships are a form of social organization. McCall (1970) stated that what makes a relationship social is the reason for its existence. The form that social relationships takes is related to some extent to the perceptions that participants hold about themselves and others involved. As interactions proceed in a social relationship, role expectations of the participants may very well change. In social relationships in which roles are known and the behaviors associated with these roles are used by participants, social interactions tend to be more structured than in situations where roles are ambiguous. Social interactions tend to focus on knowledge of person, whereas social relationships focus on roles, role behaviors, and expectations.

Social Structure

Social structure may be defined as the patterns of social activities or arrangements that exist over a period of time with regularity and uniformity and organize much of social life. These collective patterns have a unity that makes them greater than the sum of patterns that an individual develops for social living. Durkheim expressed this basic fact of social life in the following way:

> A whole is not identical with the sum of its parts. It is something different, and its properties differ from those of its components parts. . . .
> By reason of this principle, society is not the mere sum of individuals. Rather, the system formed by their association represents a specific reality which has its own characteristics. . . . (Durkheim, 1964, pp. 102–103)

Social structure grows out of social processes. These are the interactions, interrelationships, communications, and feelings that are generated and emerge from recurring social relationships. The establishment of social relationships assumes that participants create a body of shared ideas. Social structure brings order and meaning to these ideas and is necessary for enriching the human experience. Although there is stability in social structure, there are also opportunities and pressures to change. Together, the stable and changing parts of relationships provide opportunities for learning, personal growth, self-actualization, and involvement with people in other kinds of relationships.

The concept of social structure may have another meaning, one that relates to categories used for classifying members of society. The structure of society in this sense is thought of as being stratified, that is, there are layers or levels in society in which people are placed on the basis of some characteristic. These layers, or strata, may be arranged as a hierarchy and people assigned to them on the basis of wealth, power, social esteem, education, and social and economic power. People who are born into and grow up in one stratum have vastly different kinds of experiences, opportunities, expectations about careers and jobs, and marriage possibilities than people born in another stratum. For example, a child born of wealthy parents who are among the socially elite in a community has different kinds of opportunities open to him or her than does a poor child from the same community; in addition, the rich and the poor child will have different kinds of personal and family life experiences that shape attitudes, world view, and preparations for life.

The placement of individuals in any kind of social structure category endows them with the stereotypes associated with the category. For example, the phrase *welfare family* carries certain pejorative meanings. To be labeled *poor and from the wrong side of the tracks* evokes certain kinds of stereotypes associated with a certain social class.

Social position is another concept related to social structure. It places an individual, family, or group in respect to other positions in some particular social system and context. Social position always involves reciprocal relationships. This means that a person in one position experiences being in that position vis-à-vis another person in another social position. An example will illustrate this reciprocality. The President of the United States and her or his family occupy the position of "first family" in relation to all other families. This position sets it apart from and makes it different from other families in many ways, so long as one spouse in the family occupies the role of President. When a new President is elected, the old first family finds this social position no longer accorded to it. Their position is now redefined in relation to other families who have been first families, while the new first family realigns its position in relation to the new social reality.

Assignment to social position is based on many factors over which people have no control. Age and sex are two examples. Assignment to a position may also be on the basis of achievement, competition, or by virtue of powerful connections or kinships. Some positions, such as that of wife or husband, are acquired by legal acts, while others, such as king or queen, are acquired by birth.

The concept of social position identifies a place in social space. It is related to but separate from the concept of role. Everyone occupies a social position of one kind or another from the time of birth. As people grow older, they occupy many different kinds of social positions, some at the same time. The social position that people occupy determines to a large extent the nature of their participation in organizations, relationships, and living activities. Social positions endure because they help people to organize their relationships and situations. As such, they are the small building blocks on which groups, organizations, and families organize.

Role

The concept of role interrelates many of the complex aspects of relationships that make up the fabric of group living. Roles link social, cultural, and personal values, beliefs, expectations, and behavioral systems of individuals as they adapt and cope in situational aspects of daily living.

Role has many definitions. From an interactionist perspective, it is concerned with the reciprocal relationships that evolve between people who occupy particular social positions. In role relationships, people have to adapt their behavior and reactions to what they think other people are going to do (Lindesmith et al., 1975; Lindesmith & Strauss, 1968).

Role relationships evolve within patterns of *anticipated* behaviors and expectations. These patterns, in turn, help to structure personal relationships and social positions. Role behaviors have stability as well as variability, thus allowing for behavior to evolve on the basis of interactions and interrelationships. Even the more stable aspects of roles associated with social positions change over time because roles are dynamic and undergo expansion and redefinition. An example is the role of the nurse. This role has some enduring behaviors that have persisted over time, namely, caring and nurturing activities and assisting the physician in the technical aspects of medical care. Other aspects of the role of the nurse have undergone profound change in a very short time through expansions, extensions, and redefinitions. These changes have occurred in large part because of the advancement of the nursing science of health care and revolutionary changes in medical care.

The concept of role is not a unified one. Everyone has many roles and some of the behaviors used in one role generalize to others. All of the stable roles that a person uses daily may be referred to as *role sets*. These sets link behavior, thoughts, and feelings associated with past roles to present ones, thus providing for continuity in behavior and a base on which new roles may evolve.

Role has a double reference. The first is to the individual as a person; the second, to the groups in which the individual holds membership. An important link that unites these two aspects of role is the socialization process. Through socialization, individuals learn various kinds of social roles and associated behaviors and use these in interpersonal and group relationships. Roles are learned through imitation, role modeling, direct observations, and trying out the roles of others. The development of different roles involves the use of reflexive behavior. This means that a person stands apart from the self and looks at a role and its behaviors to determine their meaning and shape and, in effect, "try the role on."

The behavior of people in groups is strongly influenced by the role an individual occupies in the group. Role relationships in group settings involve negotiation and compromise vis-à-vis other members in relation to their respective roles and positions. Positions in the group may be more formal than those of role. For example, chairperson is a formal position with defined role behaviors, whereas the role of the comic is an informal one and is usually not accorded a formal position.

In a family, the role of father is a well-established one. It has some generally accepted behaviors, expectations, and cultural values accorded to it. These common aspects operate across cultures in respect to this role. For example, father, more than any other family member, is considered as "head of the family." All family members to some extent negotiate, adjust, and adapt their roles to the role of father.

All kinds of role relationships in families and groups undergo changes and create various kinds of stress. Harmonious role relationships in families and groups tend to produce group integration and cohesiveness—the sense of closeness and unity that draws people together. Competitive and conflictive role relationships tend to pit member against member in their efforts to adapt, cope, and achieve individual and group goals.

Cardwell (1971) linked several concepts together that are often associated with role. Under role, he defined three subconcepts: (1) role playing, (2) role taking, and (3) role definitions. These subconcepts have been abstracted from the social psychological symbolic interaction perspective. This perspective borrows meanings in relation to role from drama.

Role playing is defined as a wide variety of acts within a range of acceptable activities that may be acted out with considerable variation. Role playing unfolds as situations change and new behaviors become more desirable than those being used. It is creative when it departs from the established or usual ways in which roles have been enacted to discover new meanings and new patterns of behavior.

Role taking is a process of interpreting the role of others. It involves an evaluation and an interpretation of another person's behavior. Lindesmith and colleagues (1975) described role taking as the "putting on of another's role at a symbolic level." A common-sense way of saying this is the mental exercise we use to "try something on for size." A person, by imagining or actually using the gestures, postures, words, and intonations of someone else and by drawing upon one's understanding of another person from past experiences, evokes in himself or herself responses that are approximate to those of the other person. Role taking operates in all social relationships.

Role definitions are defined by Cardwell (1971) as the expected behavior patterns or plans of action that are associated with particular social organizational positions. Role definitions evolve as guidelines for people to use when they interact and relate.

Biddle (1979) identified five assumptions that underlie most of the different concepts of role in social psychology:

1. "Some" behaviors are patterned and are characteristic of persons within contexts (i.e., form *roles*).
2. Roles are often associated with sets of persons who share a common identity (i.e., who constitute *social positions*).
3. Persons are often aware of role and to some extent roles are governed by the fact of their awareness (i.e., by *expectations*).
4. Roles persist, in part, because of their consequences (*functions*) and because they are often imbedded within larger social systems.
5. Persons must be taught roles (i.e., must be *socialized*) and may find either joy or sorrow in the performance thereof. (Biddle, 1979, p. 8)

Various social roles are necessary for daily living and working in formal and informal social organizations. Role performances are cued to expectations from significant others in various contexts. The learning of new roles occurs as individuals move from position to position, grow and develop from infancy to old age, and occupy a specific role such as wife, mother, or father. Where roles are not too well defined, a considerable amount of negotiation, communication, and accommodation has to take place before successful interactions and relationships occur. This lack of structure means that roles have a high probability of changing and evolving into something new and different. Where roles are clearly defined with specific prescriptions of behavior, there is little need or opportunity to negotiate changes until the prescriptions come to be questioned.

Inherent in all role relationships is the matter of authority. It may be less apparent in many role relationships but it is present and influences role behavior of participants. For example, one kind of authority is the control of needed resources by direct or indirect means. This confers an advantage in role relationships to the holder of power as it provides greater bargaining power and the possibility of coercive actions against the lesser power holder. An example of this inbalance of authority in role relationships with which all nurses are familiar is the way in which hospital resources are controlled by hospital and medical professionals. Nurses constantly find themselves on the defensive in the never-ending process of negotiating and renegotiating for needed resources to provide effective and safe professional nursing care.

Adaptation and Coping

Adaptation and coping interrelate a number of things that are involved in adjustment, survival, and growth. Both are basic to all living systems and are used in interactions with other systems and with environments. Adaptation depends on the social, cultural, and personal systems of humans and shapes the efforts people make coping with life. Coping refers to modes of actions that people use in trying to get along in daily living.

Adaptation has been described by White (1974) as the master concept that links together coping actions and the tasks with which one needs to cope. Adaptation is a complex and continuing process. It is the process through which the organization of the self and the groups in which social life occurs is modified to make a better "fit" between physical and social environments and individual needs for growth, development, and self-actualization. McGrath (1970) stated that adaptation specifically refers to the relationships that have to be managed between physical and social demands on people and the resources that are available to deal with these.

Three components of successful adaptation at the personal level have been identified by Mechanic (1974): (1) capabilities and skills needed to influence and control the demands made of a person and the pace of social and environmental demands; (2) motivations to meet the demands that become evident in the environment; and (3) capabilities to maintain a state of psychological equilibrium so that an individual's energies and skills may be directed to meet external, in contrast to internal, needs.

White (1974) defined adaptation at the individual level as a dynamic process involving compromises that take into account the simultaneous management of three tasks: the securing of adequate information, maintaining satisfactory internal conditions, and having some degree of autonomy and freedom of action. A balancing process has to be learned over time to keep the three tasks on an even keel. White believes that mastery, coping, and defense are necessary to effect compromises and manage the three tasks. He views *mastery* as the use of adaptive efforts to handle complex cognitive and management problems. *Coping* refers to adaptation efforts under relatively difficult conditions. *Defense* is a response to danger or threat but it is not the same as defense mechanisms as these are interpreted in psychodynamic theories.

Adaptation requires a cognitive organization of reality. This organization takes into consideration the task of securing the right kind and amount of information about environments because this information must serve as a basis for action. Cognitive organization of reality is facilitated by positive support from groups that a person values and that enhance the person's self-image.

Information about environments considers the social demands placed on people and the resources and relationships in the environment that facilitate or retard their meeting such demands. Information should be obtained about whether people want to meet social demands and possible alternatives to such demands should be ascertained. But more is needed for adaptive behavior than information. Internal organization of the cognitive, physiological, and emotional systems of people has to be brought into balance so that adaptive behavior can be organized and used. For example, if a person feels overwhelmed by anxiety, behavior can become disorganized despite adequate information. In addition to securing adequate information and maintaining a balanced internal organization, the use of adaptive behavior also requires that people have adequate autonomy and freedom of action. This requirement is recognized and expressed in a common-sense way by the expression: "Keep one's options open." This recognition is also evident when more than one way is explored by which actions may be directed to handle problems and situations.

Cultural change is also part of the adaptation process. People adjust to changing environments by deliberate acts or gradual alterations of the routines of living. In these ways, the patterned ways of life are changed. Change occurs through modifications or by innovations. As changes in patterned ways of life take place, changes also take place in characteristic forms of behavior, values, attitudes, the self-images that people hold about themselves, and the ways in which these images are maintained. Adaptation at the cultural level involves learning to cope with particular environments, technology and knowledge, different values and attitudes, and the way in which these change the views people hold about themselves and self-regard.

Goldschmidt (1974) noted that man is an adaptive being and has to learn to cope with many kinds of environments. However, this dynamic and changing process does not negate the fact that there are some continuities over time in personal behavior, even in environments that are disharmonious and dysfunctional. Although people are not infinitely flexible in coping with changes in environments, they are able to make adjustments of a significant and far-reaching kind. These adjustments bring about institutional, attitudinal, and personality changes that conform with the external circumstances of life.

Goldschmidt holds that culture is the adaptive mechanism in man for handling the diverse conditions in which he lives. This mechanism is expressed by individuals through both the means for exploiting the environment and the pressures by which personal self-aggrandizement are held in check and channeled. This means that each person has a symbolic self with which he or she has to be concerned and that each person must learn to cope with different kinds of external events that require different kinds of socially accepted behavior. Adaptations are necessary to preserve and enhance an adequate sense of self.

Central to the concept of adaptation is the process of appraisal, that is, making perceptions that sort out potentially harmful, beneficial, or irrelevant events or situations. Lazarus and colleagues (1974) found that appraisal involves not only a response to the perception of some threatening condition, but also to potential avenues of solution or mastery. Coping strategies and emotional responses flow from appraisals and reappraisals of people, events, and situations. The appraisal process relies on definitions of situations.

Adaptation has a biological component and, in the long view, concerns the survival of the species and the complexities involved in maintaining conditions favorable for populations to survive. Adaptive survival strategies are learned in social settings and involve both the self-organization of the individual and the ability of families and other kinds of primary groups to provide opportunities for members to learn appropriate responses.

At the biological level, adaptation involves a complex set of interactions that take place when stress or threat are perceived or experienced. Stress stimulates the release of an adrenocorticotropic hormone (ACTH) from the anterior lobe of the hypothalamus. With continued stimulation, this causes the activation of other cortical hormones. Stress, through cortical and sympathetic nervous stimulation, causes the production of norepinephrine and epinephrine and helps to prepare the individual to respond to fight or flight. This complex biopsychological and social process is reflected in a number of physiological indicators such as increased heart and pulse rates, higher blood pressure, and heightened activity levels.

An understanding of physiological adaptation was advanced by Selye (1956) when he presented the General Adaptation Syndrome, a theory of how human beings handle stress. This theory unified several more limited formulations, research, and clinical observations. Selye proposed that three phases of activities occur when individuals are stressed: the alerting or getting ready to act phase that activates the sympathetic nervous system; the phase of resistance and increased level of psychological functioning necessary to deal with the stress; and the phase of exhaustion. More recently, Selye (1977) focused on understanding the role of stress both positive and negative, as a necessary aspect of living.

The abilities of people to cope with environments are related to the effectiveness of solutions that their culture provides and the skills that are developed in educational, work, social, and family experiences. Coping is also related to the kinds and strengths of motivation people have, the incentive systems that help to channel the directions that motivations take, and the ability of people to maintain psychological comfort. Comfort depends on a person's inner resources as well as on social support systems in the environment. Because adaptation is so complex and involves interrelationships between social, cultural, and personal systems, all of these have to be taken into consideration when trying to understand how people adapt and cope.

Coping is often used in an intuitive sense to denote particular kinds of behavior used by a person to handle particular situations. Definitions of coping are confounded by diverse meanings that have been developed over the years, many of which come from the social, behavioral, and psychiatric sciences (Pearlin & Schooler, 1978).

Coping has been used to mean the same thing as defense mechanisms in the sense that these are conceived of in psychoanalytic theories of human behavior. These two kinds of strategies are, however, not the same. In 1974, White called attention to the need to understand a distinction between these responses. He noted that there is no doubt that defense mechanisms are attempts at adaptation, but in a sense, they are adaptive devices gone wrong. In the short run, defense mechanisms may work and be adaptive because they defend the self. In the long run, successful adaptation has to be based on a broad array of coping strategies. These have to address many aspects of reality in ways that allow people to grow, develop, and self-actualize. Defense mechanisms that successfully defend the self from anxiety and threat may be quite unsuccessful and inappropriate to cope with many life events. For example, denial is a major mental mechanism used by people in defense of self. But of what value is denial as a defense for a person who is drowning? Behavior more relevant for a person at such a critical time is to have some coping abilities that can be used to survive in water. This example helps to distinguish different kinds of adaptive behaviors, two of which are defense mechanisms and coping strategies. Both of these kinds of behaviors address two different kinds of efforts to get through the trials, tribulations, and stresses of life. The realities of living require a range of different kinds of behavior so people can make for themselves the best "fit" possible in different kinds of environments.

Lazarus and his colleagues (1974) stated that coping is problem-solving and is used by people when the demands they face are (1) highly relevant to their welfare and (2) tax their adaptive resources. Coping efforts occur in both situations and emotional contexts and there are always positive or negative feelings involved in such efforts.

Mechanic (1968, 1974) viewed coping as the learned behaviors and problem-solving capabilities that people learn in the process of meeting life's demands and stresses. Coping includes the application of learned skills, techniques, and knowledge. White (1974) saw coping as the responses made by people to fairly drastic changes or problems that defy familiar ways of thinking and doing.

As a concept that is essential to the practice of community mental health nursing, coping is defined as all the efforts that people use to get along in daily living. These efforts fall into patterns in which two major modes of action seem to be dominant: (1) actions that interrelate self and environment; and (2) actions that function primarily through psychological processes.

The interrelationships and connections between adaptation, determinants of coping, and coping modes are shown in Figure 5.1.

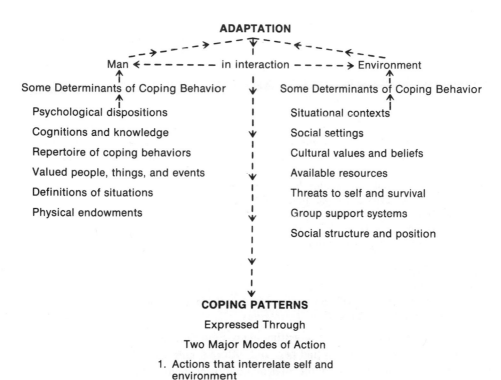

Figure 5.1
Model of adaptation and coping

The adaptation and coping diagram shows adaptation as the general, or master, concept that embodies the process of coping as humans and environment interact. Coping behaviors are expressed primarily through two major modes of actions.

Determinants of coping that people "carry with them" are social, behavioral, and physical in nature. They include the ability to define situations; cognitions and knowledge; psychological dispositions; emotional values attached to people, things, and events; and the behavioral repertoires of coping responses that have been learned from birth. Physical strength, special abilities and disabilities, and general state of health have a direct bearing on how people learn to cope.

From the environment, important determinants of coping are the situational contexts and social settings in which activities take place, cultural values and beliefs, and threats to self-esteem and survival. The presence or absence of group support systems is a major factor in being able to cope effectively. Resources of certain kinds from the community are crucial for effective coping, particularly when threat to self is real. These range from resources that meet basic human needs for survival to family and group support systems. Placement of people in social strata and social positions is an important factor in coping in that it sets to a large extent the conditions under which coping responses are learned. For example, life situations in which chronic stress and deprivation are the norm have a tendency to create a high level of anxiety in people. Coping responses learned under such conditions tend to be ones that are defensive in nature and stereotypical in response.

The strength and competencies learned for coping interact with factors in the environment to shape particular responses. To focus on only one side of the coping equation or ignore the interactions between man and environmental determinants of coping is to minimize the realities of what is involved in the complex process of coping.

In the process of coping, people call upon learned patterns of behavior that have been effective as well as those that have been less than effective in the past. Innovative responses have to be developed through problem-solving if situations are to be dealt with more effectively. Situations tend to "pull" a person toward using psychological and interpersonal solutions as modes of coping. In general, if a situation cannot be changed, people will try to effect some kind of inner change of a psychological nature in order to cope. If a situation can be changed, direct actions are usually brought into play. The choice of coping actions depends in large part on how people define situations and appraise the gains or threats that might result from them.

Coping behaviors represent a holistic response to life situations. The modes of action common to the human experience show a variety of activities and concerns that make up this integrated response to living.

Actions That Interrelate Self and Environment

Actions that interrelate self and environment include a number of coping strategies. The following are examples of such strategies:

- Using routine patterned ways of getting along until they are not effective
- Problem-solving activities to find new and different kinds of solutions
- Testing approaches to control the environment or changing or controlling one's own behavior in response to environmental demands
- Seeking support from others
- Seeking information and feedback
- Practicing successful coping efforts

- Seeking instructions and advice
- Seeking suggestions and explanations
- Using satisfying and comforting activities to formulate and promote one's self-image and self-esteem
- Evoking and using the help of others to relate in different ways to others in environmental conditions
- Planning for and anticipating problems
- Mobilizing resources under stress; being able to get second wind
- Rehearsing and trying out new solutions to problems
- Learning new skills and approaches to problems and situations
- Avoiding problem situations
- Attacking and being aggressive, verbally or physically

Actions That Function Primarily through Psychological Processes

Coping involves subjective strategies that bring about changes in thoughts, feelings, and perceptions. A number of these kinds of actions are identified:

- Defining and redefining situations to arrive at new meanings
- Appraising threats to self
- Maintaining one's self-esteem from actual or perceived sources of threat
- Reappraising situations as new information becomes available
- Setting priorities in terms of energy and efforts
- Developing a sense of personal autonomy and self-confidence to handle problems and situations as balanced against rewards to be achieved
- Thinking of alternative actions to problems and situations
- Insulating against defeats by an inner dialogue with oneself to minimize the importance of the experience and maximize the learning that comes from the situation so that it can be generalized to future problems and situations
- Controlling the demands of others and the environment by withdrawal, being nonresponsive, and interpreting such demands to exclude self-involvement
- Deploying and rationing attention, energy, and effort
- Differentiating sources of fear while receiving comfort from others
- Internalizing a feeling of comfort and associating this feeling with the image of the comforter and using this image to comfort someone else
- Fantasizing what one would do if———
- Submitting to feelings of helplessness, apathy, and noninvolvement
- Withdrawing emotions and thoughts
- Using psychological defense mechanism to excess

Lazarus and his colleagues (1974) proposed that coping through use of problem-solving efforts is related to the kinds of responses that are provided to a person by others and obtained from the environment. This group of researchers believes that when conditions exist that pose little or no threat or gain for people, coping activities tend to be flexible, reality-oriented, and rational. On the other hand, when conditions exist that evoke frustration, stress, and heightened emotions, coping activities shift to more rigid, primitive, and less adequate and realistic efforts to handle the situation. Under such conditions, the more routinized patterned responses come into play and are ineffective in coping. Lazarus and his co-workers have not indicated how threats in situations relate to stimulation of novel responses to enlarge the coping dialogue. Crisis theory predicts that in such situations, people can learn new responses if professional counseling and guidance are provided.

Coping involves cognitive appraisal of situations and events as well as the degree of threat. Perceptions are the basis for actions even though appraisals may be inaccurate. The mode of coping may be to use routine patterns of actions or it may require a different strategy that evolves from problem solving. Specific coping responses are variable and considerably influenced by the situation facing a person. Such responses are also influenced by the environment that people have grown up and lived in. For example, street-wise children in urban ghettos learn coping strategies and use support systems to maintain street activites—both legal and illegal—that most children never experience in their lifetimes.

The perceptions that people hold about their environments are important to know because coping behavior does not depend on accurate perceptions of reality. People will seek to cope on the basis of whatever reality they make, accurate or not. This basic assumption of social psychological theory is important to understand. Mechanic (1974) believes that many times misperceptions of reality aid coping, energize involvement and participation in life's endeavors, and alleviate the pain and discomfort that distracts from successful efforts to cope. For example, coping on the basis of misperceptions of reality is not unusual in serious illness. This may be the only way people can handle information that provides the brutal truths that pose threats to self, to others, and to life itself. Misperceptions may be a way of controlling information until terrible truths can be accepted and handled. Another example of this phenomenon occurs in mental illness. Patients experiencing certain kinds of mental problems misrepresent and grossly distort reality. As bizarre and maladaptive as these misrepresentations are, they serve as a basis for motivation and action, influence numbers, kinds, and quality of relationships, and structure the immediate environment and life space for such patients. Interventions try to change such distorted perceptions.

Modes of coping are essential to adaptation because they interrelate psychological, social, and cultural factors and are the behavioral expressions of efforts to manage self and environments in interaction. These modes are influenced by constant interchange and the fact that new factors influencing adaptation have to be assessed and managed as part of an ongoing coping process.

Coping, as the holistic response that people make to personal, environmental, and social pressures, cannot be handled by reflexes or organized skills. It involves attribution of meanings to situations, judgment, and problem solving, as well as struggles, trials, and a persistent focus of energy and effort toward achieving goals.

The process of reviewing with a person or family the efforts to cope is quite often a revelation. This is true because efforts at coping are frequently not recognized by the people who make them. Too often, what is recognized and focused on is the cumulation of unsuccessful or less than successful efforts. A review is a helpful first step in the learning process. People begin to see their efforts to cope in different ways and redefine situations in ways that use more effectively their abilities and capabilities.

Coping strategies may be analyzed in terms of their effectiveness for recurring and unusual problem situations. What is effective coping for one of these kinds of situations may not be appropriate for another kind of situation. Skills and abilities can be taught but most of all people have to be helped to learn how to use problem-solving approaches.

White (1974) once suggested that effective coping and adaptive efforts are those that have successful conclusions. This after-the-fact kind of evaluation continues to be one way in which efforts to cope can be judged.

SOCIAL PSYCHOLOGICAL PRINCIPLES OF BEHAVIOR

Social psychological principles of human behavior take into account multiple dimensions of the human experience. They consider how and under what conditions an individual interacts and copes. An assumption underlying all the principles is that the behavior that people use at any particular time is the best adaptation and coping possible under given circumstances.

> *Principle 1: Human beings are distinctly human and have the capacity to develop behavior in the process of adaptation and coping that puts them above and apart from other animals.*

One of the most important behaviors that humans alone develop is the ability to communicate through verbal symbols. Humans and humans alone, are capable of using symbols from the past to deal with the present and to predict the future. This ability to communicate makes possible the uses of communication symbols as the basic social process.

Communication literally makes it possible for individuals and groups to have a "common meaning" or understanding with one another. Through communication, social interaction becomes possible, group activities are encouraged, and people are able to have a social life.

Communication has the capacity to influence and control the behavior of human beings. It is also the means by which past and present events involving human experiences are integrated and transmitted to others so that each person does not have to always start anew without benefit of what previous generations of humans have learned. One generation stands on the shoulders of the previous one and builds on the existing bases of knowledge and skills. Competencies are passed on from one generation to another about how to have growth-promoting social relationships as well as how to maintain and advance social and cultural roles, norms, and values.

Another distinct kind of human behavior is the ability of a people to reflect back on themselves the results of the appraisals of their own behavior. This means that people can be objective about their thoughts, feelings, and actions, by "standing back from the self." A person can step out of herself or himself and take the role of another and evaluate her or his behavior from that standpoint. These evaluations are used to guide future behavior.

A third distinction of the humanness of behavior concerns the unique ability of people to develop lasting, loving, and caring relationships for other people. They accept the responsibilities for the care and well-being of persons close to them for many years. These relationships are bonded together by love and affection that are mutually satisfying and meet basic human needs of being loved and needed.

The development of these unique abilities in humans requires social environments that foster the growth and development of people and provide socialization experiences so that each new person will be humanized to hold human values and rights. To become human means that a person learns to use commonly shared symbols, to communicate, and to accumulate knowledge and experience. Being human also means a person can define situations, hold lasting and loving relationships, assume responsibility for self and others, and acquire the ability to reflect back on self about his or her actions. These abilities foster autonomy and independence of self. In this complex and unfolding process, interpersonal, family, and social relationships interact with the biophysical aspects of growth and development to create an individual who is both unique and a social member of a family, community, and society.

> *Principle 2: Cultural and social systems provide the symbols and patterns that people use to define situations and organize thoughts and behavior essential to relationships.*

Human beings are cultural as well as social, psychological, and physical beings. The prevailing culture and subculture in which one is born begins to have its influence long before the actual birth of a person. For instance, there are subcultures in which the birth of a son is considered a necessity for family continuity and survival, while daughters are devalued and experience different kinds of relationships in the family. They may be considered as a chattel, useful to exchange for wealth or other things that the family needs or wants. Once the sex of a child is established at birth, social expectations are set into motion in relation to roles, position within the family, and relationships. The organization of self in children of both sexes is influenced by what happens to them in these early relationships. This includes how they are valued, whether love is expressed, role modeling and role expectations, and the opportunities provided for them to develop some individuality. The avenues open to the child of a particular sex vary from culture to culture and family to family.

Just as the organization of the self, or personality, arises in part from the culture, so does the mind. Personality and mind develop in conjunction with each other and are not separate entities. Each has social, cultural, and cognitive dimensions that integrate to form a unity with society. Communication, social and interpersonal contexts are crucial factors in the development of both personality and mind. The development of self-control of behavior occurs in social and cultural contexts because some kinds of standards of conduct have to be "taken inside," or internalized, by human beings.

The mind simply does not emerge because of some innate potential. Because human beings are born, live, and die in group contexts, the human abilities to communicate, think, and develop cognitive pathways are related to socialization experiences. These abilities are related to new relationships and challenges that require different and new ways of coping and the internalization of values that help to organize and give meaning to significant experiences. Over time, people learn that there are views other than their own. Gradually, with maturity the realization develops that in order to get along and be effective in groups, consensus and compromise are necessary in respect to many facets of working and living. The necessity of having to cope with different situations and relationships helps the individual develop cognitive, affective, and problem-solving processes.

The mind is social in another sense. Through use of cognitive abilities, people learn to "talk to themselves" as well as to others. This form of internal reflection, or silent conversation with oneself, is an indication that significant symbols are being used by the individual. This kind of communication is not to be confused with non–reality-based experiences such as hallucinations.

Understanding the social and cultural meanings of experiences is especially important in community mental health nursing because social and cultural patterns of living, health, and nutritional practices have profound influences on health and mental health behaviors. Such patterns and practices have to be identified and understood in terms of the purposes they serve members of particular cultures and subcultures and why they continue over time. Many of these are embedded in religious beliefs and strong sociocultural mores. From a health standpoint, if changes are desired, it is necessary to pay close attention to the definitions or explanations of what the behavior means to the individual or family. Furthermore, it is useful to explore what some of the consequences might be if changes are made and decide whether change would be better or worse for the persons involved, considering the benefits that might accrue. With the advent of modern medicine and technology, cultural gaps between traditional folkways of handling health care problems and scientific approaches are always present. These gaps are reflected in quite different conceptions about health, illness, care, treatment, and the consequences of being treated by modern medicine.

Principle 3: Families and other primary socialization groups provide the essential experiences that are necessary for the growth and development of self-actualization of individuals.

The physical and emotional nurturing that all people need in infancy is the process that links the neonate's physiological, personal comfort and his or her social needs to the interplay of the world around him or her. The infant and young child are unusually sensitive to comforting as well as disrupting experiences that are provided by adults during mothering and nurturing activities. Tension is transmitted from the mother or significant other to the infant through muscle activities and the tone of the voice as they are held close and nurtured. Tensions are also communicated by touch. Regardless of how these early experiences are felt by the infant, the social identity of the child as a separate person begins to evolve.

Essential nurturing and mothering experiences take place within a cultural framework of values, beliefs, and child-rearing practices. For example, breast-feeding practices of mothers are influenced by the cultural values and expectations placed on such activity and on the mothering role.

Early in the socialization process, the infant experiences pressures and directions to learn ways of behaving. These are the first efforts of adults to shape the infant's behavior to conform with parental needs and their ideas about roles and expectations. The baby soon comes to understand that there are limits to certain kinds of behavior that can be employed to try to meet her or his needs and desires. What the baby does not know until he or she is much older is that these limits and expectations about appropriate behavior are rooted in familial values, norms, and practices. Over the years of growth and development from infancy to childhood, new family members have to face a series of changing roles and relationships in relation to self and to other family members.

Socialization patterns and practices influence the development of the organization of self in its personal and social dimensions. People learn to act and respond in the contexts of family and other kinds of primary groups that form emotional bonds, and acquire necessary social behaviors and role relationships. The learning of communication, which is basic to the use of symbols, is essential for developing mature cognitive processes and the means for communicating with other people.

Peer groups and the family continue to be important in different ways in the growth and development of the individual self through childhood, adolescence, and adulthood. In the many diverse experiences in which people participate, characteristic modes of coping are learned. A major developmental need is self-actualization, that is, the development of autonomy and a personal identity of self that is, for the most part, independent of a group identity. At the same time, self-identity remains linked to the support values and beliefs of the peer groups. These groups remain important in a person's life from then on because they are sources of support and help to stabilize the concept of self one holds about oneself.

> **Principle 4:** *Coping is learned through the interaction of individual abilities, social and cultural factors, and the situational contexts in which experiences take place.*

This principle recognizes that in trying to adapt and cope, people are proactive, active, interactive, and reactive in their relationships with others and in their attempt to exert control over environments. In general, people try to manage their coping behavior on the basis of conscious and rational perceptions and evaluations of reality. Adaptive behaviors and coping patterns are learned through role modeling and imitation, curiosity and discovery, and use of cognitive and affective abilities to meet hour-to-hour and day-to-day demands of personal and social relationships.

Interactions between humans and environmental systems are generated as people perform the activities and maintain the relationships necessary for life. People go about their business of facing challenges, trying to manage relationships in ways that are satisfying, and controlling to a certain extent their life situations. These efforts require the use of reasoning, logic, problem solving, risk taking, and concern for others. The learning of coping and adaptive behaviors in this complex life process occurs in many contexts, and at every turn chance and unanticipated factors may alter effective coping and individual motivation or pose threats to self-esteem. Data about these interactions must be included in the base from which community mental health nursing makes clinical decisions.

> **Principle 5:** *Definitions of situations help people appraise events and experiences to determine relevancy to their well-being and activate coping.*

Situational contexts are the social settings in which ongoing human events take place, and they have considerable variability. This variability introduces an ongoing or emergent kind of information process. The definitions people make of such situations provide the information needed to assess comforts or threats to self and to decide how to cope with particular experiences at particular times and places involving particular people. This does not mean that only unusual and atypical information is involved in definitions of situations. It does mean that most human experiences involve situations that occur in frameworks of learned roles and relationships and these have to be modified to get a fit between a particular situation, events, and people that the person has to cope with.

Definitions of situations have a subjective component. This component is part of the appraisal of reality and it helps motivate people to act, react, and interact. Subjective definitions of situations are unique to the people who make them because of the standpoint from which they are made. The subjective component of definitions is an essential aspect of understanding what views and feelings a person holds. Subjective definitions also provide information that is otherwise not available about why people think other people act as they do (Maloney, 1971).

The objective component of definitions of situations is made by people somewhat removed from the immediate situation and provides another dimension to the reality of what is happening. "Objectifying" a situation is an attempt to hold in abeyance or not to consider the intense emotional aspects of relationships and events until they can be reconceived in broader contexts. A common-sense way of saying this is: "I need to back away because I can't see the forest for the trees."

Situational contexts not only have variability; they also have instability because some relationships that exist in a situation may be temporary. Even so, such contexts exert powerful influences on the ways in which individuals learn to cope and adapt. Specific events that occur in situational contexts limit or facilitate the options one has to use. Whatever the choices, the actions taken begin to generate and set into motion the selection of coping responses, feelings, beliefs, and ideas about self, which in turn influence the role through which behavior is expressed.

An example of how powerful the influence of contexts on behavior can be may be seen in crisis situations. Crisis situations involve subjective definitions of situations. These definitions evoke responses from the person involved that may not be adequate to handle the crisis event. For example, when the crisis situation is defined as overwhelming, a sense of failure or inadequacy may be experienced, with coping efforts falling back on repetitive learned patterns. These are usually not effective for coping with the situation at hand. Crisis theory holds that this is the time to help people learn new ways of coping. The situation is redefined, and individuals are assisted in using new behaviors to handle it. When this happens, the people involved experience a sense of control over events and are able to cope. Then, when a new crisis situation occurs, they will use the past experience to define it and try out the previously learned coping behaviors. If these are effective for handling the situation, it may not be defined as a crisis. But without knowing how a situation is defined by a person, it is difficult for a nurse to know whether a crisis exists for that person.

The dependence of people on definitions of situations to motivate behavior and understand their emotions may be reduced under some conditions. Bem (1972), after reviewing a body of research on this phenomenon, concluded that a person comes to "know" their own attitudes, emotions, and other internal states by inferring them from observations of their own overt behavior or the circumstances in which behavior occurs. Bem suggested that once people know this about themselves, they tend to deduce their internal states from their own overt actions and judge them on the basis of a feeling of inconsistency between attitudes and action. When there is a feeling that attitudes and actions are consistent and clear-cut, there is no need for a person to infer from overt behavior their attitudes and emotion. The situation is being handled; that is enough feedback.

> **Principle 6:** *Current patterns of behavior are emphasized in relation to their effectiveness in situations of daily living.*

A major assumption of this principle is that current behavior is influenced by things, events, and relationships. The effectiveness of patterns of behavior used in daily living situations is a measure of coping and of achieving satisfactions in life. This means that the nurse is concerned with recent experiences and the conditions under which modes of coping occurred. The behavior that people use at any particular time is the best possible synthesis of past cognitive, emotional, and experiental learnings. Coping patterns indicate how a person copes irrespective of the historical reasons of why or how such patterns developed. Assessment of such efforts is an essential source of data for evaluating current levels of functioning.

Emphasis on present behavior patterns further directs the community mental health nurse to find out how people define and perceive current reality. In this process, there is a need to consider how personal and family relationships and community support systems are used to cope with situations. Stable patterns of coping, feeling, and adapting are the basis for coping with current experiences. Temporary or rapidly changing coping efforts may be interspersed with the more stable efforts. Once a pattern of responses is recognized, it can be assessed for effectiveness and new coping skills learned as needed.

Principle 7: Maladaptive or deviant behavior is usually identified as such when a person is not able to perform social roles, maintain social and personal relationships, and achieve psychological comfort.

Maladaptive behavior has a likelihood of developing in social groups where interactions create situations that lead members to develop distorted roles, thoughts, feelings, and relationships. In such situations, reality testing becomes impaired, and the individual may focus on discrete bits and pieces of experiences without being aware of the broader contexts and interrelationships involved. Definitions of situations are distorted, and they motivate actions and interactions that are often not perceived by others as appropriate. At some point, people begin to relate to the confused person on the basis of this distorted and inappropriate behavior. This sets into motion a cycle of mutual reinforcement that may be very difficult to diminish so that more adaptive patterns of behavior can be established. Unless interventions occur, the person experiencing difficulties in reality testing and control of behavior receives feedback from a mutually reinforcing system that does not provide the information needed to learn corrective actions.

Maladaptive behavior has social, psychological, and situational dimensions. In addition, bizarre behavior may have psychopathological content and dynamics. Because social and situational factors contribute to the development of abnormal behavior, they must be considered when clinical therapeutic interventions are designed.

Maladaptive behavior is not viewed as mental illness of the psychological structures of the personality, nor is it conceived of as a medical illness like any other illness. Rather, it is considered to be dysfunctional and inappropriate coping and adaptation processes in life situations. These responses may be temporary or become more or less permanent. If maladaptive behavior is labeled mental illness, powerful forces are set into motion to confirm this label. For example, learning the deviant role of mental patients in response to the expectations of others is a major factor in the persistence of such behavior.

SUMMARY

A social psychological view of human behavior places an emphasis on the social and cultural determinants of behavior. Socialization, the basic process for humanizing the young, teaching them the essential competencies needed to survive and achieve satisfactions in loving relationships, work endeavors, and coping with life, occurs for the most part in primary groups. The family system is the most important of such groups and is the milieu in which the organization of self evolves and support for continued growth and development is provided.

A social psychological perspective about the development of a personal self and essential social competencies uses particular meanings for certain basic concepts. Five important ones are socialization, cultural and social systems, social structure, role, and adaptation and coping.

A model of adaptation and modes of coping consistent with the social psychological perspective of behavior consolidates a number of ideas and views. In efforts to adapt and cope as humans and environment interact, there is a synthesis of the strengths a person has developed and the conditions in the environment that have to be managed that is expressed in modes of coping action. Two dominant modes are those that interrelate self and environment and those that change feelings, thoughts, and definitions. This model of adaptation is both practical and useful in community mental health nursing as a way of organizing assessment data, identifying problems, making clinical decisions, and evaluating outcomes of nursing interventions and actions.

REFERENCES

Baron, Robert A., and Bryne, Donn. *Social Psychology: Understanding Human Behavior*, 3rd ed. Boston, MA: Allyn and Bacon, 1981, chapters 7 and 10.

Bem, Daryl J. Self-Perception Theory. In Berkowitz, L., ed. *Advances in Experimental Social Psychology*, vol. 6. New York: Academic Press, 1972, pp. 2–57.

Biddle, Bruce J. *Role Theory: Expectations, Identities, and Behaviors*. New York: Academic Press, 1979, chapters 1–3.

Blumer, Hubert. *Symbolic Interactionism*. Englewood Cliffs, NJ: Prentice-Hall, 1969, pp. 173–175.

Cardwell, J. D. *Social Psychology: A Symbolic Interaction Perspective*. Philadelphia: F. A. Davis, 1971, chapters 1–6.

Durkheim, Emile. *The Rules of Sociological Method*. Solovay, Sarah A., and Muller, John H., trans. New York: Free Press, 1964, pp. 102–103.

Feldman, Phillip, and Orford, Jim. Overview and implications: Toward an applied social and community psychology. In Feldman, P., and Orford, J., eds. *Psychological Problems: The Social Context*. New York: John Wiley & Sons, 1980, Chapter 13.

Geertz, Clifford. Ritual and social change: A Javanese example. *American Anthropologist* 59:32–54, 1957.

Goffman, Erving. *The Presentation of Self in Everyday Life*. Garden City, NY: Doubleday, 1959, chapters 1–2.

Goldschmidt, Walter. Ethology, ecology, and ethnological realities. In Coelho, George V., Hamburg, David A., and Adams, John E., eds. *Coping and Adaptation*. New York: Basic Books, 1974, pp. 13–31.

Grace, Helen K., and Camilleri, Dorothy D. *Mental Health Nursing: A Sociopsychological Approach*. Dubuque, IA: William C. Brown Co., 1981, pp. 37–41.

Kluckhohn, Clyde. The study of culture. In Rose, Peter I., ed. *The Study of Society: An Integrated Anthology*. New York: Random House, 1967, pp. 74–92.

Lakin, Martin. *Interpersonal Encounter: Theory and Practice in Sensitivity Training*. New York: McGraw-Hill, 1972, pp. 29–54.

Lazarus, Richard S., Averell, James R., and Opton, Edward M. The psychology of coping: Issues of research and assessment. In Coelho, George V., Hamburg, David A., and Adams, John E., eds. *Coping and Adaptation*. New York: Basic Books, 1974, pp. 249–315.

Levinson, Daniel J., Darrow, Charlotte N., Klein, Edward B., et al. *The Seasons of a Man's Life*. New York: Ballantine Books, 1978, Introduction and chapters 1–3.

Lindesmith, Alfred, and Strauss, Anselm. *Social Psychology*. New York: Holt, Rinehart and Winston, 1956, Chapter 1.

Lindesmith, Alfred, and Strauss, Anselm. *Social Psychology*. New York: Holt, Rinehart and Winston, 1968, chapters 1, 11, and 14.

Lindesmith, Alfred, Strauss, Anselm, and Denzing, Norman. *Social Psychology*, 4th ed. Hinsdale, IL: Dryden Press, 1975, chapters 1 and 14.

Maloney, Elizabeth. The subjective and objective definitions of crisis. *Perspectives of Psychiatric Care* 9:257–268, November–December, 1971.

McCall, George J. The social organization of relationships. In McCall, George, ed. *Social Relationships*. Chicago, IL: Aldine Publishing Co., 1970, chapters 1 and 2.

McGrath, J. *Social and Psychological Factors in Stress*. New York: Holt, Rinehart and Winston, 1970.

Mechanic, David. Social structure and personal adaptation: Some neglected dimensions. In Coelho, George V., Hamburg, David A., and Adams, John E., eds. *Coping and Adaptation*. New York: Basic Books, 1974, Chapter 3.

Mechanic, David. *Medical Sociology*. New York: Free Press, 1968, pp. 302–310.

Miller, Daniel R. The study of social relationships, situation, identity, and social interaction. In Koch, Sigmund, ed. *Psychology: A Study of Science*. New York: McGraw-Hill, 1963, pp. 642–645.

Mullen, Edward J., and Dumpson, James R. *Evaluation of Social Intervention*. London: Jossey-Bass, 1972, chapters 6–10.

Pasquali, Elaine, Alesi, Eleanore G., Arnold, Helen M., and Debasio, Mary. *Mental Health Nursing: A Biopsychocultural Approach*. St. Louis: C. V. Mosby Co., 1981, chapters 2, 3, and 4.

Pearlin, Leonard I., and Schooler, Carmi. The structure of coping. *Journal of Health and Social Behavior* 19:2–21, March, 1978.

Selye, Hans. *The Stress of Life*. New York: McGraw-Hill, 1956.

Selye, Hans. *Stress without Distress*. Toronto: McClelland and Steward, 1977.

Sundeen, Sandra J., Stuart, Gail W., Rankin, Elizabeth, and Cohen, Sylvia. *Nurse–Client Interaction*. St. Louis: C. V. Mosby Co., 1981, pp. 134–151.

White, Robert W. Strategies of adaptation: An attempt at systematic description. In Coehlo, George V., Hamburg, David A., and Adams, John E., eds. *Coping and Adaptation*. New York: Basic Books, 1974, pp. 47–68.

6 DEVELOPMENT OF PERSONAL ORGANIZATION: THE SELF

INTRODUCTION

A social psychological approach to human behavior requires special consideration of how a person develops a self, a personality. A basic assumption of social psychology is that the self is primarily organized by social experiences and learning. Therefore, it is necessary to understand the relationship between the personal development of self, the structure of self, and the phases of development.

The development and organization of the self are grounded in the interactions and relationships that occur in the normal course of being born, growing up, and becoming an adult. These basic human relationships involve a host of social, biological, and cultural factors and shape the psychological development of the self of each person. This holistic view considers a human being as a person with biogenetic, social, psychological, moral, and spiritual dimensions having infinite potential for self-actualization. The sum of all of these constitute the wholeness of a person relative to a particular time and stage of development.

A human being is basically a social person and, as such, cannot stand alone and maintain a wholeness of self. Because the development and organization of self and achievement of selfhood are so closely linked to social experiences and meaningful relationships and communications with other people, all of these have to be maintained on a continuing basis. What people are and what they want to become depend to a large extent on relationships with other people. These also depend on the development of adaptive and coping behaviors that effectively deal with life situations and relationships and the inner strength that is needed to cope with events over which little or no control is possible. People do have unique abilities and creative potentials as well as common concerns and needs, and all of these are used to develop adaptive coping responses. Such responses help to influence or control the quality of life events, social relationships, and living.

The concept of self is important in social psychological theories of behavior. Lindesmith and co-workers (1975) noted that people are not born with a sense of self, other, or social situation. A cardinal task of parents or significant others in care-taking roles is to change the socially neutral infant into a symbolically functioning human being. Lindesmith and his colleagues viewed the organization of the self as: (1) a set of more or less consistent and stable responses on a conceptual level that (2) exercise a regulatory function over other responses of the same organism at lower levels. The self is an organization or integration of behavior imposed upon the individual by societal expectations and demands.

The organization of self changes over a person's life span and takes on new and different sets of responses as new life tasks have to be dealt with. As old ideas and responses are given up or delegated less importance, new ideas and responses are formulated and integrated. Throughout this never-ending process, there is continuity and constancy by having one's own name and sense of personal identity.

Cardwell (1971), in an effort to prevent the concept of self from becoming elevated to an independent entity, described the self as the set of all descriptions and concepts held by people about themselves. He made the point that people do not have "selves" that they carry around with them. Rather, people have ideas or notions about themselves that are the result of learning through interactions with others and participation in experiences that occur during lifelong socialization.

The development of self, or personality, has been conceptualized in many ways. Some theories emphasize social factors, others emphasize factors arising from within the individual. Nearly all theories of self have focused on stages of development in early childhood and up to early adulthood. The social psychological perspective that emphasizes symbolic interaction is used to describe how the self develops. Other social psychological perspectives are presented, most of which are congenial to the perspective that development and organization of self are in large part dependent on social experiences. Recent formulations of adult growth and development and organization of self address socialization over the life span.

SOCIALIZATION AND DEVELOPMENT OF SELF

Socialization, the complex process through which each new individual takes in, or internalizes, the culture in which he or she is born, prepares people for roles and develops a concept of self. Very early in life, each person has to learn that social and cultural values and expectations are translated into general and specific social roles and relationships. These, in turn, are related to consistent and stable responses expected from others. These responses integrate conceptual, social, and behavioral levels of feelings, thoughts, and actions.

The human self is not something that people are "born with," it is "made" (Parsons & Bales, 1955). This means that the self is not innate and does not develop from a genetic blueprint that is based on universal primitive drives and tensions located within the psychic infrastructure. Social development of the self occurs in stages and phases, which, in the early years, interrelate developmental tasks and skills of personal, social, and physical growth and development. The development of the self begins with the nurturing relationships and activities that are provided by the mothering one.

The family, as the major social system in which primary socialization of the young takes place, is the milieu in which the basic physical, personal, and social necessities of survival, growth, and development are provided. This is a critical role in the development of human beings and makes the family the most important social setting in the development of both the young and adults.

The modern nuclear family has been described as having two major functions: (1) the primary socialization of children to be members of the society in which they are born, and (2) the stabilization of adult personalities (Parsons & Bales, 1955). These basic functions interconnect the relationships parents have with their children. If the family is reasonably effective in meeting the two functions, then a social setting is created in which children are reared by secure and mature parents. Family and cultural values are inculcated in the young. Children experience a sense of security and comfort and know that they are valued members of the family. Under these kinds of conditions, growth and development in all dimensions of health provide optimal opportunities for children and adults to achieve mature selfhood and self-actualization.

A major characteristic of the family is that it is a setting in which children can invest intense emotional energies. Dependencies can be safely fostered for a short while, then parents have to begin the process of helping the child to develop more autonomy and independence. The child has to achieve independence by separating from dependent relationships.

The development of a personal organization of self cannot be understood outside of the family or primary group settings in which much of this development occurs. The family as an interacting social system is a very special kind of primary group because it is where adaptation is learned and early patterns of coping tested. In this setting, children must be socialized not only to function in the family system but to reach out to other groups and individuals. This requires participation in different kinds of roles in different kinds of social systems. All of these experiences are essential for the development of self.

Socialization of the young sometimes occurs in primary groups other than families. Children may be reared in various institutional settings. At best, it is difficult for these settings to provide the special intensive relationships that are possible in a family. Although the physical needs of the child may be more than adequately met, the child's social and psychological needs may not be met to the extent that emotional and social growth are impaired. Intense mothering relationships and needed stimulations may not be available at the times or in the form they are needed by the infant or young child.

In institutional settings such as children's homes, small group homes, and foster families, children occupy different kinds of roles, status, and positions from those experienced by children in natural families. Hence, children reared in these settings find it difficult to have the same kinds of experiences as children reared with parents and siblings. If a child cannot be reared in her or his own family, a surrogate or foster family that can provide as many of the essential relationships of the family as possible is usually more desirable than placing infants and young children in institutional settings.

Families that successfully socialize their young help them to develop caring relationships with parents and siblings. These relationships are rooted in common experiences and collective memories that bind the family together as a unit.

ORGANIZATION OF THE SELF: AN INTERACTIONIST PERSPECTIVE

The personal organization of self emerges in large part from social experiences that include definitions made by others. Communication, symbolic gestures, and roles are ways in which these definitions are conveyed to help a person develop a self. Society and self join to form a unified and dynamic whole. This concept is associated with but not limited to theories emphasizing the importance of symbolic interaction in the development of the self (Mead, 1943; Lindesmith & Strauss, 1956; Stryker, 1964; Meltzer, 1966; Blumer, 1969).

The self is an organization of feelings, attitudes, and experiences. The use of this organization makes it possible for people to respond to their own communication. People then act toward themselves in the same way as they act toward others. People may praise, blame, encourage, be disgusted with, or punish themselves. When this is done, people are actually objects of their own intentions and actions. All of us have experienced "talking to ourselves" about something we did or did not do as well as made value judgments about our actions.

The social and psychological organization of the self begins at birth. The just-born infant is sensitive to light, touch, and sound. Recognition of these sensitivities has altered the milieu in many delivery rooms and the immediate postdelivery care of the newborn. For example, LeBoyer (1976) recommends a dimly lit delivery room so that the infant in the first extrauterine moments is not subjected to harsh glaring lights and loud noises. Immediately after delivery, he places the baby in the mother's arms so she can stroke, touch, and coo to the infant to begin the establishment of maternal–infant bonding. This early establishment of an emotional attachment between the newborn and its mother is now recognized as an essential relationship that, if not well-developed, has implications for the future physical and emotional development of the child.

Early mothering experiences with the infant are both verbal and nonverbal. If the mothering one is tense when touching or holding the infant while providing nurturant activities, then the infant experiences discomfort and unease in an undifferentiated way. This discomfort is communicated nonverbally through muscular tension. Most of us have observed infants being startled by loud noises and then comforted by cuddling, rhythmic patting, and soft whisperings. These are usually successful in bringing about a cessation of crying, kicking, and flailing behaviors. Conversely, we have all seen infants who fail to be comforted by mothering behaviors and are sometimes placed alone in a crib to cry out anger and frustration.

The Structure of Self

The structure of self develops in concert with the physical and social growth and development of infants and starts as basic needs are met. These needs become the vital pathway through which social and psychological organization of the self begins to develop. At first, there are diffuse and unorganized feelings and experiences because the self is undifferentiated. As infants are cared for and nurtured, they are also being taught how to be human. This humanizing process starts early as infants are encouraged to develop individual activities for which they are rewarded; at the same time, as the demands and needs of infants are met, the needs and desires of others are taken into consideration. At this early age, the development of a personal self-identity and of a socially responsive human being go hand in hand.

The structure of the personal self is conceived of as having two distinct aspects: the "I" and the "me". The "I" part of the self organization develops first. It consists of the unorganized aspects of the human experience, such as biological needs, impulses, and creative potentials. These sources provide some of the energy that propels a person to action. In the infant and young child, these undirected tendencies and actions have to be brought under control and in line with the expectations, norms, and values of others. Energies have to be curbed and channeled into accepted actions or squelched.

The "me" aspect of the self-organization develops later. It is mostly social in nature and represents the organized set of attitudes, definitions, understandings, expectations, and meanings common to the social group in which the child is a member. These standards are the yardstick by which a person regulates her or his own behavior. Such standards, directly and indirectly, link the individual, group, and society.

There is a dynamic relationship between the two aspects of the self. The "I" is spontaneous and provides for creativity. The "me" is a regulator and provides direction to behavior by channeling energies toward attainment of goals. These two aspects have to be brought into some kind of harmony; however, the degree to which behavior associated with one or the other is valued and encouraged in a family may have considerable variation.

Stages of Development of Self

The development of self involves the acquisition of attitudes, competencies, skills, and knowledge at particular stages. The ability to develop emotional relationships is an essential competency and is necessary for people to achieve selfhood and have meaningful relationships with significant others. Failure to achieve certain competencies with peers, adults, and authority figures at particular times may leave a person with deficiencies or gaps in the repertoire of essential competencies. These basic competencies are needed to develop more complex and varied relationships and skills. Deficiencies in the repertoire of essential competencies become part of a general impoverishment in the area of personal, interpersonal, familial, and social relationships, all of which are necessary to fulfill basic roles and relationships and to learn more complex coping competencies. With each succeeding stage of development, this impoverishment becomes more pronounced. Assessments of developmental tasks and skills usually indicate these deficiencies.

Individuals have to develop the ability to respond to their own communications and intentions in order to reach full selfhood and actualization. This ability involves standing back from oneself and reflecting back on one's behavior by using available information to guide one's actions and is called *role taking*. Role taking means that a person is able to take the role of another, stand back from self, and examine his or her own actions. An example of this crucial competency may be cited. A young daughter decides to play the role of mother. In this process, she takes the role of her mother and admonishes herself for having smeared mother's lipstick on the bedspread. In effect, the child talks back to herself and uses her observations to step apart from her real self.

A distinct quality of humanness is the ability to develop intense and loving relationships with others. This important dimension begins at birth with the mothering one. As physical, biological, and social psychological growth occurs, the kind and quality of interpersonal relationships change. These changes present a constant challenge to individuals to grow and enlarge the scope of interrelationships, many of which have different purposes and require different kinds of emotional investment. The personal organization of the self is closely associated with the development of the ability to take the role of other. Three stages are involved in this process.

The Preparatory Stage

A few months after birth, infants start to imitate the behavior of others without understanding what they are doing. This use of imitative behavior is necessary because infants do not have the neural, physiological, psychological, and social development to do otherwise. Through imitation, infants soon learn that certain behaviors done by parents can also be done by them. Some of this behavior gets rewards and some does not. The ability to imitate behavior and development of the awareness that rewards and punishment are meted out for different kinds of behavior set the stage for the development of more complex behavior in different kinds of interpersonal contexts and situations.

The Play Stage

Play begins when the young child learns to actually "play" the role of others. This play acting is essential because in the process the child "tries on," if you will, another role.

This process involves the development and use of sophisticated cognitive and social competencies that go beyond those needed to imitate behavior.

In the play stage, the formation of the self begins as children learn to act toward themselves to influence their own actions and intentions. Observations of children in this stage show that they often speak of themselves in the third person. Children may stand back and say of themselves, "I'm a bad girl (or boy) because I left the yard without permission."

Play-acting behavior indicates that the child is playing the role of others. In this play stage, the child's perceptions of roles are unstable. They are not clearly organized and may be inconsistent with one another. For example, mommy and daddy are more likely to be viewed as two distinct people who provide and do specific things for the child rather than as parents, which is a general role. A unified viewpoint of self has not yet evolved. The child cannot yet stand apart from herself or himself and take the role of another person in a way that combines specific aspects of roles to form a more composite or general role such as parent.

The Game Stage

The game stage is the third stage of development of self. It represents the time when the child arrives at a unified conception of self. During this stage, the child learns how to handle a number of roles at one time in group situations. This becomes possible because she or he is now capable of abstracting the common or general factor from a number of roles. This process makes it possible to develop a generalized role that represents viewpoint(s) common to a group. Once a person has achieved this ability, it is possible to conduct oneself in a consistent and organized fashion.

An example of this phenomenon is the development of the role of mother by a woman. The content of the mother role is developed for the most part from experiences with her own mother, observations and experiences of other mothers, expectations that respective families have about the role, popular stereotypes, and views from significant others. From all these sources presenting particular roles of a mother, the woman develops for herself a general role of motherhood. This composite role allows a mother to behave with consistency over many different kinds of situations because her definition of motherhood has been internalized.

Language and communication are important processes in the development of the self. Language is the basis for using significant and abstract symbols that make human beings distinctly human. The meanings of symbols come to be internalized through membership in various kinds of social groups and provide definitions for appropriate conduct.

Motivational Energy

Motivational energy is related to the development and organization of the self. From a symbolic interactional perspective, sources for motivational energy come from the individual, society, and interactions generated in interpersonal and group relationships. From within the individual, some energy comes from certain basic biological impulses such as hunger, the need for oxygen, sleep, and other basic essentials and the unorganized potentials in the "I" part of the self. From society, some energy comes from values and beliefs, definitions of situations, expectations of others, and the guides that person follows in relation to specific actions. From interactions, energy is generated as human beings interrelate in groups and participate in social networks in the process of daily living. The total energy from all these sources is more than the amount that each person needs to establish and maintain interpersonal and group relationships for achieving social and personal goals. The extra energy is then used for creative activities and self-actualization.

Not all behavior involves the self. Involuntary and automatic behaviors involve few, if any, of the dynamic and changing aspects of self. Examples of such behavior are eye blinks, ritualistic behavior, and learned patterns of behavior that are used so frequently they no longer require involvement of emotional and cognitive processes. Many of the "necessary things" we do as part of daily living are done with little or no thought. These kinds of actions reduce the amount of time and energy a person has to expend to get through a day of activities. For example, we do not have to make a conscious effort each time we put on our shoes to determine which shoe fits which foot.

Relationship of Mine, Self, and Society

Development of mind depends on relationships that integrate self and society. Mind is the perceptive and thinking part of the conscious self. It develops in conjunction with the self through social, personal, and interpersonal relationships, language, communication, and all kinds of experiences. The mind grows in social and cultural dimensions as well as in cognitive and emotional ones. All of these dimensions help shape the ways in which a person thinks, organizes thoughts, influences opinions and values, and shapes the perceptual frameworks and categories that are used for organizing reality and defining situations. These actions are the direct links between mind, self, and society.

Through interactions and communications with significant others, people gradually acquire a set of values, beliefs, norms, and standards of conduct common to a group and society. This process is called *internalization*. It is one of the basic processes by which "yardsticks" get inside the heart and head of individuals and guide much of individual behavior.

Selfhood

Selfhood refers to those important aspects of the personal organization of the self that have been achieved. People internalize many aspects of the society in which their selfhood has been organized and developed, thus making them an integral part of it. With selfhood, people are able to use the creative energies from the "I" to work toward self-actualization. People develop the strictly human and unique ability to step apart from the self, appraise actions, and then use these appraisals to change their behavior.

In mature selfhood, the "I" and "me" have integrated motives, feelings, attitudes, beliefs, perceptions, and ways of learning. This integrated whole includes the patterns of adaptation and coping that have been learned. Although there is consistency and constancy in beliefs and patterns over time and across different situations, there continues to be present in the self an openness that permits new learning and discovery of experiences to occur. This openness of self continues throughout life.

The acquisition of selfhood also means that a person has a personal organization from which to make decisions about his or her own behavior. Instead of being passive players in the stresses and presses of daily living, people are active and interactive participants. They monitor their own behavior, influence others, and control to some extent the environmental forces that impinge on their lives. Inherent in these competencies is the assumption that people who have achieved mature selfhood have a considerable amount of behavior under conscious awareness and management. This is true because they have information that emerges in the interactional process that can be used to judge present behavior and project future courses of action. In this process, people use a general set of expectations, definitions, and standards for guiding behavior. These guides keep people from being mere spectators and reactors to interactional, situational, and environmental demands.

ORGANIZATION OF THE SELF: AN INTERPERSONAL PERSPECTIVE

Social psychological perspectives of personality development differ in their emphasis on particular aspects of human development. Interpersonal theory emphasizes the kind, quality, and process of interpersonal experiences in one-to-one relationships.

An interpersonal theory that has been very influential in mental health and psychiatric nursing is the one developed by Sullivan (1953). Sullivan defined personality as a relatively enduring pattern of interpersonal situations that characterize human life. This view was influenced by the ideas of social psychologists and anthropologists who emphasized a perspective that the growth and development of people and their existence require interchange with environments and other people for full growth to take place.

The personalities of individuals are considered to be representative of the common culture in which they are socialized rather than a result of unique interpersonal events. Although socialization experiences with significant others vary from culture to culture, they are translated in all cultures to roles and patterned interrelationships. Such roles and relationships have to be experienced and learned at appropriate times during different developmental eras in order for more complex and extensive ones to evolve in subsequent eras.

Central to Sullivan's theory of personality development is the assumption that mental health and mental disorder have to be considered in the context of interpersonal situations. Patterned responses, both adaptive and maladaptive, are learned during socialization in interpersonal experiences. The learning of these patterns begins in infancy and becomes increasingly more organized as a person grows older.

The Self-System

A self-system has to be developed by each person. This is the organization of experiences that come into existence in order to help a person secure satisfactions in life without having to experience uncomfortable levels of anxiety. The self-system develops out of interpersonal experiences that in the past have aroused anxiety as a person tried to meet the basic needs of security and satisfaction. Such anxiety-producing experiences are basic to all human relations and involve both rewards and punishments. Sullivan considered his concept of the self-system to be similar to the concept of self that characterizes a symbolic interactionist view.

Structure of Self

Interpersonal theory postulates three aspects in the structure of self. Early organization of the self-system centers on the development of a "me." This development is closely associated with interpersonal responses that meet an infant's basic needs for survival and early mothering experiences. These experiences are the basis for the more refined development of a general concept of me into three different aspects: the good-me, bad-me, and not-me.

Good-me is the first aspect of the me that develops. It is related to the satisfactions that the infant experiences with the mothering one. At this stage of physical, social, and interpersonal development, experiences are in a prototaxic mode, that is, symbols are not used. Communication is felt through empathy, tenderness, tenseness, and other kinds of feelings that impart a message to the infant. Good-me develops to become the "I" part of the self.

Bad-me is the second aspect of the self and develops in the context of interpersonal relationships that produce an uncomfortable degree of anxiety. With the infant, anxiety is initially experienced as tension in the arms of the mothering one. The discomfort becomes associated with a vague sense on the part of the infant of not feeling "good," of feeling that something is not right. In time, the child associates this feeling with the belief that she or he is bad.

Not-me is the third aspect of the self and develops from the not-understood aspects of interpersonal relationships. Such relationships are associated with intense anxiety and are unclear in their meaning because of the distorting effects of anxiety on definitions of situations and reality testing. A person is not able to make clear connections between feeling intensely anxious and the events and relationships associated with the anxiety, so experiences become distorted. When a person experiences in interpersonal relationships feelings of bad-me and not-me, he or she is using what Sullivan called the *parataxic mode*. This means that experiences are interpreted in a private and autistic way without validation from others and become subject to distortion and bizarre interpretations.

In time, the three aspects of the self-system integrate into a generalized self. The self-system is an integral part of the self and operates to ward off uncomfortable anxiety in interpersonal relationships. An inner-oriented alerting and warning system signals when an uncomfortable increase of anxiety is being experienced. Upon such signaling, the self-system activates interpersonal strategies such as distancing to minimize or avoid anxiety. Anxiety may be decreased by converting the experiences from distorted fantasies to reality-based ones. Sullivan called this process *experiencing in a syntaxic mode*. This way of experiencing reality is characterized by one person communicating with another with symbols that both persons understand and that have common definitions and meanings. This kind of communication encourages validation of experiences.

In protecting the self against anxiety, the self-system acts to minimize changes in the interpersonal relationship process. Distortions in interpersonal relationships and communication are difficult for people to correct because their self-systems move to protect and close out of their awareness what is happening.

Three kinds of defenses help the self-system to achieve protection of the self: dissociation, parataxic distortion, and sublimation. Dissociation involves the exclusion from awareness of anxiety-provoking experiences and impulses. Parataxic distortion involves unrealistic changes in experiences to make them more tolerable and less anxiety producing. Sublimation involves the exchange of unacceptable goals associated with certain needs and impulses to goals that are socially acceptable (Maddi, 1968).

Anxiety

Anxiety is a major concept in interpersonal theory. At a moderate level, it is a positive factor in learning. At a high level, it becomes a disruptive force because it causes distortions of reality, particularly in interpersonal relationships. These distortions become an integral part of major social, interpersonal, and psychological problems that a person may experience.

Anxiety may be experienced in grades or levels. As the level of anxiety increases, the ability to realistically evaluate interpersonal experience decreases; learning is impaired; attention becomes more selective about fewer things and events. At the same time, the individual may have little awareness of the impact that anxiety has on his or her interpersonal relationships and the kinds of evaluations and definitions of situations that are being made.

Motivational Energy

Motivational energy is both biologically and interpersonally generated. Interpersonal theory postulates that energy to propel actions arises from biological requirements and psychological needs that have to be met in order to survive and to achieve satisfaction in interpersonal relationships. Another source of energy comes from the multifaceted self-definitions and self-appraisals that a person makes about experiences on the basis of approval and disapproval of others. This feedback helps a person use actions that achieve feelings of security and minimize anxiety.

Sullivan suggested that in the realm of personality and culture, tension has two important aspects: as potential for action and a felt state of being. The felt state of being comes from social and interpersonal experiences rather than innate tensions. Both kinds of tensions are transformed into energy that is expressed in both overt and covert behavior.

Emergence of Mind

The emergence of mind was not explicitly discussed by Sullivan. He did say that the organization of social and interpersonal experiences is related to learning, which in turn depends to some extent on how much anxiety a person experiences. The more anxiety that a person feels, the less is his or her ability to discriminate, pay attention, and be objective about the situation and experience. A small amount of anxiety increases alertness and facilitates learning. A high level of learning occurs when people use their cognitive processes for educational purposes. Learning also takes place through trial and error, by use of rewards and punishment, and through imitation.

Social factors related to the development of the mind focus on the development of language and symbols. The utterings of the infant, which sooner or later become words that are heard from adults and imitated, are praised and rewarded as they approximate the cultural way of saying things. The gestural aspects of speech are learned as well as the verbal. Both language and gesture become linked to interpersonal relationships and help to develop the competencies to develop and maintain these. Through language, experiences may be validated by obtaining a consensus of views and opinions from others. Language is necessary for logical thinking and helps an individual organize perceptions of self and reality.

Phases of Psychosocial Development

Interpersonal development of the individual occurs in psychosocial phases. These phases identify the kinds of interpersonal competencies a person needs to develop at different times in growing up. The acquisition of certain interpersonal tasks and skills in one phase is preparatory to the learning of new ones in the next phase.

The Phase of Infancy
Infancy starts at birth and continues to 1 year or 2 years of age. The most important interpersonal relationship at this phase occurs between the infant and the mothering

one. This relationship develops around the necessity of meeting the infant's needs for survival. These needs are experienced as tensions and discomforts. The mothering person, in providing physiological relief, also provides psychological comfort, closeness, and relief from anxiety. This association in a diffuse way results in feelings of closeness that become attached to the mothering person.

The mothering one may create anxiety rather than satisfaction and comfort in the interpersonal relationship. When the mothering person is upset, angry, or anxious, the infant experiences these feelings through the tenseness of muscles in the arms and body of the mother and through psychological feelings experienced through empathy. An anxious or angry mother is not relaxed. The baby feels the tenseness and tries to avoid the anxiety that develops as a result of this unease and discomfort. Common ways for the infant to respond to this sitation is to refuse nourishment, refuse to be comforted, or become apathetic.

Very early, the infant learns to seek satisfying experiences from the mother and to avoid anxiety-producing ones. Because the range of behavior of the infant is limited, it is not long before avoidance behaviors take precedence over approach ones. These experiences play major role in the development of patterns of responses involved in adaptation and coping. Such experiences and the feelings attached to them are also used in the development of the personal organization of self: the good-me, bad-me, and not-me. The pattern of responses learned as the basic needs of infants are met incorporates meanings and symbols about such relationships with significant others.

During the time before the three aspects of self fuse into one, other facets of interpersonal relationships are learned. Late in infancy, the baby begins the development of dynamisms, or learned habitual patterns of responses, that are used in interpersonal situations. The dynamisms become incorporated in the child's developing self-system and become *security operations*. Once developed, these operations serve as mechanisms to avoid anxiety-provoking interpersonal situations.

During infancy, Erickson (1963) suggested that attitudes of basic trust versus attitudes of mistrust have to be worked out. Both attitudes begin in infancy and arise from interpersonal experiences around nurturant activities. He believed that if basic trust develops as the dominant attitude, core strengths of drive and hope are accentuated.

The Phase of Childhood

Childhood covers from 2 years to 5 years of age. The major focus of interpersonal relationships during this era is learning to become more independent of the mothering one, learning to play, and communicating with other children. The child starts to use words in association with gestures. Learning nonverbal behaviors such as facial expressions, pantomimes, melodies, and rhythms of speech are important as they later become part of more complex communications. In experiences, some verbal responses are rewarded more than others. The child tends to retain responses that are rewarded. Gestures and speech are eventually used together to help the child validate experiences and use logical thinking through talking things through. This era in interpersonal theory roughly corresponds to the play stage previously described in the symbolic interaction theory of personal organization of the self.

During childhood, the good-me, bad-me, and not-me become fused as one, but the self is not closed to further development. The self-system can be changed by experiences with peers and significant others. Additional skills and abilities are rapidly learned. Socialization pressures the child to learn new and appropriate behaviors for novel situations involving people other than mother and members of the family.

Autonomy versus shame and doubt are basic attitudes that have to be handled in this phase of development. This resolution is related to the development of independent behavior and freedom of expression without a loss of basic trust and self-esteem. If autonomy develops, the outcomes are a sense of self-control and will power (Erickson, 1963).

The Juvenile Phase

The juvenile phase covers the years from 5 to 8. Major changes in the number and kind of interpersonal relationships take place as children leave home to go to school. They become involved in peer relationships oriented around age-related activities and "best friends." During this era, children are exposed to many adults, all of whom will have expectations about their behavior.

Children quickly learn that the standards of conduct sanctioned in the family may be viewed quite differently in the school and other social situations. The opinions and views of parents, which up to now have not been questioned, are now called into question. Competing and conflicting views are put forth as alternatives by others. Children soon recognize that their relationships with parents and siblings are changing in many ways. The values, beliefs, views, and actions of peers may suddenly be more important than those held by adults—even adults whom the child loves. This juvenile phase has been described by Sullivan as the time when the child "becomes social."

During this era, the force of authority in situations is encountered. Because competing and often conflicting demands arise in various kinds of situations, accommodation and compromise have to be learned in order to develop and maintain satisfying interpersonal relationships. Children also have to learn to focus attention on things to achieve goals. When this happens, it means a person has learned to "tune out" distracting stimuli, a mental operation that facilitates problem solving.

The basic attitudes that the child must cope with in this phase are initiative versus guilt. Through various experiences, children learn that they have the energy and ability to engage in a broad array of new and different activities and interpersonal experiences. These new experiences alter old relationships. For example, aggression toward siblings and parents may be openly expressed and a withdrawal from interpersonal closeness may occur. Children have to learn that their love for their parents must now be channeled to other pursuits and parental relationships take on a different kind of closeness. This change in love objects may be frightening and frustrating but it frees the child to become independent of infantile needs and relationships so that development can go forward without excessive guilt. If initiative develops as the dominant attitude, the child develops a sense of direction and purpose (Erickson, 1963).

The Preadolescent Phase

Preadolescence covers from 9 years to 12 years of age. In this period, the maturing child encounters new kinds of interpersonal relationships that have to be mastered. Close and intimate relationships with chums or pals usually of the same sex are important during this era. Collaboration is a major task that has to be learned. Patterns of intimacy developed at this time set the stage for more enduring love relationships in later phases of development.

A recent phenomenon during this phase of preadolescent development is interest in the opposite sex that includes sexual intimacy. Although preadolescent girls and boys continue to develop peer same-sexed interpersonal relationships, the ability to "make it" with a member of the opposite sex seems to have become a valuable experience. This has resulted in the use of sexual relationships for meeting a number of social and psychological needs associated with uncertainty about self and gaining acceptance by others. These changes in sexual behavior have resulted in a preteenage pregnancy rate that is making a generation of girl-women into biological but not sociological and psychological mothers.

The self-system during this time is open to change. Pal and chum relationships are important for sharing ideas and information. They are also confidants for checking out private views and experiences with a nonthreatening person. Failure to develop peer relationships and related competencies at this stage of development can result in loneliness as the person grows older and lacks the confidence and competency to establish meaningful relationships.

The social and interpersonal competencies learned in this phase are similar to the ones described as occurring during the game stage of development of the self in symbolic interaction theory. People need to have learned to extract generalized rules from situations and be able to take the role of the other by this stage of development.

Erickson (1963) proposed that the basic attitudes that the young adult has to deal with in this phase of development is industry versus inferiority. Emphasis is on learning to gain recognition by producing things rather than by direct attacks and aggressive acts. The danger at this time of development is that a person will acquire a sense of inadequacy and inferiority, especially in school. In the best sense, the outcome for resolution of the two basic attitudes is the development of methods to function in roles in the world of work and relationships with other people.

Adolescence

This phase of development covers from 12 years to 18 years of age. The interpersonal relationships that matter during early adolescence are those developed with members of the opposite sex. These are truly sexual in nature and may involve emotionally meaningful intimacies that have the potential for lasting relationships.

The establishment of meaningful heterosexual relationships is both satisfying and anxiety-provoking. The meeting of a person's sexual desires with a partner requires that a person has to come to grips with intimacy and give up some security of self. In establishing heterosexual relationships, there may be a fear of failure to live up to these situations. If heterosexual relationships provoke considerable anxiety, then a person may avoid trying out relationships with other persons as well as avoid situations that might lead to their development.

During these years of development, conflicts between the basic attitudes of identity and role confusion become a paramount concern (Erickson, 1963). Young adults experience physiological development and changes that contribute to major alterations in body image and sense of self. Many of the conflicts and issues that caused friction in earlier years and were resolved in some measure may now be reawakened and replayed with significant others. Such conflicts may become almost adversarial. The self-identity of the young adult becomes rapidly integrated and embodies inner drives, tensions, desires, aspirations, achievements, and social role experiences. Role confusion may occur and there can be temporary overidentification with individuals who are viewed as heroes and heroines. There is experimentation in relationships that involve "being in love." The positive outcome of experiences by the end of these critical years is the learning of a sense of devotion and fidelity to others and for others (Erickson, 1963).

Adulthood

Important interpersonal relationships are those that have to be faced and handled as the adult leaves home and enters the world of work, study, and possible marriage. The successful negotiation by adults through these new challenges depends to a large extent on whether relationships in earlier stages of development were successful and provided satisfactions. In the adult world, the person has to go forth and stand ready to establish new roles, relationships, and challenges.

In adulthood, Erickson (1963) identified the basic competing attitudes that young adults experience as intimacy versus isolation. There is an active search for identity of self and intimacy with others. Ambivalent feelings range from a desire for close relationships on one hand and avoidance of intimacy and a seeking of isolation on the other. A capacity to affiliate and love is a desired outcome for adults and this is an essential achievement if the person is to continue personal growth and development in ways that actualize and satisfy.

The adult has to come to grips with attitudes of generality versus stagnation (Erickson, 1963). This concern relates to the establishment and guiding of a new generation. Erickson suggested that the failure to generate new members of society (have children) is stagnation reflected as self-love.

In late adulthood, a person has to cope with the dilemma of ego integrity versus despair. Ego integrity integrates the feelings of triumph and achievements the person has experienced. There is dignity and pride of self in relationships with children. The use of wisdom to assist others in developing and implementing new ideas is a source of satisfaction. A lack of or loss of ego integration may come from unsatisfying experiences and create despair, futility, and a wonderment of what life is about.

ORGANIZATION OF THE SELF: A PSYCHODYNAMIC PERSPECTIVE

One of the most widely used perspectives of the development of the self, or personality, is that developed by Freud (1933). This theory has been revised over the years by clinicians and theorists. In mental health, it continues to be influential even though its adequacy for application to many problems has long been questioned. The perspective is psychosocial but differs in major respects from the more social psychologically oriented theories. It is included primarily for comparison and reference.

The development of personality, or self, is based on certain kinds of assumptions. Behavior occurs as a result of unconscious determinants. The personality or self develops through responses to primal instincts and the extent to which desires are gratified. The basic core of the personality is set by the age of 7. Humans, in their need to meet their instinctual desires, are ever in conflict with society, which sets limits on the ways in which these needs can be expressed. Because of the permanent influences of early life experiences, humans are not too open for continued growth and actualization for the remainder of their lives.

Maddi (1968), in his classic and perceptive comparative analysis of personality theories, pointed out that Freud's view of humans postulates a basic tendency to life that is based on maximizing instinctual gratifications while minimizing punishment and guilt. This assumption is a basic tenet of psychodynamic theory, which holds that a number of instincts are common and innate to all people. These instincts are rooted in biological needs and are the mental representations of somatic processes. Biological deprivations convert somatic and biological processes into mental terms, thus the source of energy for motivated behavior is within the individual.

Freud's emphasis on instincts led him to adopt a determinate view of behavior. This means that behavior is caused by energies from innate drives and previous experiences of which a person has become unaware. Instinctual drives, or innate psychological energies, are generated within the psychic infrastructure. Freud did include situational events along with instinctual drives as motivators of behavior. However, situational events were considered primarily in terms of how they are sought and used for tension reduction (Ford & Urban, 1965). People can escape from situational events but they cannot escape from the energy sources generated within their own personalities, and these seek and find behavioral expressions in one way or another.

Freud proposed that three inborn instincts govern behavior: the pleasure, reality, and compulsion principles. The pleasure principle operates to achieve pleasure through tension reduction. The reality principle operates to achieve tension reduction (pleasure) by appropriate interactions and situational events (reality). The pleasure principle assumes that instinctual drives cannot be directly expressed by impulsive and self-gratifying actions in groups and society, so socially acceptable and organized behavior has to be substituted. Obviously, the pleasure principle and reality principle operate in concert. Both, however, may be overridden by the compulsion principle. Compulsive repetitive behavior is not necessarily tension-reducing or satisfying in nature. This kind of behavior serves to organize, or master, a flood of sensations that if allowed to be expressed in a disorganized fashion would neither reduce tensions nor achieve satisfactions. The purposes of the inborn principles are to: (1) reduce tensions, (2) accommodate behavior to situational events, and (3) repeat already learned behavior to get excess stimulation under control.

An important aspect of behavior is the link between instinctual gratifications and punishment and guilt. Instinctual gratification is to be maximized, whereas punishment and guilt are to be minimized. As instincts push from within for expression, such expression may engender both punishment and guilt. A set of defense mechanisms, that is, responses that defend against anxiety, is used to accommodate these two mutually conflicting goals. The defense mechanisms are developed through life experiences in infancy and childhood and used when anxiety threatens. In effect, in this theory of personality all or nearly all behavior is defensive in nature.

Instincts are of two kinds: eros, or life instincts, and thanatos, or death instincts. Life instincts are directed toward self-preservation and procreation. The death instinct is directed toward destruction and is in opposition to life-maintaining energies. Aggression toward oneself and others with a desire to destroy is a part of this instinct.

The Structure of Personality

The personality has three parts: the id, ego, and superego. They make up the psychic infrastructure of the personality. The *id* is the oldest part and is a collective name for primitive biological urges, impulses, and the energies these generate. Procreation and self-preservation are basic id functions. The *ego* is the part that deals with reality testing. It arises in part from the id and in part from social and interpersonal experiences. The primary functions of the ego are to modify drives from the id and channel them into socially acceptable modes of expression. This process helps a person learn psychosocial adaptations that are necessary to cope with reality. The *superego* is the third and last part the personality develops. It is an observer and evaluator of ego functions and compares behavior with codes of conduct that are a part of the conscience, or internal value system a person holds. The superego internalizes behaviors that evoke punishment and rewards; thus, it can become rigid or weak in carrying out its function in controlling and regulating behavior. Balance has to prevail between the three parts of the personality in order to prevent or correct neurotic or psychotic behavior.

Stages of Development of the Personality

The personality develops through four major stages. In the early stages, there is a major emphasis on the kind of behavior that is learned in infancy and early childhood and carried over to behaviors used in adulthood.

Infancy is the time for the *oral stage* of development. Gratification of biological needs are met by sucking behaviors, thus the mouth becomes an important zone of oral gratification. As sucking assuages biological needs and discomforts, satisfactions are experienced. Over time, the use of oral behaviors is transferred to other objects for obtaining satisfactions for other drives and needs. Around 8 months, the infant adds biting, an aggressive kind of behavior, to sucking.

The child next goes through the *anal stage* of development. This stage centers on eliminative functions: how they are controlled, and the feelings experienced by the child and the mothering one around toilet training. Punishment for failures evokes fears and an undue need in the child to please the parent. Rigid and harsh toilet training regimens are thought to lead to patterns of excessive cleanliness, a need for order, and submissiveness in the adult.

Behaviors associated with gratification in the oral and anal phases of development may be retained throughout adulthood. Where pronounced, people may be labeled as having oral or anal types of personalities.

Childhood begins by the end of the second year. By then, the child has developed a surprising array of behaviors: language, partial control of eliminative functions, motor activities, and ways of obtaining attention from others. Relationships extend beyond the mothering one.

During childhood, the *phallic stage* of development takes place. About 3 years of age, pleasures and satisfactions are derived from stimulation of the genital region. This interest continues to about 7 years of age. A major conflict of this stage is that which occurs between a parent of one sex and a child of the opposite sex. This conflict is called the *Oedipus complex* and is characterized by the attraction the child holds for the parent of the opposite sex and rivalry toward the same-sexed parent. Inadequate resolution of this conflict is thought to cause problems in adulthood by a person of one sex having difficulties establishing relationships with a person or persons of the opposite sex.

In late childhood, the interests of the child extend considerably beyond parents and the family. Peers become important, particularly those of the same sex. Important social and interpersonal competencies are learned; values acquired from parents and others are tested by the child outside the family with many different people.

Adolescence is a period of rapid and changing social and physical growth. There is physical development of the sex organs. For the girl, menstruation begins; for the boy, sexual activity with ejaculation occurs. Development of a sense of self, or self-identity, is very important during this period. It is accentuated from feedback from others, particularly peers. The conflicts that occurred during the Oedipal period are aroused, relived, and resolved by establishing sexual relationships with members of the opposite sex.

Adulthood is reached when a person is mature and has developed a clear personal identity, is independent and autonomous in behavior, and is willing to establish relationships and be responsible for others. Psychological adulthood is not thought of as occurring at any particular age, and some persons may never attain this state of development.

Motivational Energy

Motivational energy comes from two sources: one within the person and one in society and groups. In psychodynamic theory, energy from both of these sources merges within the person to become psychic energy, which is expressed in social experiences as behavior. Behavior is purposeful, goal-directed, and occurs in response to inner needs and dictates.

Ford and Urban (1965) described Freud's picture of humans as basically an ugly one, pushed by demonic, destructive, and animalistic forces. Such forces are fueled from a reservoir of energy that exists in the individual. Humans are "full" of emotion of which they are unaware, of behavior directed toward ends that are not consciously intended.

Mind and Society

The relationship between mind and society is complex. Individuals strive to satisfy inner needs and desires, whereas society sets constraints about those that may be expressed. In Freudian theory, the mind seems to evolve in part from the id. Ego and mind seem to be interchangeable concepts. The ego differentiates from the id as life experiences occur that focus the person to use behavior other than responses to basic needs, emotions, and desires.

Maddi (1968) stated that in Freud's theory of personality, the ego is the part of the mind that is composed of thoughts and perceptual processes involved in recognition, rememberances, and actions that are used to satisfy instincts. The mind is the bridge between somatic and metabolic processes and the intelligent actions and interactions that constitute living.

Mental life is divided into kinds of awareness and responses: preconscious, conscious, and unconscious. Preconscious responses are available to a person's awareness or can be called up and made conscious. Consciousness is a sense of awareness of self and of the environment. It is thought to develop through successive integration of biological and psychological development with the highest level of integration occurring at the psychological level. Unconsciousness is the part of mental life that is not available to awareness. It represents psychic energies, desires, forces, and motivations that determine behavior. Unconscious determinants of behavior are thought to become conscious through special techniques such as free association, hypnosis, dream analysis, use of drugs, and analysis of purposeful forgetting, mistakes, and amnesias.

DEVELOPMENT OF THE SELF: ADULT PERSPECTIVES

Inherent in a concept of self is a self-identity. *Self-identity* is defined as a synthesis of personal, interpersonal, and social experiences that organize the feelings and views that a person holds about herself or himself. This synthesis covers the feelings of self-esteem, physical mastery, social prestige, group identity, and pleasure in various activities. These experiences are related to cultural and social realities about traditional and contemporary roles of men and women in society. Increasingly, it is recognized how much traditional roles are changing and responsibilities associated with such roles are altering the functions of men and women in both the home and work place.

A social psychological conception of human growth and development holds that the self continues to develop and to remain open to growth as long as a person lives. One of the major contributions that nurses make as health care providers is to help adults develop a more optimistic view and awareness of their potential and of their abilities to continue to grow and change throughout life.

Traditionally, theories of personality have focused on the intensive development of the self in the first decade of life. Some theories such as Erickson's (1963) have addressed adulthood in very general terms. An assumption of most theories is that by the time adulthood is reached, essential relationships, competencies, and patterns of coping and adaptation are established. Because such patterns are supposed to be stable and resistant to change, they determine much of the behavior of people in their adult years and for the remainder of their lives.

Over the past few years, the idea that continued development of self across the life span has increasingly been promoted. Theories of development for adults are becoming more complete as research becomes available. In recent theories, attention has been given to the differences in continued adult development of the self for women and men. Only now is it being recognized that different-sexed adults have different kinds of developmental and identity crises and growth marks from 20 years to 60 years of age. Research and theories that support this view of adult development are social psychological in perspective because they take into account multiple interactions of personal growth needs, social factors, and cultural roles and expectations on the development of the self.

Sheehy (1976) made a contribution to our understanding of adult development of the self by identifying a series of predictable social and psychological passages through which women and men must travel to reach mature adulthood. These life passages occur over a period of several years during which major changes occur in life goals, personal relationships, and self-identity. One of the most important findings by Sheehy has been the identification of the dyssynchronization of roles and needs for continued self-growth of women as compared to those of men.

Sheehy views the years between 18 and 50 as being at the center of the life process for the life span. During these years, there is an unfolding and flowering of maximum opportunity and capacity. In her research she found that after the years of 18 to 20 there was little in personality theories about this growth process.

Adult personality theories consider growth over the entire life cycle. The human being is open to new actualization experiences and capable of development. The identification of passages that need to be traversed through adulthood are related to significant tasks, roles, and changes in aspirations and expectations that have to be achieved on each passage.

Levinson (1978) conducted a longitudinal study of the ups and downs in the lives of men from the ages of 18 to 47. He identified basic principles that govern this period of development for men. As in earlier years, men continue to have developmental periods during which specific tasks are achieved and related competencies learned. As the man completes tasks and masters competencies in one developmental period and moves to another, he starts to work on new tasks and competencies. In this process, a new support and relationship structure has to be established. Levinson calls these *life structures* and found that a life structure for a particular period does not last more than 7 or 8 years. At that time, the sequence starts anew around the tasks and competencies that the man needs to learn and use in the next period of growth.

Sheehy's (1976) concept of passages means that there is a strategic interplay of stable periods and critical turning points in one's life. Instead of the concept of passages, Levinson uses the idea of a "marker event" to define particular events that bring about or signify a notable change in a person's life. Developmental periods are demarcated by changes that begin within the individual and end in major changes in roles, behaviors, and expectations.

Crucial shifts in thinking about one's place in the life structure that has been constructed signal that changes are starting to take place within a person in relation to his or her self-concept, self-identity, and self-actualization. The next stage of development is underway. Shifts and changes that may occur in relation to age, sex-related experiences, peer experiences, family relationships, aspirations, and other events may cause upheaval. Such upheavals affect at least four areas of perception: (1) in the interior self in relation to others; (2) in perceptions of time; (3) in the proportion of safeness and danger felt about one's life; and (4) at the intuitive level a feeling that one is alive or stagnating. In earlier research, Neugarten (1968) identified the major changes that occur in middle life as: shifts from external to internal values, shifts in time perspective, and shifts to compensate for losses. The changes in perceptions of self proposed by Levinson as a result of upheavals and that signify marker events are related to this earlier research.

Differences in Development of Self for Men and Women

Using primarily the work of Levinson (1978) and Sheehy (1976), some principles of adult development for men and women are identified. These have been consolidated from various sources in order to understand better growth and development of the self and self-actualization and some differences in these processes for men and women.

Around the age of 20, individuals leave home and begin the processes of career development and setting up a family. At this time of life, it is important for young adults of both sexes to come to grips with what they want "to be, to do" and set about mastering ways in which their goals can be reached. There are, however, some young adults who resist peer pressures, cultural demands, and social expectations by not making such commitments. The life process for this group of adults may proceed in quite different ways from adults who make career and marriage commitments.

For adults who decide what they want to do or do what they are supposed to do, the process of achieving goals is different for men and women in several respects. Men put their energy into developing a career. If married, women are expected to provide the support structure to free their husbands from most if not all of the realities of daily living so that they can pursue their career goals. Women are expected to be care givers and provide necessary support systems to their husbands. The woman's role and work is to focus on these tasks. Any aspirations, career goals, and dreams held by women in the late teens and during college years are given up or put away in favor of supporting the career of their husbands. Women do this because there continues to be powerful social and familial values that focus on two major options: marriage or career. Society has done very little to help women achieve both of these goals by providing adequate support structures women need for child care, career counseling, and educational opportunities.

Men do not experience this career dilemma. If children arrive, it is very difficult for couples to work out two careers during these early years, so the pattern is for women to forego theirs. By the end of the second decade, dyssynchronization between the needs for personal growth and career advancement for wives and husbands, and to a large extent, men and women who may not be married, are evident.

An important passage occurs between 28 and 32 years. There is a centering, or focus, away from what a person is supposed to do and a movement to what she or he wants to do. Psychological shifts that involve the concept of self occur within a person and involve the concept of self: "Me" starts to take on as much value as "others," reasoning and intellect are recognized as inadequate to solve all problems, and questions are raised about marriage and other commitments.

During the brief span between 28 and 32 years, men feel more confident in their careers and begin to be bored with their wives serving as substitute mothers. Husbands begin to exert pressures on wives to get them to broaden their experiences, but in doing so, they send a double message: "I encourage you to do something for yourself—but don't mess up my support structure." The wife's willingness to risk testing this double message has little basis in experiences that are grounded in accomplishments. Women sense that making serious efforts to improve their education and develop their careers will not be supported by their husbands. But a woman's inner self strives for achievements and a broadening of experiences. If they act on their inner longings and actively pursue the expansion of self and career, serious problems may arise in the marriage. On the other hand, some husbands may accept this move with a feeling of relief because it lessens some of the responsibilities that were accepted in marriage.

During the third decade, roots are put down, homes are purchased, and dreams are converted to goals. Men, in achieving their goals, may have to be mobile, and this prevents the occurrence of a stable family and community rooting. This failure often causes social and psychological anguish and upheaval for the wife and children.

At the same time, there continues to be stirrings in the woman to do something about her career, to broaden her life. Being a care giver for husband and family is no longer enough. Personal integration of self and meaningful experiences have occurred to a degree that both marriage and career responsibilities can be tackled if risks are taken.

The mid-thirties is a time when women in particular become conscious of a sense of time running out. The last child goes off to school, her sexuality reaches its peak around 38 years of age, and the working world is reentered. It is the time when women will try to find more intimate and satisfying relationships, or seek a new husband, or just up and leave husband and home. It is past high noon for her on the reproductive time clock. In short, a general reassessment of life occurs and the woman wants something for herself in her own right.

Turning 40 is a marker event for men. It has implications for further career advancement. Redefinitions of earlier dreams have taken place. Somewhere along the way, the man starts to examine his life in the way the woman did in the thirties. There is a shift away from pouring all one's energies into a career and advancement. A redirection of energy focuses on other people and their problems. The man is now caught between this interest and the need to continue putting his time into career activities. He knows that time and attention placed on the new activities will not collect achievement points in the corporate world and gain career advancements and promotions. If the costs for incorporating these new activities become too high, the man may find himself locked into his job because of less energy and commitment being applied to it.

During this time of redefinition for men, the woman is getting ready to advance her career. Where the man may be experiencing staleness in his career, the woman begins to experience enthusiasm and unlimited energy. To some extent, she is set free from past confusions and responsibilities. Men often express envy at these qualitites in their wives during this time.

In many respects, the positions of husbands and wives, and men and women, are the reverse of what they were the previous decade. Some of the challenges that have to be met by the 40-year-old man are: (1) recognition of his emotions at a time when his wife has grown so that she is not dependent on his expression of these for her; (2) reaching out to his children just when they no longer need him; and (3) wanting to have satisfying endeavors, a revival of purpose, just when he is stagnated in his work. Then, around age 45, a restabilization occurs. Priorities are sorted out. A sense of renewal or a sense of resignation emerges. Around 50 and beyond, mellowing and warmth occur. Men come to grips with their essential loneliness. And it is possible for meaningful relationships to be established with his mate—if she has had the chance for her own development and is still in the marriage.

Shifting Gears

Continued development of the self in adulthood may occur in other ways. Another perspective used to describe midlife crises in terms of the development of self is called "shifting gears" (O'Neill & O'Neill, 1974). This husband and wife team define shifting gears as a response to crises that challenge the external and internal givens in our lives. Shifting gears usually requires the rearrangement of some of these givens. Gear shifting is a series of interrelated events that need not necessarily be in the order of the steps described but all of the steps are integral for a shift to new life directions.

Shifting gears involves several steps. An *awareness* must first develop, either gradually or suddenly, that presages a vague feeling of discontent. This awareness has to become intense enough that a person becomes conscious of it. Once this happens, *evaluation* along several dimensions takes place. At this point, the person comes to realize the past cannot be changed but the future can. To move forward, *exploration* of a number of alternatives takes place. These must be considered in terms of short-term and long-term goals. Priorities have to be set as to what is essential for one's happiness for the future. *Experimentation* with new arrangements and experiences follow. If satisfied that things will work out, the person must *make a decision* to cut old arrangements, which mean *action taking* and *letting go*.

The O'Neills (1974) propose a concept of creative maturity. This is defined as a self that finds security and an integration of the life plan. In order to shift gears to grow toward self-actualization and self-directed change, they propose seven keys to help one develop a stand in life:

1. Don't ask permission	Do it
2. Don't report	Check things out with yourself, not with others
3. Don't apologize unnecessarily	This tells others your are a self-diminisher
4. Don't recriminate yourself	The missed opportunity syndrome keeps you from moving forward
5. Don't say: "I should or I shouldn't"	Ask why or why not
6. Don't be afraid to say "no" or "yes"	Act on what you think or feel
7. Don't put yourself completely in the hands of another	Be a self-determiner*

When people manage themselves in terms of what they want, a clear sense of priorities

* From *Shifting Gears*, by Nena O'Neill and George O'Neill. Copyright © 1974 by Nena O'Neill and George O'Neill. Reprinted by permission of the publisher, M. Evans and Co., Inc., New York, 10017, p. 219.

is developed. In this process a greater sense of self-value, self-esteem, and self-identity is developed.

DEVELOPMENT OF THE SELF: LATE AND LATE LATE ADULTHOOD PERSPECTIVES

Levinson (1978) collected his research on men who were in their late forties. The conceptual framework that was developed to guide this research was extended to consider the entire life span although data on older subjects were not collected. The formulations for late adulthood are consistent with the concepts of changing life structures and changing purposes for living in late adulthood and late late adulthood.

Levinson's provisional view of changes in the organization of the self and in life aspirations during late adulthood is useful because it provides continuity in development of self across the life span. He envisioned that in the early sixties, middle adulthood comes to an end and late adulthood begins and continues until 85 and beyond into late late adulthood. Levinson's conception of these periods of a person's life is optimistic because it can be a fulfilling season.

Marker events, such as illness and retirement, may speed up and shape the process of moving into late adulthood. Over the years there have been changes and a steady decline in various aspects of personal and social health but a person does not become old overnight. A number of social and personal events do mark the movement toward an older age: approaching retirement, the death of friends and colleagues, persistent aches and pains, and health problems that require activities to be curtailed or changes made in life style.

Social practices assist the person in late adulthood to connect age with relationships as well as with events. People refer to the older adult as "older citizen," or "senior citizen" or "golden ager"—all of which are designed to set a particular person in late adulthood apart from younger persons. These descriptions have a negative connotation, although this is not fully appreciated. Physical appearances also change and take on characteristics associated with old age, and these evoke easy labels of "grandpa" or "little old lady."

Using Levinson's perspective, the person in late adulthood has to construct a new life structure. This is necessary in order for the individual to develop new life satisfactions, activities, and relationships. A major developmental task is to establish connections and relationships with younger people. Being a wise elder includes sharing experiences that require the person to move from a center role to one that is more supportive and sharing.

Retirement is a major turning point in adult development. Irrespective of whether a person dreads or looks forward to retirement, it is still necessary to give up the relationships, aspirations, and activities associated with work. Much of the life structure of adults is organized around the world of work, so people do not simply stop working. Retirement alters in a drastic way the organization of daily living and relationships. Failure to develop a new life structure has serious implications for the physical, mental, and emotional health of the retiree and her or his spouse and close friends and family members. At the same time, if a new life structure is developed, new roles evolve, and new relationships and interests are established. This can be a time for creative renewal and learning.

A second developmental task that has to be achieved in late adulthood is achieving a balance between social involvements and self needs. In this phase, adults can look back and see where they have made their contributions to society and can now make self-growth and self-actualization more primary.

With the lengthening life span, Levinson takes note of late late adulthood, 80 and beyond. Obviously, developmental needs and creativities during this era are meager for many people. During this time of life, infirmities are obvious and major illnesses may be debilitating. The life structure shrinks. There are few significant relationships and health problems and the vicissitudes of daily living take up one's time and energy. Instead of creating a new life structure for another era of living, the adult now has to come to grips with the reality of dying—life is ending.

In late adulthood and late late adulthood, changes occur in both biological and cognitive spheres. Although biological infirmities may be expected as an essential part of aging, there may be considerable variation in cognitive abilities. Craig (1976) pointed out that adult cognitive development tends to be less dramatic in scope and depth than childhood development and that in late adulthood, continued development depends more on life experiences than maturation. Cognitive changes in adulthood involve certain value judgments and theories about oneself (Flavell, 1970).

One important cognitive change that usually occurs in late adulthood is the decreased ability to problem solve in situations where past experience is not relevant. New tasks that involve problem solving for which the adult cannot use previous experience may be hard to master. Efforts are often made to compensate for this decreased ability by choosing new tasks that use the accumulated knowledge acquired from life experiences. Coping in this manner imposes constraints on seeking new experiences and finding enjoyment in seeking solutions to novel problems and situations.

Uhl (1981) called attention to the fact that as a result of being considered old in our society, the elderly share certain conditions and characteristics: shared grievances, segregation by society into special communities, and retirement at ever younger ages. By late adulthood, these conditions lead to social and personal experiences that promote disengagement from interpersonal and intimate relationships and meaningful activities. Furthermore, there are social pressures for such relationships to occur only with other older adults and for lessened contacts with younger people. This situation prevents, or minimizes, the chances for adults to achieve one of the major tasks of this era: that of balancing relationships between young and old.

Late adulthood and late late adulthood are natural biological phases of growth and development of the human species. A considerable amount of the anguish experienced by adults during these years is a function of health and social, economic, and interpersonal factors, most of which have the possibility of modification. Changes in social stereotypes about the aged and aging and provision of more accessible and enlightened services to this age group of citizens would greatly assist their continued development and shift the focus from survival and endurance through the late late adulthood period. Such changes would allow the continued development of the self and assist in maintaining health so that the adult would not require sick care services and institutionalization. For example, Snider (1980) found among a sample of older adults that education, knowledge level, and prior use of health services were more relevant to current use of such services than were age and health status. And Ferraro (1980) found that in late adulthood, self ratings of health are related to age. Adults in late late adulthood, while reporting more health-related problems than people in the late adult era, were more positive in rating their own health. These and other studies are beginning to provide the kinds of information that are needed for health professionals and citizens to change their expectations about late adulthood. Older adults may have quite realistic views about themselves, their health status and needs, and what is needed to continue their development of self.

Late adulthood and late late adulthood are phases of growth and development when the organization of the self continues to change. Social and cultural expectations about these periods of life are major determinants of the physical, emotional, and mental problems that adults experience. More optimistic conceptions of what can actually be achieved by adults in this era would make it possible for people to understand the importance of life structures and the need to construct new ones in order to achieve satisfying and actualizing experiences. Just as the world of work was the major organizing force during the productive years for both men and women, social reality after retirement can be constructed in ways that enhance and promote continued personal growth and satisfactions.

SUMMARY

The organization and development of self can be considered from several perspectives. Each perspective has basic concepts, phases of development, and a structure of self. Such perspectives include interactionist, interpersonal, life structure, and psychodynamic views. All of these are social psychological theories although they have quite different assumptions and concepts.

A symbolic interaction perspective postulates a self that is organized from social experiences and consists of two parts: the "I" and "me". The "I" is the creative aspects of the self and is based in part in biological drives from which it derives energy. The "me" is social in nature and represents an organized set of attitudes, definitions, expectations, and meanings common to groups in which membership is held. The crucial experiences of role taking, role making, and taking the role of the other are important processes in the organization of self. Selfhood is achieved when a person can stand apart and reflect back on herself or himself and adopt a generalized role of other. Definitions of situations and feedback from significant others are essential for the continuing development of the organization of the self throughout life.

An interpersonal perspective of behavior emphasizes developmental tasks and skills necessary for social psychological growth to occur so that progression to higher levels of functioning will occur. A psychodynamic perspective emphasizes the role of inner drives and unconscious forces in personality development. Perspectives of adult development focus on the need to build and rebuilt life structures in order for growth and development to continue through major life transitions. Adult men and women move through stages of development in different ways and at different times over the life span, and this must be recognized in order to plan for opportunities for growth for both sexes.

REFERENCES

Blumer, Herbert. *Symbolic Interactionism*. Englewood Cliffs, NJ: Prentice-Hall, 1969, pp. 62–77.

Cardwell, J. A. *Social Psychology: A Symbolic Interaction Perspective*. Philadelphia: F. A. Davis, 1971, pp. 77–85.

Craig, Grace. *Human Development*. Englewood Cliffs, NJ: Prentice-Hall, 1976, Chapter 4.

Erickson, Erik H. *Childhood and Society*. New York: W. W. Norton, 1963, pp. 247–251 and 273.

Ferraro, Kenneth F. Self-ratings of health among the old and the old old. *Health and Social Behavior*. 21:377–383, December, 1980.

Flavell, J. H. Cognitive changes in adulthood. In Goulet, L. R., and Baltes, Paul B., eds. *Life-Span Developmental Psychology: Research and Theory*. New York: Academic Press, 1970, pp. 248–250.

Ford, Donald H., and Urban, Hugh. *Systems of Psychotherapy: A Comparative Study*. New York: John Wiley & Sons, 1965, Chapter 5.

Freud, Sigmund. *New Introductory Lectures to Psychoanalysis*, translated by W. J. H. Spott, New York: Norton, 1933, pp. 15–24, 25–40, 149–169, 286–320, and 392–411.

LeBoyer, Frederick. *Birth without Violence*. New York: Knopf, 1976, pp. 51–79.

Levinson, Daniel J., Darrow, Charlotte N., Klein, Edward, B., et al. *The Seasons of a Man's Life*. New York: Ballantine Books, 1978, chapters 1–3, 5–6, 9–10, 13–18, and 20.

Lindesmith, Alfred R., Strauss, Anselm L., and Denzin, Norman K. *Social Psychology*, 4th ed. Hinsdale, Ill., Dryden Press, 1975, pp. 300–311.

Lindesmith, Alfred R., and Strauss, Anselm L. *Social Psychology*. New York: Holt, Rinehart and Winston, 1956, pp. 371–441.

Maddi, Salvatore R. *Personality Theories: A Comparative Analysis*. Homewood, IL: Dorsey Press, 1968, chapters 2 and 6.

Mead, George H. *Mind, Self, and Society*. Chicago: University of Chicago Press, 1943, pp. 10–13.

Meltzer, Bernard. *The Social Psychology of George Herbert Mead*. Kalamazoo, MI: Center for Sociological Research, Western Michigan University, 1966, pp. 13–20.

Neugarten, Bernice. The awareness of middle age. In Neugarten, Bernice, ed. *Middle Age and Aging*. Chicago: University of Chicago Press, 1968, pp. 93–98.

O'Neill, Nena, and O'Neill, George. *Shifting Gears*. New York: Avon Books, 1974, pp. 70–71.

Parsons, Talcott, and Bales, Robert F. *Family, Socialization and Interaction Process*. New York: Free Press, 1955, pp. 10–33.

Sheehy, Gail, *Passages*. New York: E. P. Dutton, 1976, chapters 5, 6, 11–13, and 15–17.

Snider, Earle L. Factors influencing health service knowledge among the elderly. *Health and Social Behavior* 21:371–376, December, 1980.

Stryker, Sheldon. The interactional and situational approaches. In Harold T. Christensen, ed. *Handbook of Marriage and the Family*. Chicago, IL: Rand McNally, 1964, pp. 129–143.

Sullivan, Harry Stack. *The Interpersonal Theory of Psychiatry*. New York: W. W. Norton, 1953, pp. 110–111.

Uhl, Joan. Caring as the focus of a multidisciplinary health center for the aged. In Leininger, Madeleine, ed. *Caring: An Essential Human Need*. Thorofare, NJ, Charles B. Slack, 1981, Chapter 12.

PROFILES OF FAMILIES AND INDICATORS OF MENTAL HEALTH

INTRODUCTION

Social psychological theories of behavior have been established in previous chapters; these include basic concepts, principles, and perspectives by which the organization of self is developed. These ideas are now used to consolidate relevant concepts and principles for community mental health nursing applications in clinical practice.

In the last part of this book, clinical applications focus on preventions with adaptive, or healthy, functioning families. This emphasis was selected to demonstrate applications because of the relative paucity of models in this particular aspect of clinical practice. The conceptual framework that has been elaborate for community mental health nursing, however, applies to more than just adaptive functioning families. It may be used to organize clinical practice with various kinds of primary groups, stressed and distressed family systems, and modified for mental health nursing in community settings.

Abstract concepts linking theory and clinical practice are more easily used if they are provided with referents. Such referents have been developed in the form of models of family functioning with characteristics summarized in profiles of adaptive or healthy, stressed, and distressed family systems.

Community mental health nursing, in its clinical practice aspects, is oriented to provide professional care and services to primary groups in which people spend a large part of daily living activities. The most important of these are primary socialization systems, or families. These systems are milieus in which intense kinds of learning experiences are provided, thus having a great influence on the kinds of things that are learned as well as on the emotional and mental development of members.

Families are charged by society to socialize members by providing them with the opportunities to learn essential social, interpersonal, and cognitive competencies necessary for problem solving, coping, obtaining satisfactions in relationships and at work, and achieving selfhood. This charge requires special kinds of milieus in which there are interactions, relationships, and support, and where members are emotionally involved with each other.

In the field of mental health and psychiatric care, understanding adaptive or healthy functioning family systems and identifying characteristics of such functioning have not been areas of major interest. Families that have been most often examined are those that are known to have severe dysfunctions and system pathologies that contribute to the development and maintenance of emotional and mental disorders. For example, various social, system, psychological, and communication pathologies have been identified in family systems, such as distorted communication processes and patterns, diffuse and inappropriate roles and functions, and scapegoating mechanisms. All of these have received considerable attention from mental health clinicians. The bias in mental health toward interest in families with major pathologies and psychiatric problems has limited clinical perspectives and roles. It is unfortunate that healthy family systems have been assumed to be virtually nonexistent by many mental health clinicians.

Healthy family socialization systems, if not of special interest to mental health clinicians, have for some time been of interest to professionals in the fields of human development, family life, and social work. These disciplines have developed programs of various kinds and tried approaches designed to strengthen the quality of family life and optimize humanization and socialization of children and adults. Research and theory developed from healthy family functioning perspectives have contributed a great deal to the development and application of preventions that help families develop and maintain climates, or milieus, that facilitate the mental, emotional, social, and cognitive growth of their members (David, 1979). In recent years, a few mental health clinicians have conducted research on the identification of factors related to healthy family functioning and the relationship of these factors to the mental and emotional health of family members (Lewis et al., 1976; Lewis, 1980).

The relationship between mental and emotional development of members of family groups and effective family functioning has long been recognized. Many things, however, affect the mental and emotional health of people. Therefore, it has been difficult to come to grips with what, if anything, could or should be done to foster the development of systems and climates that would increase the probability that emotional and mental health of people could be more actively promoted and enhanced. In recent years, the research on healthy family functioning and the influence of social environments on behavior and health, the effectiveness of teaching social competencies to families and their members for coping and managing more effectively, and the influence of family education on health and mental health have all contributed to the development of a body of knowledge and experience that can be used by the community mental health nursing. Such knowledge and experience can be used to refine and expand the scope and direction of clinical nursing practice in this special area. One impact of such an expansion is to more clearly define the leadership and clinical roles of community mental health nursing in providing preventions in mental health. This advancement is comparable to the leadership and community care roles public health nursing has provided in preventive health supervision since the turn of the century.

Community mental health nursing can expand its clinical theory and practice in different directions by using research findings on preventions relating to mental health that have been published in recent years. The discipline can make a considerable contribution to mental health by providing leadership in the delivery of primary preventions to healthy families and to other kinds of primary socialization groups that play a key role in the socialization of people across the life span. Clinical practice in this area will accelerate the refinement and development of a variety of approaches by which preventions in mental health will come to be usual rather than exceptional therapeutic activities.

The comprehensive community mental health nursing assessment is the primary source of data from which the community mental health nurse initially makes judgments and clinical decisions. One part of the assessment is to judge the level of family functioning and the competence of the family to socialize members. Family strengths and potentials are noted. From these data, the nurse makes recommendations about the need for preventions or interventions.

In order to assist the nurse in the assessment counseling process, indicators are identified that may be used to obtain data about the mental health of family and daily groups and their members. Profiles of healthy, stressed, and distressed families and some characteristics of functioning are described to help the nurse relate specific behaviors to family systems in interaction.

INDICATORS OF MENTALLY HEALTHY FAMILY SYSTEMS

Indicators, or criteria, that may be used to assess and make judgments about the competence, level of functioning, and mental and emotional health of families, or primary socialization group systems, are used in conjunction with the conceptual framework for community mental health nursing. Concepts and research from mental health, family and group theories, the community, and the world of work have been synthesized to develop a comprehensive set of criteria. The value of each indicator in making judgments about the emotional and mental health of socialization group systems is not precisely known. The relative contribution of each indicator to overall mental and emotional health of family systems and members has to be examined in a system-in-interaction context. The comprehensive assessment provides data that gives a holistic view of family functioning. The use of clinical nursing and mental health experiences help nurses make decisions about the overall level of family and group functioning and particular aspects of functioning that have relevance for mental and emotional health.

Family and primary group socialization systems data are collected about basic interrelationships and opportunities for growth from a holistic perspective. On balance, if the level of family functioning is adequate or more than adequate to meet the needs of individuals in the system and to maintain the system, the system may be judged to be a reasonably good to excellent one for carrying out its primary socialization objectives. This judgment can be validated through different kinds of feedback from observations, from accounts of members in terms of their perceptions and experiences, and from data about family functioning that describe recurring patterns, relationships, problems, and particular experiences. The frequency with which different kinds of experiences recur, particularly those that are found to be stressful and frustrating by members, usually indicates interaction or relationship tensions. These usually vary in intensity and the way that they have an impact on various members. In such cases, it is useful to identify with family members the things that seem to be causing stress and frustration, hear how they experience their impact, and determine how or whether problem solving to bring about changes has been done. Unfortunately, it is impossible to predict or generalize with accuracy how many or exactly what kinds of stressful experiences have to occur before these start to have serious and permanent effects on family members and systems. As Lewis and his colleagues (1976) noted, there is no one single thread that can be used to predict what makes healthy families healthy but there are a cluster of behaviors that seem to be present in such families. In community mental health nursing, it is necessary to obtain information about a lot of "threads" that make up the dynamics of family life and living. This information has to be organized and evaluated to determine the major clusters of behavior and how close these parallel the profiles of healthy, stressed, or distressed family systems.

Two basic functions of families and primary socialization groups have been considered throughout, namely, socialization of the young and stabilization of adult personalities that include the organization of self. In 1964, Mabry stated in more specific terms what primary socialization groups have to ensure: biological reproduction, emotional development, socialization for members, organization of roles and relations with the community, and maintenance of social contexts for health care. For both adults and children, socialization group systems have to make provisions for continued growth and development across the life span. The indicators for judging the emotional and mental health of families and other primary socialization groups that carry out family functions have to consider whether these basic functions are met. Successful socialization means that the conditions necessary to ensure that people have opportunities to develop emotional and mental health are present in family environments.

Because family socialization systems help to create conditions that influence the development of emotional and mental health problems, such systems also have the potential to create conditions that influence the development of emotional and mental health. The effects of family system functioning on members are reflected in individual behavior and system relationships, both of which are greater than a simple summation of the behaviors or tendencies of the individuals who are system members (Speer, 1970). Cromwell and Thomas (1976) noted that because people are essentially relationship-oriented and interactional creatures, a focus on individual self-actualization neglects the use of family potential resources, strengths, and efforts to prepare for a social existence.

Behavior settings at the small group level, such as families and other kinds of peer groups, have structural, physical, social, and system properties as well as personal system characteristics of individual members, and these interact as people live together. In interaction the different systems contribute to the emotional, mental, and social development of competencies that people need to cope as well as to foster individual development. Interactions also influence whether family systems meet their goals for their members. The climates created in these small interacting social systems act as a buffer between the needs of individual members and the roles and relationships in the family system. For example, Moos (1976b and 1979) found that continued interactions between members in small interacting social systems and acceptance of the system's organization produce a stable pattern of relationships. Stability in family roles, functions, and relationships helps members create certain kinds of environments. These factors interact so that particular kinds of behaviors and attitudes are both caused and knowingly adopted. Thus, environments in which people spend a considerable amount of time make a difference on how they develop an organization of self and related behaviors.

Healthy and adaptive family functioning does not just happen; it occurs as the result of efforts of members in these systems. Adults usually do not consciously structure family organization, roles, and responsibilities when new family systems are established. New family systems tend to be set up on the basis of how member's own families were organized and these new family systems are managed with built-in modifications that address particular concerns and desires of adult members of the new family. Over the last two decades, family systems have had to accommodate major social changes and different kinds of expectations about families. Today, families quite often need assistance in examining their family organization and structure in order to determine whether goals and objectives are being achieved as effectively as possible and to explore some of the effects of family functioning on members. Families may not recognize their strengths nor use their potential to advantage.

A number of sources have been used to identify social and psychological indicators of healthy families. In this context, daily living groups and community linkages are considered. The indicators are consistent with models of mental health and community mental health nursing that are based on a social psychological perspective of behavior. To apply the indicators in the assessment counseling process, the community mental health nurse obtains information, engages in interactions, and make observations of families. These are assessed to the degree that the behaviors identified describe system and member functioning in terms of interrelationships, roles, interactions, functions, outside-of-family relationships, and general social climate. These data help the nurse to arrive at an informed clinical judgment about the status of a particular family and its level of functioning. The ability of the family to provide the conditions needed to develop and maintain the mental and physical health of members, experiences and resources needed for cognitive development, and involvement in social networks and community activities is a part of this clinical judgment.

Indicators

Indicators that may be used for orienting collection of data, observations, interactions, and information about social contexts are identified for primary socialization groups. These indicators are appropriate for small group systems:

Indicator 1. Families or primary socialization groups as interacting systems encourage development of intimate, loving, and supportive experiences between parents (or parents and surrogates) and children, between siblings, and between parents without a loss of personal identity and sense of self for each person (Minuchin et al., 1967; Minuchin, 1974; Moos & Moos, 1976).

Indicator 2. Families or primary socialization milieus have a climate in which members are accorded respect; consideration is given to individual views, opinions, and unique abilities; and there is acceptance of both positive and negative feelings about people, events, and things without undue punishment or negative valuation (Moos & Moos, 1976).

Indicator 3. Families or primary socialization groups have interrelationships and roles that provide opportunities for members to learn basic social and interpersonal competencies for handling conflict—clarifying communications through "checking out," using consensus, collaborating, and cooperation—and also to learn the competencies a person needs to cope, achieve, and master and to exercise control of self and environment (Bateson et al., 1956; Satir, 1967).

Indicator 4. Families or primary socialization environments foster the development of emotional attachments among siblings, peers, parents, and grandparents yet encourage detachment to the extent that emotional attachments can be formed with significant others outside the family or group system (Whitaker, 1972; Boszormenyi-Nagy, 1965; Bowen, 1966).

Indicator 5. Families or primary socialization groups have a sense of cohesion and identity that is used to foster development of individual identity, autonomy, and self-actualization of members (Moos & Moos, 1976; Otto, 1963).

Indicator 6. Families or primary socialization systems have a set of cultural values and beliefs and social norms and expectations that are inculcated in members and that foster the development of family identity, self-identity of members, and achievement of goals for members.

Indicator 7. Families or primary socialization milieus provide opportunities to participate in cultural, intellectual, and political activities and to routinely develop social and problem-solving skills (Moos, 1976a).

Indicator 8. Families or primary socialization systems maintain kin relationships, social network supports, and community activities in order to support members in daily living and recreational activities and during times of stress and crisis (Pattison et al., 1975; Otto, 1963).

Indicator 9. Families or primary socialization groups integrate in community life, hold a community identity, and participate in the concerns and life of the community through social, recreational, school, and religious activities.

Indicator 10. Families or primary socialization groups have a general structure of roles, relationships, communication patterns, and values and expectations for the family or group as a whole yet permit variations from this structure in order to meet the mental, emotional, social, and personal needs of members (Bowen, 1966; Satir, 1967; Toman, 1976; Moos, 1976b; Jackson, 1965).

Indicator 11. Families or primary socialization groups have characteristic patterns of organization for handling daily stresses, tensions, exercising authority, organizing living activities, making decisions, and setting directions for the good of all members; this organization is flexible and can be modified and changed in order to effectively handle crisis situations (Ackerman, 1966; Aponte, 1976).

Indicator 12. Families or primary socialization groups as socialization systems have defined roles, responsibilities, authority lines, and expectations about family members (Lederer & Jackson, 1968; Spiegel, 1957; Minuchin, 1974; and Satir, 1972).

There are other indicators of adaptive, or healthy, family or primary socialization group functioning that the community mental health nurse may add to this list. Information about the ones cited provides a comprehensive amount of data about such systems and the relationships, values, and coping patterns within them. The indicators orient data collection and analysis within an established framework that can be used to make clinical judgments about the impact of the various factors on the emotional and mental health of families, other kinds of primary socialization systems, and their members and to make an overall evaluation about level of functioning.

In the case of distressed families experiencing emotional and behavioral problems such as child abuse, family violence of one kind or another, psychiatric problems of family members, or general role disorganization, additional data would be needed about the nature, extent, and social contexts of such problems. Such information would include the warping of roles and relationships of adult and child members, and patterns of coping and their effectiveness, particularly when families are under stress. Of concern also are the effects on members of being a part of and trying to cope with problems that have a devastating impact on the human spirit, self-identity, and each person's feelings of worth as well as of trying to ensure personal safety and basic survival. When the physical safety of the family and its members is at stake, the community mental health nurse may have to obtain emergency legal, social, or special volunteer services to provide assistance. As previously noted, the professional nurse generalist refers families, groups, and clients with such serious problems to a clinical nurse specialist in community mental health nursing.

INDICATORS LINKING DAILY LIVING GROUPS AND FAMILY SYSTEMS

At appropriate ages, members of families and other kinds of primary socialization systems establish roles, relationships, and activities outside these systems. Two such outside settings are school and the work place. Therefore, the kinds of daily living groups associated with these settings have important influences on the development of self of people, ways of coping, sense of achievement, and general feelings of satisfaction that people come to hold about themselves and their contributions.

Daily living groups in employment and school settings and groups organized around recreational activities are primary groups in which socialization continues to take place. Groups in these settings are not primary socialization groups in the sense that families, surrogate families, and other kinds of groups organized to care for people as substitute families are. Primary groups in daily living do not have as their primary functions the socialization of the young and stabilization of adult personalities. Whereas love, affection, and legal, social, and moral commitments tend to bind family groups together, other kinds of primary groups are held together by primary common interests around which relationships develop.

The organization of daily living and interest groups differs in structure, roles, relationships, and the interactions through which their goals are attained from those established in family socialization systems. These groups, as systems of peers, teachers, and authority figures, operate by different sets of rules, roles, and responsibilities.

The amount of time that children spend in school and that adults spend in work settings each day is usually more than the total amount of time both age groups spend in their families. Thus, experiences in daily living groups contribute to the development of the organization of the self, individual autonomy, mastery, and control in social contexts in which people other than parents and siblings have to be considered and where diverse values, roles and functions operate.

Work settings, as high-impact social environments, have a tremendous influence on the health and mental health of people. Work roles and experiences are of critical importance to adults because they occupy the central place in daily living activities. These responsibilities and the structure of the work place define roles, relationships, and daily work routines in direct ways for the adults involved and in indirect ways for the adults and children closely related to the working adult. Organizational and primary group relationships established in the work place are the most constant pathway through which adults relate to community and thence to society. Relationships formed at work also have a major influence on continued development and maintenance of self-identity and organization of a stable self-concept for individuals.

A major link between work and mental health is job satisfaction, which contributes to mental well-being. Job satisfaction is related to the feeling of achievement and level of personal stress that comes from work-place responsibilities and relationships. Relationships provide information through interactions that may or may not nurture and support self-esteem, self-actualization, autonomy, and pride of work, all of which are tied to job satisfaction, position, status, and economic rewards.

Stress and dissatisfaction at work influence the effectiveness of coping dialogues and other kinds of physiological, behavioral, mental, and emotional responses in the worker. These behaviors and associated feelings and attitudes cannot be shed as the worker leaves the work place; thus, they are carried to family and other primary groups. By the same token, the social and behavioral roles and coping responses used in primary socialization settings and the resulting tensions are transferred to the work place and its roles and relationships.

Both family and primary peer group systems in work settings are very important for continued promotion and maintenance of positive mental health. In such groups, adults receive support and confirmation of a sense of personal identity and worth in work groups. In turn, healthy functioning family systems provide milieus that continue the development of social and personal competencies promoting and maintaining the mental and emotional health of individuals in the work place.

School settings are also high-impact social environments that influence ongoing socialization of children and young adults. Age, maturation, and developmental phases influence the cognitive, emotional, and communicative tasks and skills enhanced and developed in these settings.

The basic social and problem-solving competencies that children have developed when they enter school are related to their ability to handle the frustration and stress in relation to expectations about school. One of the links between basic social competencies and mental and emotional health—not to mention progress in school—is the ability to establish relationships. When children can interact and relate to other children in quite diverse situations, a growing sense of self-assurance, a feeling of being able to act independently, and a sense of autonomy develop. When social relationships can be established, the interactive feedback provides the child with information about self and an awareness of others. Communication is facilitated. As social competencies develop and grow in each of these areas, the business of handling school work, peers, and authority figures becomes less stressful and frustrating. Interrelationships among social, cognitive, emotional, and interpersonal skills mean that deficits in one area have an impact on growth and developmental in other areas.

The social climate in classrooms for children has long been known to make a difference on learning basic knowledge and skills, although the exact nature of these relationships continues to be difficult to specify. It is also known that the development and adaptation of children are significantly shaped by a very few high-impact social environments such as families, schools, churches, and communities (Cowen, 1977). Moos (1974a and b) indicated that the social climates within which individuals function have important influences on their attitudes and moods, behavior, health, overall sense of well-being, and social, personal, and intellectual development.

Educational settings are high-impact social environments. Moos (1974 a, 1974 b) found that milieus having a high number of relational qualities, particularly cohesion and expression of caring, encourage the development of high self-esteem, increase satisfaction and comfort, and decrease irritation and depression of people in these environments. Environments high on personal development dimensions such as autonomy and problem solving also show positive effects on learning. For example, competition seems to foster development if it is not too great. It should be noted that any generalization about the relationships of social climates to learning and adaptation has to take into account a particular child's needs. The classroom environment and teaching–learning processes that promote growth and development for one child may not be as effective for another child because of individual differences.

Young adults entering college settings continue to be in high-impact social environments that influence the development of social competencies, self-esteem, and autonomy. In these settings, the high-impact environments are not necessarily classroom experiences but peer group living.

Indicators

Indicators that may be used for orienting collection of data and making judgments about experiences in daily living groups are identified. These indicators are appropriate for small peer group organizations:

Indicator 1. Daily living groups provide opportunities for members to develop different aspects of roles, responsibilities, and coping behaviors in school, work, and recreation settings.

Indicator 2. Daily living groups accord each member regard and respect as a person by providing positive feedback that becomes part of the organization of a self and a group identity.

Indicator 3. Daily living groups provide opportunities for members to accept responsibilities for self and to assist others in their mental, emotional, and social development.

Indicator 4. Daily living groups provide opportunities for members to expand and inculcate social norms and standards, cultural values and beliefs, and related behaviors beyond those learned in families and primary socialization groups.

Indicator 5. Informal and formal groups in work situations help members to integrate employment experiences in both their product production and social experience aspects in order to make them health-promoting and satisfying.

Indicator 6. School settings and related educational activities consider the emotional, mental, and physical needs of students according to their age and developmental phases.

Indicator 7. Work settings have opportunities for handling some of the conflict that arises between work and family roles and responsibilities (Renshaw, 1976).

Indicator 8. Daily living groups in work and school situations provide opportunities for members to develop an expanded repertoire of personal, interpersonal, and social competencies with peers and authority figures.

Indicator 9. Work experiences are developed so that social activities and peer group relationships lessen the impact of mechanization and depersonalization on the emotional and mental health of workers.

Indicator 10. Opportunities in work and school situations are provided to negotiate experiences that promote personal growth and career interests as well as ones that are tied to production or externally determined goals.

Indicator 11. Adults and children use work and school experiences to broaden their identities and sense of autonomy through participation in new experiences and extending relationships with new friends and people in social and community networks.

Indicator 12. Adults are provided with opportunities to restructure their relationships, roles, behaviors, and goals to accommodate work, personal, and family relationships.

It is assumed that people in school, employment, and recreation groups have some positive experiences in relation to each indicator. When this is the case, there is a good probability that these milieus are contributing to the development of emotional and mental health of members in positive ways. It should be noted again that there is no way to provide community mental health nurses with exact information about each indicator so that clinical judgment can be made with precision. For example, work experiences may be reported by clients seeking mental health counseling as noxious in certain familial, social, and psychological aspects. At the same time, counterbalancing experiences may be reported, such as excelling in recreational pursuits organized in the employment situation. In such experiences, respect and regard are accorded individuals and they may enjoy considerable prestige with congenial peers. Thus the positiveness of recreational experiences tends to lessen the negativeness of work experiences.

Preventions and interventions relating to emotional and mental health are increasingly being used in work and school settings. Industrial and occupational health has long focused on physical health and environmentally safe work places. In this decade, the industrial concept of health will be expanded to include programs that relate specifically to the emotional and mental health of workers from initial employment to retirement. In school settings, programs designed to help children reduce stress and frustrations and learn to more effectively cope will be expanded and augmented by new approaches. For example, projects in schools designed to help obese children lose weight and learn new eating habits have had the unexpected consequences of increasing interactions with peers who were not obese, which in turn had a positive effect on the self-identity and concept of the children who had a problem of overweight.

INDICATORS FOR JUDGING THE MENTAL HEALTH OF COMMUNITIES

The mental health of communities is an important part of the community mental health nursing assessment. The relationship of communities as entities to the emotional and mental health of clients and groups who live in them is important because of the interdependency of social systems that link families, primary groups, social networks, and institutions and services.

The mental health of the community can be assessed using several kinds of indicators, one of which is the extent it provides experiences and services that are essential for the development of emotional and mental health of children and adults across the life span. Another measure is the presence of community networks that connect families, groups, and individuals to institutions such as churches, schools, leisure organizations and activities, and employment settings. A third measure is whether there are social networks, defined as close kin, friends, and concerned others, that can be counted on for continuing support as an integral part of daily living and who can be mobilized to provide additional support and services in crises. A fourth measure is the assessment of the system of human services available to citizens in a community, particularly, local and state human services, community care-givers, and community citizens who volunteer to provide various services. There is also a need to know whether there are environmental networks in the community identifying problems not receiving attention and services locating new resources and planning community programs (Curtis, 1973). The mental health of a community interrelates the mental health of families, primary groups, and individuals through at least three major dimensions: emotional structural, and functional. The *emotional* community connotes feelings of identity and belonging in citizens and families. The *structural* community relates to primary social groups a community that relate and interrelate on a continuing basis. It includes the boundaries of the community in terms of identity, political jurisdiction, and other common endeavors; patterns of health and illness; and environmental, social, and technological conditions and resources that contribute to health and illness patterns. The *functional* community represents groups of families and people who have common interests in the community and work on alleviating problems and facilitating improvements for the good of all citizens (Archer & Fleshman, 1979).

Assessment of the mental health of the community is as important as assessment of the mental health of families, groups, and individuals. Leininger (1973) cited this need when she identified a holistic systems view of health that emphasizes an active dynamic state in which a person or community can maintain a balance in an ever-changing environment.

Indicators

The following indicators may be used for collecting data and making judgments about the mental health of the community. Factors in the indicators interface with family, group, and individual systems and with other outside groups. This group of indicators focuses on the community as a middle-level organization (see "Relationship Between Community Mental Health Nursing and Social Organizational Settings" and Table 1.2 in Chapter 1):

Indicator 1. Community provides school, health, social, and recreational services that are accessible to all citizens.

Indicator 2. Social networks in the community can be identified by families, groups, and clients to provide support during both crisis and noncrisis situations.

Indicator 3. Community has linkages between churches, schools, law enforcement agencies, and health services that help families and primary groups participate in the life of the community.

Indicator 4. Community provides services through both organized and volunteer efforts to community families and residents who are vulnerable and at high risk so that they do not become social outcasts or suffer from life-threatening privations.

Indicator 5. Families, groups, and their members identify with and have cohesive bonds with significant others in the community

Indicator 6. Groups can be identified by families and people in the community who share common interests and work on common problems.

Indicator 7. Community provides assistance to family and group systems so that they have more than the bare necessities in order to sustain life and promote health and mental health.

Indicator 8. Law enforcement systems protect life and property and provide security; political systems treat all citizens equal before the law.

Indicator 9. Community has a history of family and group systems pulling together to develop projects and services that benefit the health and welfare of all citizens.

The addition of data relating to daily living experiences in work, school, and community settings expands the base from which comprehensive mental health nursing can be planned and implemented. Groups formed in these settings are on integral part of the complex of relationships that are organized at family, social, and community levels (Aponte, 1976); as such, they contribute to the mental and emotional health of families and members.

The influence of social supports on the mental health of people is increasingly more clearly understood. Williams and colleagues (1981) found that social support and contacts are positively related to the mental health of people by interacting and modifying the impact of life events on emotional and mental health. This relationship was found to be valid irrespective of whether the number of life events was low, medium, or high. Heretofore, research had suggested that social support groups and networks were related to improvement in mental health of clients only in times of crises and substantial stress (Nuckolls et al., 1972).

Information from indicators of community mental health provides a view about the interrelationships between the community and the families, groups, and people who live in the community. Such information helps the community mental health nurse use community resources, take effective steps to mobilize family and group resources, and activate social networks to assist them in integrating more effectively into community life.

INDICATORS FOR JUDGING INDIVIDUAL MENTAL HEALTH

Indicators of mental health of individuals have been developed more definitively than those for families and communities. The mental health of individuals was the primary focus in psychiatry for most of this century and long before the social, cultural, and community aspects of mental and emotional problems became a major concern. Inherent in most theories of personality and behavior are the criteria by which the mental and emotional health of a person is to be evaluated.

Indicators of individual mental health are included to assist the community mental health nurse to maintain a sense of continuity from family and community levels of organization to the "individual as a system." In the clinical approach to community mental health nursing that has been presented, the nurse would be focusing on family systems rather than on individual systems as units of change. For nurses who prefer to orient their practice to mental health nursing, these indicators may be useful.

Indicators

Using a social psychological perspective of mental health, emotional and mental health indicators are identified. In this group of indicators, the "individual as a system" is the level of organization:

Indicator 1. Individual holds positive attitudes about self and uses information from the perception of others to evaluate and make changes in behavior.

Indicator 2. Individual is motivated to use potential to gain personal goals and achieve self-actualization

Indicator 3. Individual can relate to others in mutually satisfying and enduring relationships that involve sharing responsibilities for others in family, marital, and peer groups.

Indicator 4. Individual is able to mobilize personal strengths and coping abilities to meet daily living demands and unexpected situations without prolonged and intense feelings of frustration and stress.

Indicator 5. Individual, in progression to adulthood, learns to function with a substantial degree of autonomy, can regulate personal affairs, and organizes energy and activities to achieve self-actualization and career attainment.

Indicator 6. Individual maintains a level of general health that permits the implementation of age, sex, personal, and employment roles and responsibilities.

Indicator 7. Individual validates perceptions of self, others, and experiences in ways that are reasonably free from distortions arising primarily from his or her own psychological needs.

Indicator 8. Individual adapts to changes in social and environmental conditons by reorientation, maintaining a sense of personal identity, and mobilizing available resources to handle situations.

Indicator 9. Individual has a characteristic mode of coping that is effective for handling usual life situations and relationships and that can be altered as necessary to handle unusual situations and relationships, crises and events.

Indicator 10. Individual integrates personal goals and feelings, social norms, cultural values, situational demands, and the relationships necessary to perform satisfactorily in daily situations and role relationships and to achieve career goals and aspirations.

Indicator 11. Individual enjoys creative expression and experiences both satisfaction and challenge in new relationships and experiences in which outcomes are not known.

Indicator 12. Individual, on balance, experiences satisfactions in the activities of life and in relationships with significant others.

CHARACTERISTICS OF HEALTHY FAMILY SYSTEMS

An important assumption in mental health related to the prevention of mental and emotional problems is that there is a relationship between individual mental health and the kinds of primary systems in which people are socialized throughout life. Family systems are basic to this assumption. In order to obtain an idea of how healthy family systems are structured and organized, profiles of healthy, stressed, and distressed families and characteristics of functioning have been developed. Healthy family systems and their relationship to mental health may be considered from a number of different approaches, several of which will be described. Factors and characteristics of these systems have a number of things in common even though concepts of family functioning have been approached from a variety of perspectives.

In 1963, Otto called attention to the need to identify what he called "family strengths." He decried the lack of information and research about "healthy" or "normal" families and believed such data needed to be developed so that effective programs for strengthening family life and systems could be developed. From his research, Otto (1963) identified 12 criteria for assessing and judging family strengths. Family functioning was rated high, medium, or low on the ability to meet the following criteria:

1. Provide for the physical, emotional, and spiritual needs of the family and its members.
2. Be sensitive to the needs of each family member
3. Communicate effectively
4. Provide support, security, and encouragement to members
5. Initiate and maintain growth-producing relationships and experiences within and without the family
6. Maintain and create constructive and responsible community relationships in the neighborhood, the school, town, local and state governments
7. Grow with and through children
8. Help self and accept help when appropriate
9. Perform family roles flexibly
10. Hold mutual respect for the individuality of family members
11. Use a crisis or seemingly injurious experience as a means of growth
12. Be concerned for family unity, loyalty, and interfamily cooperation*

* Reprinted with permission from *Family Process* 3(2):329–338.

Otto concluded that in order to understand a family's level of functioning, judgments have to be made about family strengths, how these are developed, and how they are used for the good of members. The criteria address a cluster of family behaviors that are dynamic, fluid, interrelated, and interactive. Otto believed that the criteria could be used for helping families to focus on, identify, and use their strengths.

Using a different perspective, Pless and Satterwhite (1973) developed the concept of family functioning as a measure of how families as social units influence the health of members. Family functioning was defined as the way the family unit operates across many dimensions of everyday life. Principal dimensions of family functioning were identified as communications, togetherness, closeness, decision making, and child orientation. Families scoring high on these dimensions were found to have a high level of functioning and provided a milieu conducive to maintaining health. In clinical practice these dimensions may also be rated as being present to a high, medium, or low degree.

Deykin (1972) investigated healthy family life functioning and found six major areas that needed to be considered: decision making, emotional gratification, perception of crisis, response to crisis, perception of community, and response to community. Family functioning was significantly related to the kinds of antisocial behavior seen in delinquent children and to the degree of behavior change after treatment. Deykin suggested that family environments determine certain kinds of behavior in family members and influence changes in such behavior.

In 1976, Cromwell and Thomas developed a model of counseling with an array of services designed to release human potential in families. An underlying assumption was that normal healthy families need assistance to realize their potential and achieve optimal levels of functioning. Release of family potential can be achieved by activities that are preventive and educational in nature and designed to facilitate the development of latent family potential. Family potential was considered to be the underlying resources, motivations, and energies that can be released and used to change and grow, love and care, communicate, resolve conflict, adventure, create, and experience joy. The concept of family growth developed by Anderson (1974) was used to focus on family growth rather than on family problems and deficiencies. Using this approach, opportunities were found for families to increase their awareness of their unique strengths and actualize dormant capacities that improved family living and family life. For family growth, family members learned essential skills of coping with family interactions and developed an understanding of family change and development. The Cromwell and Thomas model emphasizes that the total family unit has to be considered in order to promote family development and prevention of health and mental health problems.

Hume and colleagues (1977) approached healthy family functioning and family adjustment by using an ecological psychology approach. This approach assumes that behavior is significantly affected by five major factors: (1) environmental surroundings; (2) the nature of the settings themselves, which have a profound effect on individual experiences, including the types of activities performed; (3) the number of settings entered; (4) the degree of involvement; and (5) the kind of satisfaction reported in interrelationships and achievement of goals. A focus solely on family systems was not found to be sufficient to predict low and high adjustments of families. Two major findings related to family adjustment were whether fathers participated in activities at home and the level of participation of the family in community activities. These factors were particularly related to the adjustment levels of sons. In general, highly adjusted families were involved in more social interactions that required a high level of social competency. This links social competencies to self-concept, which is linked to mental health, a connection Gladwin (1967) identified 25 years ago.

Barnhill (1979) synthesized several clinical theories of family functioning into what he called a "family health cycle." This cycle included eight dimensions of healthy family functioning: (1) individualization for family members; (2) mutuality between members that fosters a sense of emotional closeness while maintaining the identities of individuals; (3) flexibility in responding to various conditions and processes of change; (4) stability in which the family has consistency and security in family interactions; (5) clear perceptions of self and shared events; (6) clear communications; (7) role reciprocity in which mutually agreed-on behavior patterns complement the roles of members; (8) and clear generational boundaries that distinguish marital, parent–child, and sibling relationships.

Barnhill conceived of his dimensions as dichotomies that would distinguish healthy and maladaptive family functioning. These may, however, be rated as present to a low, medium, or high degree. Four categories were used to further organize the eight dimensions:

1. Identity Processes
   Individuation versus enmeshment
   Mutuality versus isolation
2. Change
   Flexibility versus rigidity
   Stability versus disorganization
3. Information Processing
   Clear versus unclear and distorted perceptions
   Clear versus unclear or distorted communications
4. Role Structuring
   Role reciprocity versus unclear roles or role conflict, and
   Clear versus diffuse or breached generational boundaries

These dimensions are interrelated and data obtained through observations, interviews, and tests may be used in combination with other assessment data to make clinical decisions. Low ratings show areas of weakness if not outright pathology in family functioning. This approach makes it possible to identify both strengths and weaknesses that can be used as a basis for preventive counseling and in other kinds of educational strategies.

Reiss (1980) summarized several findings about the competency of healthy family systems for achieving their major objectives of socialization and developed the following profile. Healthy families are open and growing systems capable of responding in innovative ways to outside challenges. They may be recognized by the following characteristics: a clear-cut power structure with opportunities for negotiation and cooperation; individual uniqueness is encouraged and respected; separation and death can be recognized and grieved with major changes in family functioning ensuing if necessary; reality can be confronted directly without the need for myths or distortions; and warmth and optimism are freely expressed, whereas negative feelings are expressed with supportive awareness of their impact on others.

In 1976, Lewis and his colleagues investigated ways of making judgments and ratings about the competence of healthy middle-class family systems by identifying interactional variables that characterize psychologically healthy functioning. Specially developed rating scales and related clinical judgments were found to be reliable for discrimination of optimally healthy from adequately competent families on 10 variables. Healthy families had certain kinds of characteristics that made them competent:

1. A number of interrelationships operated in healthy families and were expressed by differences in style and patterns such that there was no one single way to do things

2. The expectation that human encounters were apt to be caring, which encouraged a reaching out to others

3. Respect for one's own world view as well as that of others, with empathy and expressiveness as an integral part of this respect

4. A belief in complex motivations that encouraged the exploration of numerous options for doing things and solving problems

5. A demonstration of high levels of initiative and engagement in constructive reaching out in the community and in activities with others, thus generating a lot of stimuli and opportunities for social interactions and coping with diverse situations

6. A structure that related healthy family functioning to parental and marital relationships that were effective in meeting the needs of both parents where leadership was shared; no competing parent–child coalitions; a high degree of complementarity, that is, a "fit" between the various individual skills of parents and pride in each other's assets; no strong competitive pulls between parents; and closeness but clear boundaries for individual family members

7. Members demonstrated high levels of personal autonomy

8. Members appraised the reality of the family's competence accurately

9. Members were open in expression of affect with a prevailing mood of warmth, affection, and caring

10. Family interactions had a high degree of spontaneity

Lewis (1980) observed that children in his cohort of healthy families were achieving age-appropriate developmental tasks in cognitive, social, and intrapsychic realms. They were open, friendly, active, and athletic. Older children tended to have self-discipline and were productive. Younger children were less disciplined and more expressive and affectionate. These characteristics were not based on the sex of the child but on birth order. This work of Lewis is important because of the comprehensive approach taken to the identification of healthy families from clinical perspectives in mental health. Family functioning is related to having an adequate level of economic resources. In healthy family systems, resources are available and families know how to obtain additional ones.

Using an action approach to prevention in mental health, Vaughan and co-workers (1975) developed a program for family mental health maintenance that consisted of mental health promotion and primary prevention activities. The program was health-oriented and had no designated cases or patients, only families. It provided family-oriented information and orientation and education services for family mental health maintenance that included (1) family-focused consultation and education services based on the public health model, and (2) crisis intervention services. This group concluded that primary preventions could be effectively provided to families and such information, services, and suggestions would be used.

Pratt (1976) developed a model of an energized and effective family social system. Several characteristics of such a family system are described. First, there is a structure open and flexible so that it can change and modify in order to function effectively and has the ability and willingness to grow, develop, modify, and adapt in response to pressures from members and external sources. Structural flexibility is reflected in the following actions:

1. Responsiveness to emerging needs of members
2. Active exchange among members
3. Sensitivity to internal pressures for change
4. Health-training efforts
5. Receptiveness to information and ideas and readiness to change on the basis of new information
6. Activity linkages by all members to outside systems
7. Use of external and internal resources to develop coping abilities

A second characteristic of an energized family system is that the structure of the family system provides permissive ranges and alternative models of behavior as well as permitting divergences and novelty. Effective family functioning requires that members have the freedom to move around. There is also toleration and encouragement of individual variations.

A third characteristic is that there are regular exchanges between family members and other systems basic to family functioning and growth. In healthy functioning families, the community mental health nurse should expect to find extensive links with community and social systems and networks. Information from these sources introduces a variety of views. Linkages, information, and exchange with outside systems are significantly related to a family's ability to function effectively.

A fourth characteristic of energized family systems is that there is involvement with other systems having different interests and goals and creating conflicts in family systems. Conflict resolution and coping with conflict situations are integral to learning the social competencies necessary for effective functioning in both family systems and systems in the world outside the family, particularly work systems.

A fifth characteristic is the degree to which family systems integrate functions, roles, and relationships to meet individual and system needs. This requires a balancing of goals and making sure relationships and roles provide for members to have different experiences. At the same time that individuals are meeting their needs, they must also be socialized to get along in society and to function in particular roles and groups. In this respect, family systems must help members learn to "deviate" from existing norms and standards of behaviors and values so that they can learn to express creative ideas and actions.

Another approach to the concept and assessment of family functioning is to look at the impact of highly intense environments such as family systems on learning, development of attitudes, and behavior. This social ecological approach has led to the development of measurements to ascertain the interactional influences of socioemotional aspects of environments and certain dimensions of family functioning. It is premature, however, to think that it is possible or even desirable to predict what kinds of environments produce specific kinds of behavior. More to the point, certain dimensions of highly intense environments operate across a number of behavior settings and provide a perspective that is useful in community mental health nursing.

Moos and Moss (1976) identified some common dimensions in social environments of families and found that emphasis on different dimensions have different behavioral consequences for family members. Dimensions common to family environments are relationship dimensions among family members, personal growth dimensions, and system maintenance dimensions. These dimensions have descriptive statements that will help the community mental health nurse connect them to family functioning. The three dimensions with subcategories are described:

Relationship Dimensions

Cohesion	The extent to which family members are concerned and committed to the family and the degree to which they are helpful and supportive to each other
Expressiveness	The extent to which family members are allowed and encouraged to act openly and to express their feelings directly
Conflict	The extent to which the open expression of anger and aggression and generally conflictual interactions are characteristic of family interactions

Personal Growth Dimensions

Independence	The extent to which family members are encouraged to be assertive, self-sufficient, make their own decisions, and think things out for themselves
Achievement Orientation	The extent to which different types of activities (e.g., school and work) are cast into an achievement-oriented or competitive framework
Intellectual-Cultural Orientation	The extent to which the family is concerned about political, social, intellectual, and cultural activities
Active-Recreational	The extent to which the family participates actively in various recreational and sporting activities
Moral-Religious Emphasis	The extent to which the family actively discusses and emphasizes ethical and religious issues and values

System Maintenance Dimensions

Organization	The extent to which order and organization are important in the family in terms of structuring of family activities, financial planning, and the explicitness and clarity of rules and responsibilities
Control	The extent to which the family is organized in a hierarchical manner, the rigidity of rules and procedures, and the extent to which family members order each other around*

An emphasis on expressiveness and structure (control) were found to be two dimensions that discriminate quite different family climates. At the present time, the social ecological approach seems best applied by using the dimensions to make sure adequate information is obtained about family functioning. Data can be integrated with more clinically oriented information.

* Reprinted with permission from *Family Process* 15(4):357–372, December 1976.

PROFILE OF ADAPTIVE FAMILY SYSTEMS

A profile of adaptive, healthy family systems functioning at a high level includes the following characteristics:

1. There is a balance in the family system on meeting the needs of individual members through promotion and enhancement of age-appropriate developmental, mental, emotional, social, and physical tasks and competencies and the needs of families as interacting systems.

2. Family members express love and respect and show concern for each other, have a sense of family unity and loyalty, and have caring attitudes toward people outside the family.

3. Members are clear about their personal identities, have the freedom to be autonomous, and characteristically explore different ways of coping by using innovative approaches and ideas.

4. The structure of family systems is clear in terms of roles, relationships, responsibilities, authority, and decision making.

5. The organization of families is flexible and allows for changes to occur to accommodate daily living activities, rapid changes, and crisis situations.

6. The emotional climate in family systems encourage growth-promoting relationships and clear communications both within the system itself and in other kinds of group systems that have different interests, conflicts, and approaches for achieving goals.

7. Families have linkages to social networks and recreational and community activities that increase interactions outside the primary socialization system and encourage development and use of social and interpersonal competencies and problem-solving skills in a variety of relationships and situations.

8. Family functioning, as an interacting and ongoing process, is directly addressed by members without the need for development of family myths and distortions.

9. Climates in families respect member's views, encourage the exploration of different ways to do things and to solve problems, and develop ethical and moral values including the responsibility of self for own behavior, responsibility to others in intimate caring relationships, and a general sense of social responsibility.

10. Relationships between spouses set an overall family climate in which:
    a. Needs of both spouses are met.
    b. Leadership is shared.
    c. No persistent and competing parent–child coalitions exist.
    d. Each accepts other's skills and assets and feels pride about each other's abilities.
    e. Loving, close, collaborative relationship exists rather than a competitive one.
    f. Clear ego boundaries exist in each spouse.
    g. Shared and satisfying sexual intimacy takes place.
    h. Female spouse has time and energy and is willing to devote these to family; often does not work outside the home.

11. Families have more than adequate economic and other kinds of resources.

In planning preventions with healthy functioning family socialization systems, there is an emphasis on family systems with work, school, and community systems considered in terms of their influences on mental and emotional health. This emphasis is based on the assumption that healthy functioning families and other kinds of primary socialization systems are integrally related to how members of the family are supported, stabilized, learn, and carry out roles and responsibilities in the other settings. Members can be assisted to broaden their knowledge of the importance of other kinds of environments on the emotional, cognitive, and social growth and development of themselves and others in high-impact milieus. The community mental health nurse may need to conduct direct assessments of daily living environments other than family systems. In such a case, the indicators previously identified can be used and modified as need be because these criteria relate to common aspects of individual and group experiences.

CHARACTERISTICS OF STRESSED FAMILY SYSTEMS

According to the concept of community mental health nursing that has been presented, stressed family systems are essentially healthy, function at an effective rather than optimal level, and experience stress in one or more dimensions of family living. In general, children are socialized in ways that prepare them for adult roles, and adults have a measure of stable self-organization that supports trying out new roles.

Because of long-standing stresses and tensions, interactions, roles, and expectations between parents, parents and siblings, or siblings, members experience vague dissatisfactions, less than satisfactory relationships, and hesitation about expression of feelings and communications. When feelings of unease and discomfort, less than adequate communications and expressions of affection, and uncertainties about roles, functions, and authority sources persist within the family, they tend to diminish the potential of stressed families to provide milieus in which optimal emotional and mental health of members is developed and maintained.

Stressed family systems make members vulnerable to the development of mental and emotional problems. More than usual stress, that is, a higher level than is needed to promote motivation, alertness, and learning, begins to have an impact on emotional and mental health if it persists over periods of time. Stressed family systems have low-visibility problems in interactions between members and between the family and outside systems. These are reflected in identifiable variations from the mental health indicators that the nurse is likely to observe in healthy functioning family systems. These variations are usually discernible in the interaction patterns in the family, in role uncertainties, and in the marital relationships or relationships between significant others that are analogous to the marital dyad. Less open communication patterns and expression of affection and conflicts about differences in views between familial expectations, norms, and values and those that children or young adults in the family have adopted may be noted. Although such problems may be low-level in visibility, the emotional feelings about them may be quite intense.

At this point, it should be emphasized that the concept of *stressed families systems* does not relate to family systems that have major system and organizational pathologies that in turn are reflected in maladaptive behaviors in one or more family members and in the family as an interacting system. The profile of healthy family functioning suggests that a relatively small number of families characteristically maintain this level of functioning, but it is difficult to know because little or no epidemiological data currently exists about the levels of functioning of family systems in the United States. The stressed family profile suggests that a great number—probably the majority—of family systems function at this level. The concept of stressed families is intended to embody the realities of the living family environment and of getting along and learning how to get ahead and the stresses and satisfactions involved for both adults and children. In this process, there are variations in both kind and degree of stresses and strains, tensions, problems, satisfactions, and feelings of accomplishment. However, stressed families need to use their strengths to achieve a higher level of functioning.

Lewis (1980) identified what he calls *competent but pained families*, which are similar to what are called *stressed families* in the framework presented here. Both stressed and pained family systems differ in a number of ways from families with clearly defined dysfunctional problems. Lewis places such families in two categories: dysfunctional and severely dysfunctional.

Variations in the level of family functioning—that is, the climate, competence, relationships, and use of resources in these highly intense milieus to optimize the health and mental health of members—require attention and the organization of strategies by which preventions and interventions can be provided in mental health nursing practice. Ironically, in an intuitive and experiential sense, nurses have known for years that some families are simply more competent than others to carry out family, social, and personal responsibilities and prepare members for productive roles in society. The problem has been that clinical insights have not been translated into enough research that would identify what such differences are, how they could be measured, and how problems could be prevented. Thus, the concepts of adaptive, stressed, and distressed family socialization systems are a refinement of dichotomies that have long been used in nursing: healthy and sick families. The use of three levels of functioning for classifying family systems departs from this older medical model and uses different theory and research to reconceive a more effective approach for clinical nursing practice. This makes it possible to provide more definitive clinical nursing strategies that enable the nurse to help families recognize their potential strengths.

Because variations in family interactions, roles, and relationships are usually involved in stressed families, problem relationships and situations require clinical strategies that are interventive and directed toward changes in these areas. Again, it should be noted that such changes would not be of the magnitude, intensity, or even direction as those found in distressed or dysfunctional families. Examples of such families would be ones in which a member experiences schizophrenia or in which incest exists between a parent and daughter or son. In such cases, family systems and relationships have major problems to a degree that social, system, and psychological pathologies exist and involve all family members in ways that are not conducive to the development of their mental health.

In mental health literature, many kinds of family constellations are called stressed. However, a review of descriptions of such families, profiles, and problems addressed under this concept indicates that what are often called stressed families are, in fact, truly distressed families that are trying to cope with major familial, social, personal, and economic problems as well as system and member pathologies.

Stressed family systems are probably a way of life in contemporary society. Glasser and Glasser (1970) noted that where once it was thought that families were diminishing in importance, the opposite is true. Personal and social functions of the family have enlarged at the same time that these systems have had to learn to adapt quickly to the increasingly rapid rate of change experienced by all groups and institutions in society. Family systems are flexible and can maintain stability in ways that other groups cannot. In the process of adaptation to change, particularly rapid change, stress occurs, and if not too great, can act in a positive way to help in the change process.

Stressed families—or normal families that are trying to cope and having some problems in doing so—are not considered to be in crisis because of their characteristic style and level of functioning. A family system in crisis is one in which abrupt and disruptive changes in family organization, structure, roles, relationships, and socioeconomic status occurs and characteristic modes of coping cannot effectively handle the situation and the attendant personal, interpersonal, and familial problems created. The degree to which such changes are experienced as crises depends on family strengths, structure, organization, kind and extent of the crisis, and the ability of the family system to mobilize problem-solving skills. Having social competencies to handle crisis situations and using available social support systems to diminish the extent of the disruptive and abrupt changes determine to some extent whether abrupt changes create a crisis situation in the family.

Adaptive, stressed, and distressed family socialization systems all experience crises at one time or another. The strengths of family systems are important indicators for predicting how individual families will respond and for determining the kinds of assistance that would be most helpful.

Glasser and Glasser (1970) identified three features in families that help them to respond to and handle stress adequately. Such families have *involvement, integration,* and *adaptation.* Involvement refers to commitment to and participation in family life by members. Integration means the interdependence of task and socioemotional roles are blended together in ways that members help each other and work well together. Adaptation means that there is flexibility of the family in group structure and member behavior in responding to the demands of situations.

Vincent (1970) emphasized that family systems also have an external adaptive function, an aspect that is often overlooked. This function revolves around the need for the family organization and structure to respond quickly, modify, and change in response to social changes in an industrialized society. Family systems have to adapt to member's needs and to the demands of other social institutions, but they can be selective in adaptations. Vincent believes that family systems, more than other kinds of social institutions, help to bring about social changes. The reason for this belief is that families function in a social change process through the socialization function, which places family systems between individual needs and demands and the expectations of society. Competing and conflicting goals, demands, and expectations have to be mediated, modified, accepted, translated, and incorporated back into the socialization process.

Lewis (1980) provided what is perhaps the best profile to date about "competent but pained families." This profile is similar to our concept of stressed families. He identified the following characteristics in such family systems:

1. Wives felt emotionally deprived in relation to husbands.
2. Wives had physical health problems, symptoms, appeared angry, and were often on antianxiety drugs.
3. Wives formed coalitions with a child, parent, or friend who functioned as an ally.
4. Husbands were successful but detached, guarded in expression of feelings, and viewed interpersonal relationships as less rewarding than tasks achieved in relation to work.
5. Husbands recognized unhappiness of wives but assumed little responsibility for it.
6. Spouses did not have a feeling of intimacy.
7. High levels of involvement with children and a view that the family is important exist.

8. One parent is usually moderately dominant; no clear pattern of shared leadership exists.

9. Ego boundaries are distinct but there is no real closeness in family.

10. Members can accurately assess family assets and liabilities.

11. Family members have good negotiating skills and are efficient problem solvers on problems that are external to the family and that do not focus on the marital dyad and the pain involved in this relationship.

12. High level of autonomy is expected of members and they are expected to accept responsibility for individual behavior.

13. Range in feelings that are expressed in the family is restricted but members do show warmth and caring and empathy is present to a moderate degree.

14. Not too much humor and joy exist in the family.

15. There are shared goals about the family and a commitment to children.

16. Unhappy adaptations of members are accepted.

17. Children are healthy, achieve developmental milestones, and function well in social and educational settings.

18. Children cannot be distinguished from those in optimally healthy families.

Lewis raised the question of whether a high level of family functioning is necessary to produce physically, socially, and mentally healthy children. In a general sense, the answer is probably no. If this were not the case, the vast majority of people who are socialized in family settings not too dissimilar from the families described by Lewis as pained but competent would have significant mental and emotional problems—and they do not.

PROFILES OF STRESSED FAMILY SYSTEMS

A profile of the stressed family system in contemporary society shows variations from adaptive functioning family systems. Research and clinical experiences suggest that variations in functioning observed in stressed family systems as compared to functioning in healthy families occur in the following areas:

1. Relationships between spouses are strained and not as satisfying to both parties in the following ways:
   a. There is emotional distance in which a feeling of intimacy is diminished or not present.
   b. Wives are more unfulfilled and may be on drug therapy for anxiety or depression.
   c. Wives experience more health problems than husbands.
   d. Wives tend to form coalitions with an ally: mother, child, or friend.
   e. Husbands are oriented toward work and achievement with diminished interests and commitments to familial and interpersonal relationships.
   f. Husbands do not feel particularly responsible for their wives' unhappiness.

2. One parent is more dominant and sharing of leadership is not clearly defined.

3. Cohesiveness in family is low and there is little real intimacy between members.

4. There are diminished expressions of caring about members and others, less spontaneity, humor, and fun.

5. The organization of family, although flexible, experiences and handles crisis situations with increased stress.
6. Social and problem-solving competencies of members are more effective in situations outside the family than in situations that involve family members.
7. Unhappy situations and adaptive coping responses are accepted rather than actively explored to consider options for making changes.

Stress in family socialization systems need not be of such intensity and duration that it becomes expressed in psychological and behavioral symptoms by members. The focus of community mental health nursing in working with families that are stressed is to assess the level of stress, allay it, and reduce it in cooperation with the family before members develop coping responses and attitudes that are not particularly effective either inside or outside the family. The family can be helped to learn to problem solve in ways that use stress productively by learning alternative ways of handling situations and relationships. To achieve these goals, the nurse and the family can focus on patterns of family organization and ways of family functioning. Family counseling assists families to make changes in interactions and organization patterns, to identify troublesome communications and relationships, and to foster the expression of affectional relationships.

CHARACTERISTICS OF DISTRESSED FAMILY SYSTEMS

Distressed family systems have well-developed problems and pathologies that are evident in the system's organization, structure, and interactions as well as in the mental and emotional health of members. Inadequate and deviant socialization is an integral part of the interactional patterns in distressed families. Such interactions influence the kind and quality of relationships that are developed as well as the values and expectations that are learned by members and come to be held in relation to self and others.

An implicit assumption in understanding distressed family systems is that social adjustment, lack of availability of necessary resources, or the ability to accept and use these and the general socioemotional climate in these systems socialize members to have attitudes, behaviors, and health practices that do not prepare them adequately for adult roles in the world of work or even to maintain healthy family systems. The relationship between family structure and health practices has been found to be related in a number of ways by Pratt (1976). Two important ones in all kinds of family structures and organizations are: (1) the emphasis that families give to problem solving contributing to the development of sound health practices and active problem-solving efforts, and (2) the involvement of men in internal family functioning.

Severe and chronic stress and maladaptations are evident in distressed family functioning in the organization and definition of roles and allocation of responsibilities, in clarity and meaning of communications, in diminished ability to express caring and concern for others, and in marked deficiencies in familial interrelationships. This means that the potential for socialization and development of positive emotional and mental health of members is fair. Stress and maladaptations in family systems to the extent seen in distressed families mean that there are considerable disorganizations of various kinds. Such disorganizations are not conducive to having socioemotional milieus in which members can learn roles, develop mature selfhood, learn personal autonomy, and acquire other essential social, interpersonal, and problem-solving competencies that are needed to relate to other people during childhood and adolescence and to prepare for adult roles.

In 1975, Tonge and colleagues compared 33 problem families with a cohort of families who had been matched on the following criteria: both parents in the home, site of residence, age of wife, and use of social services. The purpose of the study was to determine the nature and extent of psychiatric pathology in problem families and to identify some of the effects of such pathology on social adjustment of families and their members.

In general, problem families lived in poverty and had more problems than the cohort of comparison families in most areas of family functioning. Problem families had few contacts with relatives and neighbors, were distrustful and had negative attitudes toward schools. The general level of mental health of members was impaired and there were more frank mental disorders in problem families. Children experienced more "growing-up problems" such as temper tantrums, discipline problems, and chronic physical health problems than children in comparison families. In general, children in problem families had a lower intelligence level and higher number of criminal convictions than children in comparison families. Children in problem families did not receive appropriate care and attention.

Problem families were characterized by a high level of gross marital disharmony with spouses who used aggressive behavior in marital and sibling relationships. Wives in these families were found to have more psychiatric illness and husbands took little part in social organizations outside of the home. Husbands in these families also did not seek assistance from social agencies and neighbors.

Social adjustment problems were evident in all problem families. Impairment of mental and emotional health was related to many aspects of social adjustment. Psychiatric pathology did not account for all aspects of social maladjustment. A value system held by many problem families contributed to problems. It consisted of the following ideology: Rules are ignored, discomfort is ignored, long-term consequences of actions are ignored, and education is distrusted.

In this comprehensive study, Tonge and colleagues did not find a typology of problem families. Instead, they found distressed families with a mosaic of social adjustment problems. It was suggested that there may not be such a thing as problem families—only families with different patterns and degrees of disorganization. No single pattern of maladjustment was identified in problem families.

Problem families were social isolates and became so by a process of exclusion by neighbors, which then fed into self-condemnation. Self-condemnation got worse as demoralization and social failures repeatedly occurred. As a rule, family systems can cope with failures if they are restricted to partial involvement of family functioning or to a single event or experiences in which a conclusion is expected. In problem families, personal and social failures were nearly total and members constantly had to face the accumulating effects of inadequate performance and failure. Tonge and colleagues noted that social failure—like debt—breeds a type of compound interest in that denial of failure holds back anxiety, disrupts performances of individuals, and generates the qualities of "crisis-living": apathy, impulsiveness, aggression, and decisions made only for the moment.

Psychiatric disorder in problem families had more effect on social adjustment when it was present in the male partner and the effects were greater on family relationships than in other relationships. Long-standing unemployment was often an indicator of mental problems in men. Signs of vulnerability in women were a lack of confidence, anxiety about the care of babies, and difficulties in management of money. When both marital partners experienced personal and employment stresses concurrently, the family was gravely at risk of disorganization.

Many family systems may be distressed because they have handicapped members at home for whom care is provided. Kershaw (1973) found that handicapped children in families have some special points of vulnerability that could be modified through socialization practices and changes in relationships. Handicapped children are vulnerable because their total powers of adaptation are restricted. Furthermore, too much stress over that usually experienced increases the disability. There is a need for handicapped children to learn to cope more effectively, with an understanding that while stress related to handicaps may be "unfair", it must still be managed. They also need to learn to manage dependency and feelings of inferiority more adequately. In family systems where there is a handicapped member, there has to be an accommodation of roles and responsibilities among members. These changes affect all other members in many different ways. Where the family may not have adequate resources and support, considerable stress and frustration can occur throughout the family system. The handicapped person has developmental, social, and personal needs that pose special problems for families that intimately involve every family member in their own development and self-actualization.

Lewis (1980) described "dysfunctional and severely dysfunctional families" in terms of competence and functioning. In dysfunctional families, two patterns of organization were found: dominant-submissive and conflicted. Both kinds of families showed rigidity and a fixed "is now, was then, and ever will be" quality of family life.

Lewis (1980) described a dominant–submissive pattern of family functioning as one in which one parent dominated and controlled every aspect of family life. This dominance was handled by other family members in a passive way or circumvented by acting-out behavior, usually outside the home. Both parents usually had clear ego boundaries; however, parental relationships were strained by gross inequality in power and authority. There were little closeness and intimacy in the marital dyad and between other family members, since all were distant with each other. Sometimes coalitions were present between the submissive parent and one or more children; this coalition aligned against the dominant parent.

Dominant–submissive families viewed their situation as normal and tended to blame problems on things or persons outside of the family or on one family member who was scapegoated and blamed for all wrongs. Families with dominant–submissive patterns of organization did not know how to negotiate, since the dominant parent made decisions; hence, there was a process of blaming each other instead of participating in and accepting responsibility for family decisions. Communication processes in these families were clear but the substance of messages often did not get through. The dominant parent did a lot of "mind-reading." Expressions of feelings were few. The family mood was hostile or sad. Empathy was little used and seemed not to be valued. Conflict was always present if not acknowledged.

Lewis (1980) noted that the dominant–submissive family organization pattern of functioning is occasionally seen where there is no identified patient with mental or emotional problems. It is a common pattern in families that have both children and adults with problems.

The second type of dysfunctional functioning families were ones that were chronically conflicted. Family organization was characterized by parents constantly at war with each other, with one parent trying to dominate the other and neither parent willing to accept a submissive role. This conflict involved other family members and influenced to a considerable extent the kinds of relationships that were capable of being established. Children and other members often formed coalitions with one parent and then the other. There was no closeness or trust between members. Individual ego boundaries were, however, quite clear. Families tended to deny difficulties and scapegoated each other or other persons external to the family system. Negotiation and collaboration were simply not possible around problems because of the perpetual conflict. In such highly intense environments, children cannot learn problem solving and other essential social and personal competencies that are necessary for assuming adult roles and relationships. Emotional comfort and satisfaction are at a minimum.

Lewis (1980) noted that in family systems in which there is chronic and persistent conflict, communications are moderately clear. Families communicate problems to other persons and hostile, attacking feelings are often expressed. Warm and caring attitudes cannot or are not expressed and empathy is not evident. Generally, the family mood is hostile and conflict and marital warfare seem endless.

Despite intense and persistent conflicts, these highly conflicted families are not bizarre; their members are not frankly mentally ill. However, these families do not develop family strengths in ways that support the emotional needs of members, and the socioemotional climate does not provide a milieu in which members are sustained by closeness and intimacy. Social, developmental, cognitive, and personal learning occurs in ways that diminish the opportunities for self-actualization of both child and adult members.

Severely dysfunctional families as described by Lewis (1980) were the least competent of families to support the growth and maturation of children and adults. Such families did not promote the development of autonomy in members. In severely dysfunctional families, one pattern of organization was found in which one parent was usually dominant and unstable, even idiosyncratic in his or her views, and often frankly mentally ill or on the borderline. Many of the interior family roles and relationships were similar to but more accentuated than those found in dysfunctional dominant–submissive families.

Another pattern found in severly dysfunctional families was chaos. No one member had enough influence and authority to provide the leadership the family as a system needed. There were vague, amorphous role and ego boundaries between family members. The meanings of family communications were difficult to decipher for both members and others. Families tended to avoid, deny, and rarely resolve issues to anyone's satisfaction. Clarity of expression was low and members were often unreceptive to the feelings and concerns of others. The family mood tended to be hostile, cynical, and hopeless. The fusion of individual members in some areas of functioning such as in coalitions tended to blur the extent of conflict. These families often appear strange and bizarre to others. They have poor if any linkages to social and community networks. In effect, the family system constructs their own world. Achieving selfhood and a strong sense of personal identity and learning the social and interpersonal competencies that are necessary to function in worlds other than the family are difficult if not impossible in such distressed, highly intense learning milieus.

PROFILE OF DISTRESSED FAMILY SYSTEMS

A profile of distressed family systems shows evidence of disorganization and even chaos. Affected to some extent or other are the structure, organization, interactions, interrelationships, and general sense of identity of the family. Fortunately, distressed family systems as primary socialization groups occur in small numbers in the population.

A comparison of the adaptive functioning family profile with the distressed family system profile suggests that differences in characteristic patterns of organization and functioning are so great and extensive that it is not just a matter of degree in the variations of competence in family systems that distinguishes them; rather, family relationships and patterns are different in both quantity and quality. The resources that children and adults need to develop essential competencies at appropriate developmental levels to prepare for roles in society are not usually present in distressed family systems. Furthermore, the interactive influences of disorganization and maladaptation in so many aspects of family system functioning are accumulative, reinforce pathologies in members, and are involved in developing and maintaining a family structure and pattern of organization that supports continued family system pathologies. It should be noted that not all of the indicators of distressed family systems have to be present to a great extent in order to assess families as being distressed. Rather, major dysfunctions in any part of the system can be so distressing that the family as an interacting system responds, thus causing maladaptive coping responses in members and creating a milieu that affects the development of positive mental health.

Distressed family systems differ from healthy and stressed primary socialization groups in the following areas:

1. Relationships between spouses are quite conflicted; conflicts are behaviorally expressed in different ways.
   a. Wives and husbands often have emotional and mental problems that are serious enough to be classified as mental disorders.
   b. One spouse usually dominates and controls family decision-making and actions.
   c. Little closeness and intimacy exist between spouses.
   d. Spouses may constantly battle over control and dominance.
   e. Neither spouse is able to provide the leadership the family needs.
   f. Wives experience considerable anxiety; husbands are often unemployed with a history of difficult relationships in work settings.
2. There is often a lack of sufficient economic and other kinds of resources needed for the essentials of family living.
3. Disorganization in family systems or maladaptations in personal behavior of members is evident in most aspects of family functioning: organization, structure, interactions, attitudes, and relationships both within and outside the family.
4. Few if any linkages exist with kin, neighbors, friends, and community resources.
5. Families may have members who are frankly mentally ill or have borderline mental disorders or behavioral problems or other kinds of handicaps.
6. Children have many "growing-up" problems as well as chronic physical health problems.
7. Violence and aggressive behavior may be used by both adults and children to handle problems and assert authority; scapegoating is common.
8. Family mood tends to be hostile as well as apathetic; there is little closeness and intimacy; hostile, attacking feelings are expressed.
9. Organization of the family is oriented toward here-and-now actions.
10. There is rigidity in family organization, structure, and functioning; personal autonomy and development of self-identity are not encouraged.
11. Ego boundaries between family members range from moderately clear to diffuse.
12. Coalitions are common between a parent and child or children.
13. Communications are usually clear but meanings are not always in accord with message.

SUMMARY

Indicators of positive mental health for primary socialization systems such as families and other kinds of peer groups in work and school situations show linkages between these and their relationship to positive mental health. The indicators have been selected on the basis of a social psychological perspective of human behavior. They include a broader array of behaviors than what is usually associated with mental health as conceived of from a psychodynamic perspective of personality and behavior. Indicators of the mental health of communities are identified and linked to family mental health.

Profiles and behavioral characteristics of adaptive, stressed, and distressed family systems show differences and variations in family behaviors, the extent of such differences, and the quality of relationships and life in three types of family systems. These profiles and characteristics provide a base and a means of comparison that can be used in community mental health nursing to make clinical judgments and decisions from assessment data about individual families.

Stressed family systems may be effective in providing the climates and relationships and using resources in ways that promote the mental health of members. However, the relationships found in stressed families suggest that these systems are vulnerable, particularly relationships between spouses. With both stressed and distressed family systems, interventions need to be provided on the basis of the therapeutic goals that need to be achieved with each type of system.

Healthy family systems provide milieus in which the positive mental and emotional health of members are enhanced, promoted, and maintained. Such family systems need to be identified and provided preventions that help them to recognize their strengths and their potential as milieus in which essential personal, social, and cognitive competencies are learned, children are effectively socialized and humanized, and adults can continue growth and actualizations across the life span.

REFERENCES

Ackerman, Nathan. *Teaching the Troubled Family*. New York: Basic Books, 1966.

Anderson, D. A. The family growth group: Guidelines for an emerging means of strengthening families. *The Family Coordinator* 22:437–442, 1974.

Aponte, Harry J. Underorganization in the poor family. In Guerin, Philip, ed. *Family Therapy: Theory and Practice*. Gardner Press, 1976, pp. 432–447.

Archer, Sarah, and Fleshman, Ruth, eds. *Community Mental Health Nursing: Patterns and Practices*, 2nd ed. Scituate, MA: Duxbury Press, 1979, pp. 23–29.

Barker, R. G. *Ecological Psychology: Concepts and Means for Studying the Environments of Human Behavior*. Palo Alto, CA: Stanford University Press, 1968.

Barnhill, Laurence, R. Healthy family systems. *The Family Coordinator* 38:94–100, January, 1979.

Bateson, Gregory, Jackson, Don, Haley, Jay, and Weakland, John. Toward a theory of schizophrenia. *Behavioral Science* 1:251–264, 1956.

Boszormenyi-Nagy, Ivan. A theory of relationships: Experience and transaction. In Boszormenyi-Nagy, Ivan, and Framo, James, eds. *Intensive Family Therapy*. New York: Harper & Row, 1965, pp. 33–86.

Bowen, Murray. The use of family therapy in clinical practice. *Comprehensive Psychiatry* 7:345–374, 1966.

Brown, William D. A socio-psychological conceptual framework of the family. In Nye, F. Ivan, and Benardo, Felix M., eds. *Emerging Conceptual Frameworks in Family Analysis*. New York: Praeger, 1981, pp. 176–197.

Cowen, Eli. Baby-steps toward primary preventions. *American Journal of Community Psychology* 5:1–22, 1977.

Cromwell, Ronald E., and Thomas, Vicky L. Developing resources for family potential: A family action model. *The Family Coordinator* 25:13–20, 1976.

Curtis, Robert W. Community services networks: New roles for mental health workers. *Psychiatric annals* 3:23–42, 1973.

David, Henry P. Healthy family functioning. In Coehlo, George V., and Ahmed, Paul, eds. *Towards a New Definition of Health: Psychosocial Dimensions*. New York: Plenum Press, 1979, pp. 281–311.

Deykin, E. Life functioning in families of delinquent boys: An assessment model. *Social Science Review* 46:90–102, 1972.

Gladwin, T. Social competence and clinical practice. *Psychiatry* 30:30–43, 1967.

Glasser, Paul H., and Glasser, Lois, eds. *Families in Crisis*. New York: Harper & Row, 1970, pp. 3–14.

Hume, Nicholas, O'Conner, William A., and Lowery, Carol R. Family adjustment, and the psychosocial ecosystem. *Psychiatric Annuals* 7:32–49, 1977.

Jackson, Don. The study of the family. *Family Process* 4:1–20, 1965.

Kershaw, J. D. Handicapped children in the ordinary school. In Varma, Ved P., ed. *Stresses in Children*. London: University of London Press, 1973, pp. 1–20.

Lederer, W., and Jackson, Don. *The Mirages of Marriage*. New York: Norton, 1968.

Leininger, Madeline M. An open health care system model. *American Journal of Nursing* 73:171–175, 1973.

Lewis, Jerry M. Family matrix in health and disease. In Hofling, Charles F., ed. *The Family: Evaluation and Treatment*. New York: Brunner/Mazel, 1980, pp. 5–44.

Lewis, Jerry M., Beavers, W. Robert, Gosseh, John T., and Phillips, Virginia. *No Single Thread: Psychological Health in Family Systems*. New York: Brunner/Mazel, 1976, pp. 199–217.

Mabry, J. Medicine and the family. *Journal of Marriage and the Family* 26:162, 1964.

Minuchin, Salvatore. *Families and Family Therapy*. Cambridge, MA: Harvard University Press, 1974, pp. 1–15 and 46–56.

Minuchin, Salvatore, Montalvo, B., Guerney, B., Rosman, B., and Schumer, F. *Families of the Slums*. New York: Basic Books, 1967, pp. 192–243.

Moos, Rudolph H., and Moos, Bernice. A typology of family social environments. *Family Process* 15(4):357–372, December, 1976.

Moos, Rudolph H. *The Social Climate Scales: An Overview*. Palo Alto, CA: Consulting Psychologist Press, 1974. (a)

Moos, Rudolph H. *Evaluating Treating Environments: A Social Psychological Approach*. New York: John Wiley & Sons, 1974. (b)

Moos, Rudolph. Evaluating and changing community settings. *American Journal of Community Psychology* 4:313–326, 1976. (a)

Moos, Rudolph M. *The Human Contexts: Environmental Determinants of Behavior*. New York: John Wiley & Sons, 1976, pp. 394–431. (b)

Moos, Rudolph, H. Evaluating family and work settings. In Ahmed, Paul, and Coehlo, George V., eds. *Toward a New Definition of Health*. New York: Plenum Press, 1979, Chapter 16.

Nuckolls, Kit B., Cassel, J., and Kaplan, B. H. Psychosocial assets, life crisis, and the prognosis of pregnancy. *American Journal of Epidemiology* 95:431–561, 1972.

Otto, Herbert A. Criteria for assessing family strength. *Family Process* 3:329–338, 1963.

Pattison, Mansell, de Francisco, Donald, Wood, Paul, Frazier, Harold, and Croder, John. A psychosocial kinship model for family therapy. *American Journal of Psychiatry* 132:246–251, 1975.

Pless, I. B., and Satterwhite, B. A measure of family functioning and its application. *Social Science and Medicine* 7:613–621, 1973.

Pratt, Lois. *Family Structure and Effective Health Behavior: The Energized Family*. Boston: Houghton-Mifflin, 1976, pp. 1–6 and chapters 7 and 10.

Rallings, E. M. A conceptual framework for studying the family: A situational approach. In Nye, F. Ivan, and Berardo, Felix M., eds. *Emerging Conceptual Frameworks in Family Analysis*. New York: Praeger, 1981, pp. 130–151.

Reiss, David. Pathways to assessing the family: Some choice points and a sample route. In Hofling, Charles F., and Lewis, Jerry, eds. *the Family: Evaluation and Treatment*. New York: Brunner/Mazel, 1980, pp. 86–121.

Renshaw, Jean R. An explanation of the dynamics of the overlapping worlds of work and family. *Family Process* 15:352–372, 1976.

Rowe, George. The developmental conceptual framework to the study of the family. In Nye, F. Ivan, and Berardo, Felix M., eds. *Emerging Conceptual Frameworks in Family Analysis*. New York: Praeger, 1981, pp. 198–222.

Satir, Virginia. *PeopleMaking*. Palo Alto, CA: Science and Behavior Books, 1972.

Satir, Virginia. *Conjoint Family Therapy*. Palo Alto, CA: Science and Behavior Books, 1967.

Speer, David C. Family systems: Morphostasis and morphogenesis, or is homestasis enough? *Family Process* 9(3):250–258, 1970.

Spiegel, John P. The resolution of role conflict within the family. *Psychiatry,* 20:1–16, 1957.

Toman, Walter. *Family Constellation,* 3rd ed. New York: Springer Publishing Company, 1976, pp. 117–129 and 143–195.

Tonge, W. L., James, D. S., and Hillam, Susan M. *Families without Hope*. Kent, England: Headley Brothers, 1975, chapters 4, 6, 10, and 12.

Vaughan, Warren T., Huntington, Dorothy S., Samuels, Thomas E., Bilmes, Murray, and Shapiro, Marvin I. Family mental health maintenance: A new approach to primary prevention. *Hospital and Community Psychiatry* 26(8):503–508, 1975.

Vincent, Clarke. Mental health and the family. In Glasser, Paul H., and Glasser, Lois N., eds. *Families in Crisis*. New York: Harper & Row, 1970, pp. 319–362.

Whitaker, Carl. *Process Techniques of Family Therapy*. Unpublished manuscript, University of Wisconsin, Madison, WI, 1972.

Williams, Ann W., Ware, John E., and Donald, Cathy A. A model of mental health, life events, and social supports applicable to general populations. *Journal of Health and Social Behavior* 22:324–336, December, 1981.

PART THREE

CLINICAL PRACTICE MODEL FOR COMMUNITY MENTAL HEALTH NURSING

OVERVIEW

The focus of Part Three is the application of theory in community mental health nursing. A model of clinical practice is presented that uses (1) a clinical organizing framework, (2) a comprehensive community mental health nursing assessment, and (3) a plan for applying preventions with adaptive functioning families to promote and maintain the mental health of members. These three parts of the clinical model may be modified depending on the focus of nursing practice, the population group(s) with whom the nurse is to provide therapeutic and professional mental health care, and the different "mix" of concepts and principles that a particular nurse has in her or his conception of community mental health nursing.

There are three chapters in this last part of the book. Each one focuses on an important aspect of applying theory to clinical nursing practice. The assessment and application of concepts in the area of prevention are illustrative of a general model of community mental health nursing that uses theory and research for its conceptualization and links these to the therapeutic plan and activities used in clinical practice.

In Chapter 8, a clinical organizing framework is established to link principles and concepts from theory and research to clinical practice with particular groups at the small-group level of organization. Key interrelationships are identified that relate to each group. The three groups identified concern major life experiences with which community mental health nursing is concerned: primary socialization groups; daily living groups, particularly in school and employment settings; and special groups in mental hospital settings that are used for corrective mental health experiences. Community and social networks link these systems and together contribute to the health and mental health of people and communities.

In Chapter 9, a comprehensive community mental health nursing assessment is presented complete with assumptions, rationale, and structure. This assessment is organized as a *nursing assessment* that provides the primary base for clinical practice. A secondary base concerns aspects of mental and emotional problems.

The comprehensive nursing assessment is considered to be an assessment counseling process and experience. It usually takes at least four sessions to conduct it, one of which is done in the living situation. The objectives of the assessment and for each session are established as well as the discussion of the therapeutic counseling process.

In Chapter 10, the model of clinical nursing practice is applied to adaptive functioning family systems to provide preventions enhancing and promoting the development and maintenance of positive mental health. Primary socialization systems in general are the level of organization for which applications are designed because they represent highly intense learning milieus in which preventive behaviors can be taught.

General goals related to prevention counseling for positive mental health are based on the basic interrelationships characterizing these kinds of groups. Activities and strategies related to each goal are developed to provide the nurse with structure and direction and for therapeutic use of self. More specific goals would be added to this framework as the need evolves from interactions with families.

8 | COMMUNITY MENTAL HEALTH NURSING: AN ORGANIZING FRAMEWORK

INTRODUCTION

Community mental health nursing has been defined as having a unique clinical process. The uniqueness of the process is based on a synthesized conceptual framework that has specially selected principles and concepts from nursing, mental health, and the basic and applied sciences. The focus of clinical practice is to assist families and groups in natural community settings to promote and maintain the mental health of their members and to learn how to more effectively manage emotional and mental problems they and their members may experience and to assist them to potentiate the use of strengths to realize their potential and self-actualization.

The conceptual framework for community mental health nursing, as already noted, is based on a number of concepts and principles from different sources, all of which are congenial to a social psychological perspective of behavior. From this conceptual framework, a *clinical organizing framework* has been developed to guide the application of nursing actions.

In general, the clinical organizing framework provides the structure and an approach through which the diverse concepts from different theories are organized and applied. It orients the community mental health nurse to the selection of appropriate concepts to guide assessment, preventions, interventions, use of self, and evaluation of the outcome of nursing interventions.

In community mental health nursing, the nurse has to be able to encode a considerable amount of diverse data as they evolve in the professional helping relationship. *Encoding* is the process that converts content, feelings, patterns of communication, factual information, and interactions to the language of concepts and theory from which clinical hypotheses can be made, clinical decisions arrived at, and clinical actions decided on.

The process of encoding data means that the nurse has to identify, select, and organize key pieces of information that evolve in interaction with people in order to get a sense of consistent relationships and adaptation patterns. As these relationships and patterns are recognized, different clinical hypotheses may be formulated to guide further clinical inquiries, interactions, and interventions.

The clinical process in community mental health nursing requires that nurses be able rapidly to sort and organize diverse data that literally unfolds as nurse–client interactions progress. This means that clinicians have to be acutely sensitive to and use all their abilities to see, hear, feel, and experience in order to recognize what is going on between them and clients.

An essential part of the clinical process in community mental health nursing is to have an organizing framework that provides the structure by which encoding and organizing of data can occur. Because the organizational framework is derived from a particular conceptual framework, it is the link that connects the scientific explanations of behavior and the attribution of meanings to data that may be collected as bits and pieces of information to feelings expressed, to evolving patterns in the professional relationship, and to adaptation patterns by which interpersonal, familial, and social experiences of life and living are characteristically handled. It is easy for community mental health nurses to collect a great deal of information from clients. Often, such information is collected by using a general interview format, and then the nurse experiences difficulty in knowing how to organize and evaluate the data in relation to a conceptual framework of human behavior.

The social psychological perspective of community mental health nursing emphasizes interrelationships and interactions in family systems, daily living groups, and special corrective groups. It also emphasizes the creation and emergence of new relationships, feelings, and meanings as client and nurse interact. Thus, the nurse is faced with the task of trying to capture the changing aspects of the professional relationship as well as the more constant ones. Underlying this orientation is the belief that nurses and clients engage in a process of becoming, of undergoing change and growth, of having something new and different come into existence as a result of nurse–client and nurse–group interactions. This process of becoming may be compared with that of being, that is, an emphasis on the qualities and things that a person is and has already become.

The orientation of community mental health nursing is to provide professional care and services to groups of people. It is important to note this orientation because the nurse–patient relationship is usually considered the level of organization or model at which nursing interventions and actions are directed. The dyadic interpersonal model is important and appropriate in many nursing situations. It is not, however, the model of choice in community mental health nursing, although it would be for mental health nursing. This is true because community mental health nursing involves to a large extent the socialization of people in roles and functions, norms, and cultural and familial values in relation to the development of members. This model is based on principles of nursing and learning that extend beyond and differ in some respects from those that underlie the interpersonal relationship, or dyadic model of nursing practice.

The nurse–patient dyad is ideal for emphasizing and focusing on atypical and unique problems that a particular client experiences. Nurses have developed considerable expertise and pride in their ability to "individualize" the nursing care and management of each patient or client. However, in community mental health nursing, there is a need to go beyond the basic nurse–patient model in order to orient clinical practice toward groups of people for given purposes. In this respect, data are needed about groups as interacting systems, their relationships with other systems, the handling of typical as well as atypical situations of group living, and mutual influences all of these have on the mental and emotional health of members. If such data are not part of the base from which clinical decisions are made, then the social, cultural, and situational aspects of health and mental health may not be adequately assessed and considered in designing nursing actions of one kind or another. Nurses often teach patients to learn to manage atypical and unique health experiences. Equal concern and attention have to be given to the interplay of these aspects as they occur in daily relationships with families, peers, and fellow employees.

The clinical organizing framework in this chapter has been developed for the concepts of community mental health nursing presented here. The concepts themselves are intended to guide clinical practice in both mental health and mental illness experiences. However, clinical application of the concepts is presented for adaptive, or healthy, families. Application to this area of clinical nursing practice was selected because it is relatively undeveloped and presented an opportunity to show the applicability of concepts in clinical practice in prevention counseling.

NEED FOR A CLINICAL ORGANIZING FRAMEWORK

A *clinical organizing framework* is defined as a structure of interrelated concepts, principles, relationships, and methodologies that is constructed to apply to particular phenomena. All conceptual approaches to community mental health nursing need a clinical organizing framework to guide the application of relevant concepts and principles so that clinical practice is based on the desired theoretical perspective.

A theoretical or conceptual approach to community mental health nursing can be stated without identifying the related clinical organizing framework. This approach may create difficulties for nurses because they are expected to supply appropriate practice frameworks and strategies for applications. These difficulties may be compounded when abstract concepts are expected to be used with little or no specification as to how applications can best be made and what kinds of outcomes are to be expected.

A major difficulty in developing clinical organizing frameworks are the problems that are encountered when one tries to unify a number of diverse theories into a conceptual framework for a particular discipline and its clinical practice needs. Kalkman and Davis (1972) observed that a theoretical framework for the practice of community mental health nursing is highly desirable. However, after examining a number of possibilities, these authors found that of the theories currently in use in the field, not a single one had a theoretical system that provided the understanding of the many problems encountered by the nurse and that would furnish guidelines for clinical nursing practice. Osborne (1970) stated another aspect of this problem: the need to develop a general theory of psychiatric mental health nursing that reflects the peculiar and specialized beliefs and views held by psychiatric mental health nurses.

The slow development of unified conceptual and related practice frameworks in community mental health nursing has created a need for clinicians to adapt to this situation in several ways. One is for nurses to select an employment setting in which the dominant model of human behavior and the related clinical practice framework have been established by other professionals and is congenial with their philosophy of mental care and nursing. Practice models of mental health are usually determined by psychiatrists and in some cases, psychologists. Psychodynamic models of mental functioning dominate in mental health and these have had their clinical frameworks organized and refined for over half a century in relation to therapeutic applications. In clinical mental health settings where this model prevails, it may be neither possible nor desirable to try to modify this practice framework to any extent if the nurse fundamentally agrees with this view of mental health and human behavior.

Another way in which nurse clinicians in mental health may obtain clinical practice frameworks is to combine selected concepts and principles from a number of different models of human behavior and tie these together with a unifying methodology. The methodology is usually some form of nursing process (Walker & Nicholson, 1980). This approach does broaden the theory base for nursing practice but it has some limitations. Whenever concepts and principles are taken from a number of different theories, the basic assumptions underlying them may be inconsistent and even contradictory. For example, assumptions about human behavior from a behavior modification view are radically different from those underlying psychodynamic views. Strategies used for one are not appropriate for the other.

The use of models of behavior constructed from many theories means that nurses have to resolve which meanings apply to what interrelationships and concepts. They also have to select from the various theories and concepts some principles that seem to have generality over a number of different experiences and situations. The resulting framework is eclectic, that is, a use of concepts and principles drawn from many sources.

An eclectic approach has an advantage in that concepts may be selected that have particular relevance to specific concerns and problems that patients or clients experience. It has disadvantages in that incongruences about meanings of concepts, related assumptions about human behavior, and principles of learning may minimize the effectiveness of therapeutic interventions and preventions. In this respect, Havens (1973) stated that an eclectic approach is like putting a nine-course gourmet meal in an electric blender: The product may be readily digestible but the whole is far less than the sum of the parts. Clinical frameworks constructed on eclectic models may be so individualized for a particular client or group of clients that applications of therapeutic activities may have little or no generalizability to other clients and their situations.

Still another way in which community mental health nurses may organize a clinical practice framework is to use a common-sense approach. This approach is based on life and work experiences that nurses have successfully used in personal relationships with families, groups, clients, friends, and colleagues. This approach uses both unique and common experiences from which to derive clinical nursing strategies for handling problematical situations and relationships. A major drawback to this approach is the absence of a general conceptual framework on which to base clinical nursing practice. Because of this omission, clinical data from clients and patients are "fitted" into a relatively narrow experiential framework. The inadequacy of such a framework becomes readily apparent when the needs of clients and patients differ from the experience frameworks held by the nurse. Furthermore, it is quite often difficult to integrate theory and research that might potentiate the effectiveness of nursing actions and make clear the basis for evaluation of the outcomes of preventions and interventions.

All theoretical perspectives of human behavior and of health and mental health need some kind of a clinical organizing framework if a perspective is to be used for providing direct clinical services to people. For example, theories of behavior modification have a clinical framework providing direction and a set of strategies for implementation of principles. Also inherent in this framework are the approaches used to evaluate the effectiveness of interventions to change behavior.

Clinical organizing frameworks also help to make sure that the concept of behavior stated as guiding clinical nursing practice is in fact being used. The conceptual base and clinical practice framework should be capable of being linked by overall integrating principles. These principles, of course, depend on the theories being used and the philosophy of nursing being promoted. In this clinical organizing framework, unifying principles from systems theory have been used and are consistent with the conception of community mental health nursing, a holistic concept of nursing, and a social psychological perspective of human behavior and mental health.

It should be recognized that with the multiplicity of concepts and theories that are used to develop a base for community mental health nursing practice, it is difficult under the best of circumstances to consolidate these in a coherent way. This difficulty is related to both the complexity of clinical nursing practice and the state of the art in developing integrated frameworks.

Using principles from systems theory to give the clinical framework unity, different views about the wholeness of systems need to be considered. One view is that a part of a system in interaction cannot be pulled out of the total context and independently analyzed and changed. This view holds that laws governing systems in interaction cannot be assumed to operate in like manner in each of the parts of the system. Another view holds that it is possible to account for the characteristics, dynamics, and laws of a system by examining its constituent parts and generalizing these to the system as a whole (Nagel, 1961; Putt, 1978). Both views can be used to analyze complex systems such as those the community mental health nurse usually encounters.

Mental health and mental illness are known to involve both social and cultural systems. These systems are not like biological and physical systems in several respects, two of which are important to clinical nursing practice. First, social and cultural systems have a wide range of possibilities for changing their structure and functions. This contrasts with physical and biological systems that function from genetic blueprints and are relatively limited in the range of changes that may occur in structure and function. For example, body temperature has a narrow range in which it can vary before other systems begin to experience changes in functions.

In contrast, social and cultural systems have the capacity to organize and reorganize their structures quickly and can evolve to a higher level of organization and complexity through change. These systems have more freedom and flexibility to change both structure and function, thus can move from simple to complex more rapidly than biological systems. For example, in the initial phase of organization, a group is unstable because the people who have come together may not have decided to organize. However, if the decision to organize is made, the structure of the group can be rapidly established and functions specified.

A second distinction that sets social and cultural systems apart is that they may not be as stable as biological systems, thus the concept of homeostasis has to be used with care. Many social and cultural systems are relatively unstable, inconstant, and revolutionary. They move toward the development of more complex states at a fast pace or may disorganize just as rapidly. However, as Buckley (1967) pointed out, some social and cultural systems can be relatively constant in many aspects. The family as a social system is an example.

Systems theory recognizes closed and open systems. Basically, closed systems can be specified in terms of parts that interact within predictable outcomes. An example is the chemistry of the blood in which changes in one substance cause changes in other substances. An open system has continuous interactions about which predictable outcomes cannot be made with certainty. This is particularly true when systems include social and cultural variables.

In community mental health nursing, the clinician deals with open systems such as families, other kinds of primary groups, and community and social networks. A major organizing principle from systems theory that helps to guide clinical nursing practice is that various levels and kinds of systems are always involved in exchange of energy. Information or feedback from system parts can be analyzed and given meaning with a conceptual framework. These meanings help community mental health nurses and their clients to evaluate whether goals are being realized.

In community mental health nursing, the advancement of the art and science of clinical practice depends on the development of clinical practice frameworks that are theoretically based and have the capability of being tested in clinical nursing practice. Only in this way will a body of knowledge be accumulated that determines the effectiveness of the various kinds of nursing activities. Both interventions and preventions need to be quite varied and capable of changing the behavior of people in different kinds of groups and settings. Effective approaches for bringing about changes in middle-sized and large systems need to be made more explicit or developed. Clearly, the field requires practice frameworks that are comprehensive enough to address the diversity of concepts needed to support a man and environment in interaction approach to holistic health and mental health care.

CLINICAL ORGANIZING FRAMEWORK: BOUNDARY SETTING

In a clinical organizing framework, the establishment of basic concepts and the key relationships between experiences is necessary to orient and guide the collection of the data base by assessment. From this base, community mental health nursing decisions and judgments are made and preventions and interventions are decided on. The selection of concepts and key relationships may be facilitated by *boundary setting*.

Boundary setting is a process used to select the kind and amount of data needed for assessment, organization of experiences, and selection of strategies to be used for clinical applications in relation to a particular conceptual framework. Boundary setting is defined as the placement of theoretical fences around a particular set or cluster of concepts and selected interrelationships that connect the concepts as they occur in social and family life and in the development of mental health and health of people.

Interrelationships are defined as those things, aspects, qualities, or dimensions that can be examined and predicted *only* if two or more of the parts are considered together in mutual relationships. In a social psychological perspective of community mental health nursing, the interrelationships of major concern are those between people within systems and between different kinds of systems. For example, family members have relationships within the family system. All family members interrelate with community networks, schools, and employment settings. These systems in turn interrelate with cultural systems by using particular values, beliefs, social norms, and standards of conduct.

The interrelationships that develop in groups of various kinds are important for the development and organization of the self, especially those in primary socialization systems like families. What happens in these systems determines to a large extent the emotional and mental health of members and of the family as an interacting system. Although considerable variation in roles and interrelationships may occur in family systems, there are essential ones that have to be carried out and need to be considered in every comprehensive community mental health nursing assessment.

CLINICAL ORGANIZING FRAMEWORK: BASIC SETS OF INTERRELATIONSHIPS

The clinical organizing framework considers a broad range of concepts and interrelationships and emphasizes the social and psychological aspects of the human experience. Boundaries are set to establish the key interrelationships important for a particular perspective about the mental and emotional health of people. Once boundaries are established, the wholeness of experiences can be considered with attention paid to important connections between them.

Concepts and interrelationships are established in basic sets that characterize different kinds of groups and settings. This approach is based on the assumption that there are general principles of structure, organization, and function that apply across a number of different kinds of groups, thus eliminating the need to develop frameworks and approaches that are specific to each group situation.

Three basic sets of interrelationships are identified and take into account the personal, interpersonal, social, and organizational settings in which key life experiences occur. They are (1) primary socialization groups, (2) daily living groups in school and employment settings, and (3) special groups organized for corrective experiences for mental and emotional problems.

The sets specify mutual interrelationships that link different kinds of systems: (1) cultural, in the form of symbols, values, beliefs, and mores, all of which influence our behavior in both covert and overt ways; (2) social, which includes the various kinds of primary groups in which people are socialized across the life span and which are intensive learning environments; (3) community and social networks; (4) systems of coping that people develop to handle living situations; and (5) interrelationships that connect one system to the other as people mutually interact. The sum total of all these systems in interaction contributes to the behavior and attitudes that people learn and use in coping with the multiplicities of living.

In the three sets of interrelationships, at least two kinds of data are needed in order to make an assessment about system functioning. Information is needed about stable experiences that characteristically occur over time, place, and situation, and about the less stable and more variable experiences that occur in response to unanticipated events, relationships, or situations. In reference to stable experiences, information is needed about relationships that occur in daily living situations and settings. For less stable experiences, data are needed about group and member responses to unexpected situations and sudden changes in roles and functions that evoke a need for modified or new ways of coping and handling situations.

The organization of each set of interrelationships is based on the major purpose for which each kind of group exists. Within this framework, the structure of the group is considered to determine whether opportunities are provided to foster the development of an organization of self that helps each member develop to selfhood, and the interrelationships between family and community mental health are identified. Two of the group settings are basic socialization systems in which everyone participates in the process of growing up and reaching adulthood, one the primary socialization setting, the other daily living groups. These milieus are major settings in which people learn to address the challenges that have to be faced in life if experiences are to be lived without overwhelming stress and satisfactions in life achieved. The third group setting for which interrelationships are identified is one in which corrective experiences occur for people who have mental and emotional problems to a degree that mental hospitalization is required. In each of these three kinds of settings, coping and adaptation have to take place in ways that are consistent with human developmental needs, constraints, sanctions, norms, and standards of behavior. At the same time, there is a need for people to have opportunities to express thoughts and emotions and to be creative. Both opportunities and constraints are always present in situations, but the extent to which they influence behavior may not be recognized. By taking such factors into account, the community mental health nurse has a more comprehensive data base from which to consider options about possible preventions and interventions.

The three sets of basic interrelationships of special concern in community mental health nursing are set out. Each set has significant concepts and interrelationships.

Interrelationships are posed as delicate dilemmas that have to be managed constructively in order to maintain group systems and to promote and maintain the mental and emotional health of members.

Primary Socialization Groups

Concepts

1. Families, families of adoption, and surrogate families
2. Families as interacting systems
3. Family structure, organization, roles, and functions
4. Social and cultural values and beliefs held by famlies and members for guiding behavior and community involvement
5. Social and interpersonal competencies
6. Organization and maintenance of self
7. Coping patterns
8. Community networks and resources available to family
9. Family involvement in community activities, organizations, and participation in community concerns

Interrelationships

1. Between expectations of parents or surrogates about development of warm, caring, and concerned relationships for others by members *and* whether beliefs fostered in the family promote these socioemotional qualities in members
2. Between emphasis on the development and expression of unique qualities and abilities of individual members *and* an emphasis on relationships and activities that promote close family relationships, identity, and cohesiveness
3. Between expectations that members participate in family life and contribute to maintenance of the family system *and* the needs of individual members to develop roles, relationships, and social competencies apart from the family
4. Between the need for members to develop a strong family identity *and* the need for each member to develop a personal sense of individuality, autonomy, and independence
5. Between the responsibility of the family to inculcate values, standards, and respect for the rights and views of others *and* the need to assist members to critically examine thoughts and feelings of others and self without undue punishment and negative valuation
6. Between the need to organize the structure, roles, relationships, and patterns of communications in the family to maintain it as an interacting system *and* the flexible use of these to maintain and promote the development of self and positive mental health for members
7. Between cultural values, beliefs, social norms, and behavioral standards that guide the family as a unit *and* the use of these to shape and influence the organization of self of members, family identity, and responsibility for community involvement
8. Between the expectations and responsibilities held for members within the family system *and* the expectations and responsibilities held for members in the world of work and school.

9. Between roles, relationships, and coping patterns members use in family life *and* the usefulness of these in roles and relationships outside the family setting

10. Between characteristic modes of coping by the family to handle daily relationships and tensions, deal with significant biosocial concerns and issues in family life, and establish themes for family concerns *and* the effects these have on the development in members of a self-identity, coping dialogues, and social, emotional, and cognitive competencies (Hess & Handel, 1959).

11. Between the need for members to learn to handle conflicts in group settings through use of consensus, collaboration, and cooperation *and* need for individual members to strive and compete for personal achievement, mastery, and control

12. Between activities centered on family living *and* activities that involve community networks and accept responsibility for community life (Otto, 1963; Williams et al., 1981; Pearlin et al., 1981)

Family Interrelationships

This set of interrelationships connects a number of basic familial, social, and personal responsibilities and experiences in which there are dilemmas: the needs of families as cohesive socioemotional and task-oriented systems to be maintained and responsive to changes and the needs of members to develop as independent human beings who use their unique abilities and potential for self-actualization. All of the interrelationships are handled in some way or other in family systems. Some interrelationships have a greater impact on a particular family member than others, and the impact of any conflict may be experienced with greater intensity at some times than at others. Some interrelationships have a great influence on the family system where conflicts arise about them that do not seem resolvable or continue over a period of time.

The age, sex, and general mental and physical health of each family member contribute to the way in which family relationships are experienced both directly and indirectly by each member and by the family as an interacting system. Relationships between family members provide a considerable amount of information about how the roles of members are defined. Roles also help to determine in some cases and influence in others the assignments of functions to family members. The social and emotional development of all members is connected to both roles and functions as both old and new ones are tried out before generalizing these to other situations.

Family identity and the individual identity held by each member become intertwined and act in mutually supportive ways as members seek their own interests and goals. Support includes opportunities to be with different people, to explore novel experiences, and to try out relationships and activities that have a reasonable risk of failure as well as those that may succeed.

The idea of sets of interrelationships is one way of organizing community mental health nursing, and it helps the nurse to maintain the essential wholeness of key systems and relationships. This approach considers the need for growth and development of all family members. Socialization as a growth process is a pathway by which life experiences are made available for examination and alteration and changes made on an ongoing basis.

In practice, the community mental health nurse has to judge the importance of a particular set of interrelationships in relation to the concerns or problems that are being expressed by a particular family. In each set, the entire range of interrelationships does need to be considered. This framework can be used for both intervention and prevention counseling with families and groups and modified for counseling with individuals. The consideration of the interrelationships helps to motivate families to assume responsibility for self-monitoring and self-growth.

Hoeffer (1980) suggested five guidelines that may be used to help nurses organize family counseling and guidance: (1) find out what the family considers to be the problem areas; (2) help the family set some realistic goals for the sessions with the nurse; (3) intervene in process versus content of communication; (4) keep the focus on here-and-now behavior; and (5) shift support to family members as indicated. This clinical framework focuses on primarily on the interior of the family system and does not explicitly consider the world beyond in terms of interrelationships that the family must maintain and contend with. This framework could be extended to include relationships that connect the family as an interacting system to other related ones. This would broaden considerably the perspective for clinical practice and provide opportunities to counsel family members about different kinds of growth-promoting experiences.

A considerable amount of mental health research has focused on disturbed families. Theories evolving from such work have tended to obscure the fact that such work may not adequately describe adaptive family systems. The majority of families do provide a milieu in which their members can achieve emotional and mental health. This potential can be further realized by mental health education and by teaching families how to monitor their functions and tension levels, to manage stress, and to identify unsatisfactory interactions and recognize their impact on family members (Lazar & Shapiro, 1981; Barnhill, 1979).

The findings of Lewis and his colleagues (1976) that no single thread or factor makes the difference between competent and less than competent functioning families suggest that many things have to be considered when trying to help families promote and maintain the emotional and mental health of their members and of the family system itself. One of the things found to be important in families is the way in which they organize to handle problems and whether a milieu is provided in which certain kinds of experiences are made available for members to develop essential social, cognitive, and interpersonal competencies. Another factor is whether the relationship between spouses is caring and satisfying and the degree to which their needs are met through parental and marital roles.

In community mental health nursing, the special quality of climates, or milieus, in families is a major concern. It influences the overall tone of family life and is important in contributing to the stability and cohesion within the family and helps it to maintain its identity and qualities as a special kind of primary group.

Daily Living Groups

Concepts

1. Formal and informal groups in schools, employment, and leisure settings
2. Members of these groups
3. Organizational settings in which such group activities take place
4. Situational contexts of experiences
5. Community networks and resources that connect with and contribute to groups achieving their objectives
6. Social and cultural values and beliefs held by members of groups that influence membership in particular groups and development of peer relationships, all of which influence the behavior of the groups as entities and their members as individuals

Interrelationships

1. Between roles and responsibilities of members in peer groups in school, employment, and leisure activities and settings *and* roles and functions expected of members in family systems

2. Between regard and respect accorded a person as a member of peer, work, and leisure activity groups *and* the regard, respect, and concept of self held by person about self and as a family member

3. Between family relationships and experiences that promote positive mental health behaviors in members *and* peer or work group relationships and experiences that promote questionable or deviant life styles, behaviors, and values

4. Between social norms and standards and cultural values and beliefs that guide role, functions, and behaviors in the family setting *and* the beliefs and behaviors that guide roles, functions, and behaviors in peer, work, and play groups in school, employment, and leisure settings

5. Between employer's conception of work as primarily product production *and* the worker's conception of work as a social experience in which product production occurs

6. Between organization and management of school environments on the basis of personal development of people and the acquisition and discovery of knowledge and of work environments on the basis of product production *and* the need to organize these settings and their activities to also contribute to the development and maintenance of mental and physical health of students and workers

7. Between satisfactions and dissatisfactions of workers about the conditions of their employment *and* satisfactions and dissatisfactions about conditions relative to personal and family relationships and experiences

8. Between need for children and young adults to develop and master personal, interpersonal, and social competencies with peers *and* the provision of such opportunities in school settings primarily on the basis of scheduled and structured activities

9. Between need for workers to develop a concept of work in terms of the related peer social and group experiences *and* the bureaucratization of relationships in the work place to accommodate the mechanization of the tools of production in order to achieve the goals of capitalism

10. Between need for workers to make commitments to employment roles, functions, and expectations *and* the need to accommodate such commitments when they conflict with roles, functions, and expectations of workers in family situations

11. Between need to help young adults effect the separation from parental and family influences in order to establish their own identity, independence, and autonomy in work roles *and* the need for them to remain connected to family, community, and peer groups in order to maintain continuity between the past, present, and future

12. Between need for adult family members to recognize and restructure personal and career expectations and goals as the family structure changes *and* developing the competencies to handle changes in relationships and roles that occur when new and different directions are embarked on

Interrelationships in Daily Living Groups

The primary groups in which individuals hold membership in community living, schools, and employment settings and for conduct of leisure activities have major influences on the social, emotional, and mental health of people. Achievements, personal satisfactions, and personal worth are validated by peer groups from all these settings. Recognition and reward from these sources complement those provided by the family.

Schools and Work Settings

Schools are major socialization as well as educational settings. It is in these settings that the child and young adult learns many of the developmental tasks and skills necessary for assuming adult roles and responsibilities. Children also need to learn social competencies such as concern for others, how to compete, how to use collaboration and cooperation to gain both individual and group goals, and how to experience the joy of group support and acceptance and the pain of group rejection. These competencies need to be learned and tested through interactions with both compeers and adults. The ways in which school settings are structured have a great deal to do with whether the child and young adult learn the kinds of things these learning milieus are ideal to provide.

At the same time that social competencies are being learned and tested through interactions with other people, the child and young adult must also experience personal growth and self-actualization. With each passing year, children and young adults increase their awareness and perception of their personal self and worth. They have to learn to function as both members of groups and as individuals in order to experience a sense of their potential as human beings.

The philosophy that schools hold about their role in the mental and emotional development of their students is important for both parents and students to know. The establishment of a milieu in which the application of appropriate concepts to promote the acquisition of knowledge and to enhance personal growth and development of students in classrooms and related activities is a major concern. Schools need to pay special attention to the promotion of emotional, mental, and physical health as well as provide for the rehabilitation and special learning needs of exceptional and handicapped children.

The college experience is in many ways a profound change for young adults. It is usually experienced in both positive and negative ways. Most of us can remember experiences that happened to us when we entered college and can still recall how uncertain and anxious we were during the first few weeks. The task of managing so many new and different situations in college can be quite overwhelming. College is often the first experience in which young adults have to assume so much personal responsibility and make so many decisions on the basis of their judgment and knowledge.

The young adult has many personal and social competencies that have to be developed further through interactions with young adults and authority figures other than their parents. Enhancement of the ability to function comfortably and effectively in peer and other kinds of groups continues. This enhancement occurs by testing competencies in different kinds of settings with peers of different sexes who hold different values and beliefs and who have different cultural, social, and racial traditions and life styles. Another ability that needs further development is for young people to become self-directive of their behavior, especially when there are conflicts with peer group values and expectations. The experience of standing alone against a crowd or group in defense of one's principles and beliefs is a major achievement. There is also the need to experience the establishment of meaningful adult relationships with persons of the opposite sex. And last, learning to relate in positive and growth-promoting ways with authority figures, other than one's parents, is a necessity if the world of work is not to be a series of troublesome and stressful experiences.

The use of criticism is a major competence that needs to be enhanced during adult years. A major aspect of using criticism is to help young adults realize that a person's behavior and performance is valued in both positive and negative aspects. In relation to the negative aspects, this does not mean that the individual as a person—as a human being—is negatively valued. The tendency of people to personalize criticisms of performances and behavior into criticisms of self creates a major difficulty in making a distinction between the two. Such a distinction is usually first experienced as a feeling of threat. This feeling of threat to self through criticism then has to be tested repeatedly in different life experiences before the separation of criticism of behavior and criticism of person occurs. For many people, this distinction may never happen. Criticism of behavior evokes feelings of anxiety in most people and causes a lowered feeling of self-esteem, but these effects can be offset if the person is helped to realize the place of evaluation as part of his or her total performance and shown how criticism can be used to increase self-regard.

Before joining the work force as a gainfully employed adult, individuals form peer groups of various kinds in school settings. These range in purpose and change over time depending on age, sex, and educational and career goals. In some phases of development, peer group values and expectations about behavior have more influence on a person than those expressed by the family. These peer group relationships also influence the social, emotional, and mental health of group members.

Once formal study in basic educational programs is completed or ended, the world of work becomes of primary importance to adults. The kind of job, the rewards related to it in the form of position, title, salary, benefits, and the chances of upward mobility are major indicators of status, prestige, and economic rewards. These factors all influence a person's self-identity as well as the social and work relationships that may develop in relation to work roles.

The position a person occupies in the work structure organizes to a large extent the structure of his or her work setting. Position sets up certain expectation about performance for both the worker and the employer. The influence of the work setting goes far beyond the actual situation of employment as the relationships and common interests that are developed between workers often lead to the establishment of meaningful relationships outside the work setting. For example, leisure activites bring workers together around such things as ball teams, bowling groups, and boating clubs.

Working adults spend more waking hours a day in work settings than they do in family settings when all family members are present. Thus, the stabilization of adult personalities, a major function of the family, is also related to the work experiences formed and maintained on the job.

Once a person has joined the work force, the settings in which employment takes place and the interactions that occur contribute significantly to his or her health and mental health as an employee. Sarason (1977) described the experience of work as a development, a flow of experiences, that has distinctive and varied qualities. The experience of work is a complicated and changing picture and testifies to the continuous interactions between the individual and environmental conditions. Furthermore, the work experience is a shaper of life yet as a "product" is shaped by the worker. Dewey (1934) noted that an intelligent mechanic engaged in his job, interested in doing well and finding satisfaction in his handiwork, and caring for his tools and materials with genuine affection is artistically engaged. The difference between such a worker and the inept and careless bungler is as great in the shop as it is in the studio. Dewey also noted that when work experiences bring fulfillment to the worker, these experiences become integrated within the general stream of experiences but are set apart from other experiences in that they have a special quality.

Leisure activities and related interrelationships with peers who have common interests represent a dimension of life experiences that both children and adults need. Membership in various leisure activities and kinds of clubs, teams, and troops have the potential for providing a wide variety of novel experiences with people whom one ordinarily would not meet. This is true because the nature of participation is on the basis of personal interests rather than on roles and functions associated with work or family settings, educational credentials, or professional orientations.

The interrelationships between school and work experiences, family life, and leisure activites are key connections that relate to the mental and emotional health of people. It is simply not possible to understand what happens in a family or other kind of primary group in which daily personal living activities occur without understanding the impact of work experiences on the worker and the persons close to him or her. In his book on working, Terkel (1972) observed that work, by its very nature, is violent to the spirit as well as to the body. The interviews that he conducted with workers vividly portray a search for daily meaning in work as well as earning financial benefits. The impact of the physical aspects of work settings and the social experiences that occur provide a graphic picture of how these affected the health and mental health of workers.

Groups for Correctional Mental Health Experiences

Concepts

1. Groups of patients and staff in mental hospitals, psychiatric units in general hospitals, specialized psychiatric services in retreats and homes, and psychiatric facilities in penal institutions
2. Situational contexts of such experiences
3. Philosophy of mental health care and treatment as held by the institution or specialized unit
4. Structure of the organization of professional psychiatric care for 24 hours a day
5. Provision in ward milieus for patients to test reality and express feelings with professionals who can make these experiences therapeutic
6. Organization of institutional milieu to facilitate social and personal learning and control of behavior
7. Roles and functions of families and friends of patients in psychiatric care and treatment plan
8. Organization of the total institution or organization of special unit(s) within the context of an organization that has a different general mission to achieve the special mission
9. Resources available for the institution or specialized unit to carry out its assigned mission
10. Community contacts, relationships, and resources that can be made available to assist the institution to achieve its goals
11. Social and cultural influences that impinge on psychiatric treatment goals and community life of persons recovered from mental and emotional illnesses

Interrelationships

1. Between philosophy of mental illness, professional psychiatric nursing care, and psychiatric treatment of patients *and* social organization of the psychiatric setting to provide such care

2. Between psychiatric and medical science explanations for psychiatric illness *and* more comprehensive explanations that include psychological, social, cultural, and behavioral concepts and research

3. Between opportunities for groups of patients in ward milieus to experience responsibilities for the behavior of all members in the group *and* opportunities that focus on self-actualization, personal responsibility, self-autonomy, and individual growth

4. Between a care and treatment emphasis that focuses on social roles and learning new behaviors oriented toward community living and employment *and* one that focuses on the development of individual insights and resolution of individual intrapsychic conflicts

5. Between organization of the ward milieu, to delineate differences between staff, and patient roles *and* an organization that uses daily living activities in ward settings for staff and patients as group learning situations

6. Between unique psychological needs of individuals in psychiatric settings *and* social and cultural needs for group identity and development of a sense of common sharing

7. Between the exercise of authority and social control mechanisms in psychiatric settings by administration *and* the exercise of patients of their rights at the risk of criticism to the institution

8. Between kind and seriousness of mental and emotional illnesses experienced by mental patients *and* their need for both humanistic and specialized psychiatric care and treatment

9. Between role and involvement of the family in the care and treatment of its hospitalized member *and* posthospitalization entry of the member into meaningful family, personal, and social roles and relationships

10. Between being labeled as a patient who needed mental hospitalization *and* the personal and social consequences of this label on reentry to family and community life and living

11. Between integration of community networks, resources, and relationships in the psychiatric plan of care *and* the use of these to help patients develop social competencies necessary to return to own communities as productive citizens

12. Between community perceptions of what mental illness means in terms of personal, social, and employment relationships *and* potential for establishing meaningful experiences in community living and work

Corrective Mental Health Experiences

A person has to be medically diagnosed and/or legally labeled as having an emotional or mental illness in order to be hospitalized for care and treatment. Once this process occurs, the personal and group experiences that mental patients have in corrective treatment settings exert a profound influence on the learning of new social and interpersonal behaviors, and values.

The interactions between mental patients and the staff who provide care and treatment determine to a large extent the kind and degree of behavior used both by staff and patients for coping with daily living situations and activities. This principle of interaction has been found to be valid in a number of institutional settings. They include total institutions (Goffman, 1961); therapeutic communities (Jones, 1953, 1976); community mental health centers (Sarason, 1977); and long-term care facilities (Kramer & Kramer, 1976; Stryker, 1980)

The organization of psychiatric treatment settings has also been found to have both direct and indirect effects on patient and staff behavior. The way in which ward milieus are organized also influences the availability and kinds of learning opportunities.

Psychiatric care and treatment settings tend to be organized and managed primarily on the basis of professional ideology and patterns of practice of the professional staff, particularly psychiatrists. Because the dominant orientation of psychiatry in this country continues to be based on a psychology of conflicts within the individual, group experiences that provide daily living opportunities for patients to learn new behaviors and their meanings in social contexts are not usually considered to be a major modality of treatment. Much of the learning that takes place in milieus in mental hospitals and specialized mental health services focuses on adaptation to institutional routines and activities that often have little relation to specific posthospitalization goals of learning how to cope and adapt in interpersonal familial, peer, and work relationships.

The ideology that mental health professionals hold about the care and treatment of emotional and mental disorders severe enough to require hospitalization can be identified in a number of ways. Some of these are the organization of activities and relationships on the basis of staff and patient roles, the organization of the medical and nursing care plans on the basis of particular mental diseases, and the kinds of medical, social, and psychological therapies provided to patients.

Mental and emotional illnesses are known to have social, cultural, situational, and physical components as well as psychological ones. All of these have to be considered when a psychiatric nursing care plan is developed for providing direct services to patients with psychiatric problems. The organizing framework not only has to consider these aspects of psychiatric nursing care but also key interrelationships with familial and community systems in order to provide holistic psychiatric nursing. In this respect, each psychiatric nursing care plan needs to collect data on interrelationships that exist between the care setting, the families of patients, and the contexts of community living and gainful employment the recovered patient will reenter.

CLINICAL ORGANIZING FRAMEWORK: COMMUNITY AND SOCIAL NETWORKS

In community mental health nursing, the nurse has to collect data about community and social networks in which families, groups, and individuals are linked. Community networks are the groups, organizations, and services that are available in a community to meet the needs of the citizens and draw them together to address common concerns. Although formal relationships and linkages may not always be apparent between various services and support groups, these may be expressed through informal contacts.

Social networks are the social and interpersonal contacts that individuals, families, and groups have with other people and groups in a community. Such networks develop as social relations occur with different people who have different kinds of interests and occupations. The social relationships people have with one another have the capacity to reach out to many contacts, provide information about activities and things in a community, and be of assistance to people who need social, personal, and psychological support.

Community and social networks differ from community to community as to their kind, purpose, organization, and number. There are also differences in the amount of participation in such networks by individuals and families. The community mental health nurse needs a considerable amount of information about such participation in order to assist families to use resources for their benefit and to contribute to the mental health of the community.

In some communities, services and help groups are listed in a directory. In smaller communities, ministers, older citizens, and officials are valuable informants about services that are available and people who will provide assistance.

Data about participation in social networks provide a base for determining whether families, clients, or groups are social isolates, minimally involved in community activities and concerns, or have a sense of community as an integral part of their perspective of life and living. The use of community resources is an important part of community living, yet many families are not aware of these resources. If they know of resources and activities, they do not use or participate in them for many reasons. Participation in community activities and groups is a major pathway by which support services and systems are mobilized to assist stressed and distressed families, groups, and individuals.

The sense of pride and identity held by the patient, her or his family, or significant other about their community is important information. Social and cultural values, traditions, and standards of public behavior differ within and between communities. Different ethnic and racial groups add to this diversity. Therefore, it is important to obtain information about whether the family is relatively isolated within the community or whether there are fundamental disagreements about life in the community that will have an impact on the extent a family can and will seek social support.

The importance of obtaining information about traditional values and how these are implemented in family and community settings can be appreciated by examining the practice of child abuse. In U. S. culture, the child is accorded a special value. Growth, development, and self-actualization of the child have a high priority. For a culture that highly values its children, it is indeed paradoxical to find a high rate of family violence and conflict that all too often focuses on a child or children. Child abuse and misuse are major public and mental health problems. Sociocultural attitudes and beliefs that child abuse is not acceptable may be interpreted by violence-prone families as interference and interpreted to mean that acceptance of certain behaviors by children are condoned by law. Whatever the case, the community mental health nurse needs to obtain information about family beliefs and values and how these are expressed in familial relationships in order to get a sense of how psychological and physical abuse of family members are perceived and experienced by the victims.

SUMMARY

A clinical organizing framework organizes clinical practice applications and is based on the conception of community mental health nursing. The purpose of the framework is to help link theory and practice and to guide the applications of the concepts and princiiples from the theory. An approach for establishing such a framework uses boundary setting and organization of key interrelationships into general sets. These sets characterize important interrelationships in groups of various kinds.

Relationship sets are established for primary socialization groups and daily living groups such as those found in employment and school settings. A third set of relationships is identified for corrective mental health experiences that are organized for persons in psychiatric settings who have serious emotional and mental health problems. Community and social networks link experiences within groups and to groups in other settings and activities. Principles of systems theory integrate the different levels of systems in order to obtain coherence between the many aspects of the conceptual framework and clinical applications.

The sets of interrelationships are used to organize the assessment process and structure therapeutic counseling for both preventions and interventions. These interrelationships consider many of the basic dilemmas that exist between group and individual needs and that have to be managed in a constructive way for groups to be maintained and provide support and for members to achieve self-actualization and independence.

Together, the conceptual framework and clinical organizing framework provide a basis for developing clinical practice applications of many kinds. Such structures are necessary whenever a holistic concept of nursing is being implemented because of the great number of concepts and relationships that have to be taken into consideration.

REFERENCES

Barnhill, Laurence, Healthy family systems. *Family Coordinator* 28:94–100, January, 1979.

Buckley, Walter. *Sociology and Modern Systems Theory.* Englewood Cliffs, NJ: Prentice-Hall, 1967, pp. 11–23.

Dewey, John. *Art as Experience.* New York: Minton, Balch, 1934, pp. 5 and 35.

Goffman, Erving. *Asylums.* Garden City, NY: Doubleday, 1961, pp. 5–6.

Havens, Lester L. Clinical methods in psychiatry. *Psychotherapy and Social Science Review* 17(4):16–21, February 5, 1973.

Hess, Robert D., and Handel, Gerald. *Family Worlds: A Psychosocial Approach to Family Life.* Chicago: University of Chicago Press, 1959, pp. 1–19.

Hoeffer, Beverly M. Family therapy and nursing practice. In Kalkman, Marion, and Davis, Ann, eds. *New Dimensions in Mental Health–Psychiatric Nursing.* New York: McGraw-Hill, 1980, pp. 557–559.

Jones, Maxwell, *Maturation of the Therapeutic Community.* New York: Human Sciences Press, Behavioral Publications, 1976, pp. 87–188.

Jones, Maxwell. *The Therapeutic Community.* New York: Basic Books, 1953.

Kalkman, Marion, and Davis, Ann. *New Dimensions in Psychiatric Mental Health Nursing.* New York: McGraw-Hill, 1972, p. xi.

Kramer, Charles H., and Kramer, Jeanette. *Basic Principles of Long-Term Care: Developing a Therapeutic Community.* Springfield, IL: Charles C. Thomas, 1976.

Lazar, Joan Marie, and Shapiro, Gloria Edelhauser. Working with families. In Burgess, Ann W., ed. *Psychiatric Nursing in the Hospital and Community.* Englewood Cliffs, NJ: Prentice-Hall, 1981, pp. 431–447.

Lewis, Jerry M., Beavers, W. Robert, Gossett, John T., and Phillips, Virginia. *No Single Thread: Psychological Health in Family Systems.* New York: Brunner/Mazel, 1976, pp. 199–217.

Nagel, Ernest. *The Structure of Science.* New York: Harcourt, Brace, and World, 1961, pp. 393–397.

Osborne, Oliver. A theoretical basis for the education of the psychiatric–mental health nurse. *Nursing Clinics of North America.* 5:699–712, 1970.

Otto, Herbert. Criteria for assessing family strengths. *Family Process* 2:329–338, 1963.

Pearlin, Leonard, Lieberman, Morton A., Managhan, Elizabeth G., and Mullan, Joseph T. The stress process. *Journal of Health and Social Behavior* 22:337–356, December, 1981.

Putt, Arlene M. *General Systems Theory Applied to Nursing.* Boston: Little, Brown, 1978, pp. 17–19 and 25.

Sarason, Seymour. *Work and Social Change*. New York: Free Press, 1977, pp. 20–21.

Stryker, Ruth. How to develop a therapeutic community. *Journal of Nursing Administration* 10(4):14–16, April, 1980.

Terkel, Studs. *Working*. New York: Pantheon Books, 1972, pp. xi–xxiv.

Walker, Lorraine, and Nicholson, Ruth. Criteria for evaluating nursing process models. *Nurse Educator* 5(5):8–9, September–October, 1980.

Williams, Ann W., Ware, John E., and Donald, Cathy A. A model of mental health, life events, and social supports applicable to general populations. *Journal of Health and Social Behavior* 22:324–336, December, 1981.

9 | COMPREHENSIVE COMMUNITY MENTAL HEALTH NURSING: ASSESSMENT

INTRODUCTION

The comprehensive community mental health nursing assessment is the broad plan by which data are collected about the emotional and mental health of families, clients, and communities and on which clinical decision making and management of nursing practice are based. The assessment is more than the collection and appraisal of data about selected aspects of behavior or factual information about life events and individual and family interactions. It is also an ongoing process in which interactions occur between the community mental health nurse and clients, and these interactions have therapeutic potential in and of themselves. They need to be considered as an important part of the process in which attitudes and behaviors of clients, families, and groups are examined and changed.

The comprehensive community mental health nursing assessment is a *nursing assessment*. It uses the sets of relationships in the clinical organizing framework for orientation. This framework in turn is based on the unique aspects of nursing, principles of community mental health nursing, concepts of mental health and related science principles, and research. As such, it includes not only life experience and behavioral data but also various kinds of interactive data on which nursing interventions and preventions are based. This base, in all its aspects, is very important because the interactive data represent a synthesis and summary of how clients cope, adapt, perceive their problems and situations, and view the nurse as a provider of therapeutic mental health services. Such data also provide feedback about the use of self by the community mental health nurse in the therapeutic process and the selection of appropriate nursing preventions or interventions, depending on the kind of clinical management clients may need for problematical situations.

Families and members as well as individual clients seeking community mental health care in clinics and centers characteristically participate in a traditional mental status assessment process that usually includes the following components: an intake interview in which basic biographical information is obtained and a clinical interview, which, among other things, elicits the client's perception of the mental or emotional problem that is being experienced. An initial mental status examination, collection of basic social and familial data, psychological testing and evaluation, psychiatric consultation, and a psychiatric social work assessment of social, familial, economic, and related conditions that may have a bearing on the mental health problem being experienced are usually a part of this intake process. If the need for special kinds of assessments, tests, or consultations is identified, these activities are conducted by an appropriate professional. This traditional approach to conducting a mental status assessment is based on the assumption that parts of this *general information base* can be obtained by professionals, paraprofessionals, technicians, or volunteers. More specialized parts of the assessment are conducted by mental health professionals in one of the core mental health disciplines of psychology, social work, or psychiatry.

Reiss (1980), in discussing pathways to assessing the family, called attention to differences in how assessments are paced, that is, the relationship between assessment and intervention. The traditional approach in pacing is based on the position that a thorough assessment be conducted before therapy activities are initiated.

Pacing of the community mental health nursing assessment is interactional and based on the assumption that assessment and development of relationships go hand in hand. Furthermore, it is assumed that a firm therapeutic relationship cannot be established until there is experiencing of the therapist by clients and a decision is made by them whether to develop a therapeutic process. Descriptive data and data collected in response to use of self by the nurse provide information and a perspective of functioning that is not likely to evolve in the assessment except through an ongoing interaction process.

It is quite possible that by the time a comprehensive community mental health nursing assessment is completed, the changes that have occurred as a result of ongoing interactions have helped clients to determine whether and what kind of a therapeutic relationship is needed on a continuing basis. This is especially true for healthy functioning and stressed family systems because both kinds are flexible, have many strengths, and have access to various kinds of resources both within and outside family systems.

At this point, it should be noted that the usual mental status examination does not routinely include a component that requires specialized nursing knowledge obtained from a *community mental health nursing assessment*. Yet, psychology, social work, and psychiatry routinely contribute a component of specialized knowledge to the mental health assessment process. In fact, such assessments are not considered complete until these disciplines provide information and recommendations that are based on their unique contributions to mental health care. It is indeed ironic that after the mental health team has decided on a diagnosis and clinical management plan, the implementation of the plan is often delegated to the community mental health nurse. In this respect, it is well to point out that there are major differences between a comprehensive community mental health nursing assessment and a mental health assessment or examination in which the community mental health nurse conducts one of the general components that can be conducted by any one of a number of mental health professionals or paraprofessionals.

One of the complexities of the community mental health nursing assessment is the multiplicity of levels of communication that occur in the process. Only selected aspects of verbal and nonverbal communications can be attended and clarified; this means that many aspects are not attended and even ignored. However, both attended and non-attended communications, feelings, and areas of information influence the ongoing assessment process. They relate to the information provided and the satisfaction that clients feel about the kind and quality of mental health care being received. It is neither possible nor desirable to try to attend to all the things that occur and unfold in the assessment. Because of this reality, the community mental health nurse has to use a conceptual framework to assist in the selection of basic and important communications and areas of information on which to focus in the limited amount of time that is usually available. Furthermore, the nurse should keep in mind that although it is important to obtain sufficient and relevant information in the assessment, it is equally important to begin the establishment of a relationship that will serve as the base for continued counseling should this be needed by the family or client.

In the comprehensive community mental health nursing assessment, relationships between the nurse and clients need to be regarded as being very special and requiring particular attention. The assessment can be organized so that relationships can develop and the necessary data collected. Of importance is the use of a holistic approach that helps to maintain the continuity between the various life experiences of clients. In this approach, the community mental health nurse becomes an integral part of the wholeness of the assessment experience and subsequent counseling ones. This conception of the comprehensive community mental health assessment assumes that the whole of life experiences is more than the sum of the various parts of an assessment process.

PURPOSES

The comprehensive community mental health nursing assessment is an integral part of the clinical process of nursing practice and, as previously noted, has therapeutic qualities in its own right. In this most human of relationships, the nurse has opportunities to demonstrate the application of humanistic and scientific nursing concepts that are the hallmark of caring and competent community mental health nursing care.

The comprehensive community mental health nursing assessment has four major purposes. First, a mental health data base has to be obtained about the emotional and mental health of families, of the relevant groups in which members spend a considerable amount of their time and energy in the process of daily living, and of members as individuals. This data base includes basic biographical, personal, social, psychological, and familial information. Second, a data base has to be established about the "mental health" of the community as an integral aspect of the interdependent systems that families and clients live and work in. Third, a nursing data base has to be collected that uses principles of community mental health nursing and nursing to obtain the kinds of necessary data on which to base clinical nursing practice. Fourth, the assessment process has to generate interest and motivation in people to be responsive to their own health and mental health needs in ways that promote the establishment of helping and caring relationships.

It is important for the community mental health nurse to understand the purposes of the community mental health nursing assessment in order to ensure that relevant and adequate data are collected and an appropriate relationship is developed. Furthermore, both a general mental health and a special nursing data base have to be secured and then synthesized into a community mental health nursing practice framework. The purposes of the community mental health nursing assessment as identified may be different from those to which many nurses are accustomed; therefore, it may be necessary for some reorientation to occur in relation to role and perception about assessment. This reorientation is most useful when the assessment is presented as an important and integral part of the therapeutic process and essential for professional practice of community mental health nursing.

ASSUMPTIONS

The community mental health nursing assessment is based on several assumptions. They serve as a basis for application of nursing principles and counseling approaches. The first assumption is that the comprehensive community mental health nursing assessment differs in a number of respects from the traditional mental status examination. One difference is that data are collected using a nursing perspective. This means that data are collected that are needed to provide community mental health nursing as well as data about the mental health problems of clients.

A second difference is that the assessment embodies a holistic, interactional, and caring process. This process is different from the fragmented one that characterizes the conduct of mental status assessments in most service settings. Assessments usually include several kinds of activities that are usually conducted in sequence by different professionals, clinicians, and technicians, most of whom have various kinds of specialized knowledge and skills. Emphasis is usually on the problem of the client or patient who initiated the action to seek assistance. This emphasis includes an in-depth exploration of why this client feels, thinks, functions, believes, and acts as she or he does. After a considerable amount of information has been collected about these specific matters and psychological tests of various types conducted, the data are assembled so that a team of mental health workers can evaluate the material and arrive at a tentative diagnosis and treatment plan for the individual.

A third difference that makes the community mental health nursing assessment distinct is the inclusion of information about physical as well as mental health and relationships between these aspects as they are reflected in symptoms and daily living problems. In addition, nurses have a unique knowledge and experience base for working with families and clients in groups in community settings. People who experience health care problems and have difficulty managing themselves and coping with others are in situations that create stress and have a potential to cause emotional and mental health problems. The community mental health nurse knows and understands these interrelationships between psychosocial, physical, and familial factors and their influence on mental and emotional health.

These three differences between the community mental health nursing assessment and the traditional mental status examination or mental health assessment have an intermingling effect that creates the fourth difference: The data collected is different in kind, quality, and process. Cues are picked up and explored as the nurse makes connections between the bits and pieces of physical, social, mental, and familial information that is provided. These connections are made because of the comprehensive health and mental health orientation the nurse holds, the clinical experiences in which the nurse has routinely learned to integrate concepts and behavior that relate mental and physical health, and the role of the nurse that has integral to it considerable flexibility for exploring the various dimensions of mental health in different settings and at different times. The social and professional aspects of the role of the nurse permit a considerable amount of leeway in the conduct of the community mental health nursing assessment and the therapeutic use of self. The differences in process and data collected make the community mental health nursing assessment *an assessment counseling process.*

A second assumption of the community mental health nursing assessment is that the data base has two distinct components: primary and secondary. The primary data base component focuses on the information needed to provide community mental health nursing. This data base includes information about a range of experiences and goes beyond data usually collected in a mental status examination to include information about different social settings such as the clinic, home, school, and work settings and interrelationships between and within different primary groups in which clients live, work, go to school, and play. Data are also collected in natural living situations, such as the family in interaction in daily living activities. Health and illness information and the interactions between mental health and physical health are explored. Changes in roles and responsibilities of members in families and groups have to be considered when a member becomes ill, dies, or has to recover from an extended illness as well as the influence these have on the status and position of the family and its members.

Data about usual and unusual life events and daily living situations are also included in order to identify and understand coping modes and patterns of adaptation and expectations and beliefs about mental health and mental illness. The ways in which all of these factors come together form *patterns in life experiences* for the people who are involved.

The secondary data base includes information from various kinds of tests, psychiatric mental status examinations, illness and psychiatric treatments, social and economic data, and law enforcement data. Psychiatric consultation information, recommended treatment modalities, and tentative diagnoses are included in the secondary data base.

The comprehensive community mental health nursing assessment needs two kinds of data bases because the primary data base is necessary for planning and implementing community mental health nursing, whereas the secondary data base broadens and complements this basic nursing data base and provides specialized information about particular problems. Community mental health nursing has to be provided to clients who need such services irrespective of whether the secondary data base is available. The secondary data base enhances and validates the primary one and is inadequate as the sole base for community mental health nursing.

The primary data base needed for community mental health nursing may be compared in terms of comprehensiveness to the primary data base of the other three core mental health disciplines: psychology, psychiatric social work, and psychiatry. Psychology drives its primary data base from tests of personality, mental status, and cognitive functioning as well as behavioral indicators that signify the handling of personal and life experiences with significant others. These data are based on and interpreted through use of some theory of personality or behavior. In mental health, psychodynamic theories of behavior continue to be the major conceptual framework for such interpretations. Clinical management focuses on therapies and strategies developed and used primarily by psychology. This data base is relatively selective because of the narrow range of psychological concerns that fall within the professional and legal domain of this discipline. Psychiatric social work has long been concerned with particular aspects of social and family life contributing to emotional and mental problems of individuals and families. This subspecialty of social work has relied heavily on psychodynamic theories of behavior as the basis for psychiatric social work, interpretation of data, and psychiatric case management. Thus, the data base for psychiatric social work tends to be restricted and oriented to information and intervention strategies that characterize traditional psychiatric treatment modalities in psychiatry.

Psychiatry tends to conceive of mental and emotional problems as illness of the psyche. For the most part, this discipline uses psychodynamic theories of behavior to diagnose and interpret behavior associated with mental and emotional illnesses. Clinical management is based on the medical model of illness and includes medical treatments such as pharmacological products and somatic treatments such as electric shock and psychosurgery. Therapeutic relationships may be established; however, these are usually augmented by use of various kinds of drug therapies.

Of the four core mental health disciplines, community mental health nursing is the only one that needs and uses a comprehensive data base from which to plan and implement clinical practice. It is also the discipline that tries to implement clinical services from the perspective that the life experiences of people who have mental and emotional problems have to be considered in terms of their multidimensionality and essential wholeness. Furthermore, community mental health nursing is also the only mental health discipline that characteristically uses professional roles to move from institutional to community settings, from families to individuals, and from families to groups to provide caring and counseling services as an essential part of professional nursing practice.

A third assumption underlying the community mental health nursing assessment is that it needs to be conducted by a health professional, rather than a human services professional, who can take into consideration the unified aspects of mental and physical health, provide holistic health care, and move from one setting to another to observe and participate with families and groups in daily living environments. Community mental health nursing and psychiatry are the two mental health disciplines that have had professional education and clinical training in health, illness, mental health, and mental illness. Professionals from these fields are the ones who have had clinical experiences involving observations, assessments, and therapeutic interventions that have been developed and tested in clinical management in a variety of health and illness experiences. The doctor–patient relationship, however, has developed in ways that make it a time-limited and structured encounter that focuses on selected aspects of medical concerns about mental and emotional problems. Moreover, there is an implicit assumption in the medical model of mental illness that assessment is primarily for data collection and the relationship that is established after the assessment is completed is what is important because that is when therapeutic work takes place.

The mental health professional of choice to conduct comprehensive mental health assessments is the professionally educated and competent community mental health nurse. As noted, this assertion is made in part because of the kind of professional training and education nurses receive. But most of all, this view is held because of the perspective of nursing that orients the nurse to be a warm, expressive, and caring helping professional who is concerned about the many aspects of the health experiences of families, clients, and related groups and who participates in working on these concerns. The social and professional roles of the nurse make the content and process of the clinical nursing practice unique. This uniqueness is present because community mental health nursing is based on different assumptions and focuses on different and more comprehensive aspects of emotional and mental health functioning.

The fourth assumption underlying the community mental health nursing assessment is that the nursing perspective, nursing roles, and nursing functions have been developed by nursing for clinical nursing practice. This assumption questions the practice of nursing in mental health of using roles, strategies, perspectives, and processes developed by other mental health disciplines without reconceptualizing these to incorporate nursing theory, roles, and perspectives.

Clinical nursing based on a structure of nursing relationships and roles facilitates the inclusion of the unique aspects of nursing, the application of principles of community mental health nursing, and the use of "borrowed" basic science and practice concepts that expand and extend community mental nursing practice. Judicious "borrowing" of such concepts does not warp the essential structure of nursing and practice in community mental health nursing. This warping happens only when there is adoption of the models of mental health practice from other disciplines to the extent that the very essentials of nursing are denied or ignored as not having value in community mental health nursing.

A fifth and final assumption underlying the community mental health assessment is that family and group functioning needs to be observed and participated in by the community mental health nurse in both organized care and natural social settings. Families and primary socialization groups tend to function by using their characteristic patterns of roles, responsibilities, communications, and coping in their natural environments. In other settings, these important aspects may be altered in ways that members are not aware of because of social settings. Data from other kinds of peer groups, such as those at work and school, may be collected from respondents through direct observations if these are appropriate and pose no consequences of stigmatic labeling of individuals, or in simulations and role-playing of vicarious experiences, and through descriptions by the persons involved.

CONCEPTUAL FRAMEWORK

The conceptual framework of the community mental health nursing assessment guides its application and determines the structure of the appraisal, the organization of data and relationships, and the kind of information collected and manner of collection. It also guides the therapeutic use of self in data collection and related interactional processes, the interpretation of data, the kinds of nursing interventions and preventions that may be used with clients, and the criteria used for determining the effectiveness of therapeutic nursing interventions.

It is important to understand the relationship between concepts of emotional and mental health and the indicators, or criteria, by which it is to be judged. The conceptual framework sets the particular criteria from which judgments are made about mental and emotional health as well as the kinds of data that are needed in order to make such judgments. Francis and Munjas (1976) identified this establishment of norms by which behavior is to be measured as "a low-visibility first step" in the assessment process. These experienced clinicians in mental health nursing practice emphasized the relationship between concepts of mentally healthy behavior and the standards or criteria by which it is to be judged. For example, they cited the example of Fromm (1955) who identified a mentally healthy person as one who is productive and unalienated, able to deal with reality objectively, experiences himself or herself as a unique person, loves others and holds common feelings of brotherhood, accepts rational authority, is open to new experiences throughout life, and enjoys life and living as a precious gift.

Another example of the connection between concepts of mental health and criteria for making judgments is that proposed by Jahoda (1958). From a social psychological perspective of mental health for individuals, she postulated six criteria as indicators of mental health: a balance of psychic forces, self-actualization, resistance to stress, personal autonomy, mastery of environment, and accurate perceptions of reality.

In brief, the conceptual framework of community mental health nursing focuses on mental health of families, primary groups, and communities. The mental health of individuals is inextricably intertwined with family health and is considered in the context of social settings and group milieus.

The social psychological model of mental health presented in Table 3.5 guides the organization of the community mental health nursing assessment. Of major importance are family systems as the units through which system and member changes can occur. They are behavior settings naturally created to carry out major basic societal functions (Barker, 1968), and need not be artificially created in order to have mental health preventions and interventions. Family systems data include multidimensional phenomena that encompass physical, temporal, social, affective, and behavioral aspects of this environment and the people living in it.

It should be emphasized that although family systems are the level of organization for preventions and interventions, exclusive attention to just the family system and what goes on in its interior does not generate an adequate data base for community mental health nursing. This focus assumes that the patterns of interactions and communication processes within the family system are the determinants for much of the behavior of members. Such is not the case because these systems cannot stand in isolation from their larger social contexts. Hume and co-workers (1977) pointed out the inadequacy of focusing only on family systems when trying to understand their impact on the behavior of members.

In the conceptual framework, families that characteristically have healthy or adaptive relationships and socialization responses arc analogous to what Lewis (1980) called *optimal functioning families*. Such families are high in competence by virtue of providing a high level of emotional support and other kinds of resources and experiences that encourage the development of individuality and autonomy. Families that characteristically have stressed relationships and socialization responses put members at some risk of developing mental and emotional problems. Furthermore, the scope and effectiveness of coping responses in both kinds of systems are influenced by the kind and number of opportunities available for interactions. This conception of stressed families in the conceptual framework is similar to what Lewis (1980) described as *competent but pained families*.

Distressed families in the community mental health nursing framework are similar to the ones that Lewis (1980) identified as having dysfunctional and severely dysfunctional problems. Distressed families include those that have persistent and inflexible conflicts in family organization, structure, and relationships between parents, parents and siblings, and siblings and the family and social and behavioral norms and standards of society. Problems of violence, child and spouse abuse, and drug and alcohol abuse and mental, emotional, and behavioral problems of various kinds contribute to learning dysfunctional socialization responses. These make such family and other kinds of small group environments less able, if not incapable, of providing healthy growth-promoting experiences to help members promote positive mental health and achieve adulthood and selfhood.

ORGANIZATION OF THE COMPREHENSIVE ASSESSMENT

The organization of the comprehensive community mental health nursing counseling assessment is very effective when the community mental health nurse uses both theory and experience to guide nursing practice. In this respect, several useful guides are cited that will assist the nurse to organize the assessment process and therapeutic use of self.

It should be recognized that each clinical nursing session with clients, whether with families, groups, or individuals, has both complete and incomplete aspects. In a sense, each session is a complex and complete situation in which interactions occur and are sustained for a short while; at the same time, the session is incomplete and interactions end on a note of uncertainty for both the nurse and clients. The nurse is uncertain as to whether families, their members, or clients will want to return for continued counseling, and clients are uncertain as to whether they want to continue interactions that may develop into a therapeutic relationship.

In the assessment counseling relationship, as in all complex interactive situations, the overt focus of participants may be on one thing, whereas other things are going on at a covert level. In the assessment process, the overt focus is usually on the collection of data in order to ascertain the strengths of families, assess patterns and level of functioning, and identify concerns and potential problems. If problems are present, they have to be clarified as to kind, scope, and severity. At the same time, covert activities occur in which the nurse and clients size one another up, form impressions about what is happening, and sort out feelings and perceptions about the situation.

Interactions, the face-to-face encounters that people have with one another to achieve a limited goal, have to change in both purpose and process in order for a continuous therapeutic relationship to develop. Although the assessment counseling relationship focuses on information collecting, it is at this time that the base for future counseling is established.

Each assessment counseling session usually changes somewhat in focus. These changes occur in the process of examining the patterns of coping and problem solving in connection with both stressful and nonstressful situations and because of the kind of data being collected. As patterns are examined in relation to their effectiveness for handling frustration and stress in the family, certain roles and responsibilities of members are highlighted. As emotional and mental health tensions or problems in relationships are explored, there may be painful remembrances; however, since the entire family is involved in the counseling process, different emphases evolve in the different assessment counseling sessions.

In the assessment counseling process, data that arise in the course of interaction are used by nurse and clients, often without too much awareness; thus, nurse and clients do not recognize the influences of this data on the ongoing counseling process. Data generated on a face-to-face basis by nurse and clients are a source of immediate feedback and consist of several kinds of communications: expressions, gestures, body language, posture, perceptions, impressions, feelings, and problem-solving efforts. This feedback and related cues are used to judge what is happening in the face-to-face interaction and how to structure it. This important source of data, which is always emergent, has to be recognized by both nurse and clients and acknowledged with an intent to examine and use it in the service of the therapeutic activity.

An important guide for organizing the community mental health nursing assessment is to make sure that the wholeness of client–family or client–primary group experiences is not unduly fragmented. These experiences have to be considered in the context of community and social networks in which clients participate and through which support is received and provided to others. It is this wholeness of life experiences, as they are lived in different kinds of primary groups, that provides a picture of whether the needed resources for the development and maintenance of mental and emotional health for members are anywhere near adequate.

It should be clearly recognized that the base for the establishment of a helping relationship between the nurse and clients begins at the time of the first face-to-face contact. If the groundwork is not begun at this time, then the definition of the situation by clients may result in an appraisal that minimizes participation or makes them decide to terminate the situation as soon as possible. In this initial reaching-out encounter, connections between the community mental health nurse who provides the mental health service and clients who seek such service are vulnerable, fragile in commitment, and prone to termination. It is for these reasons that initial contacts and interactions with the nurse have to be of a special kind and quality in order to minimize premature termination on the part of clients and to establish a climate for a helping relationship.

Another guide that is useful for organizing the community mental health nursing assessment is for the nurse to conduct a rapid appraisal of the family, group, or client on the basis of inspection to determine whether the assessment counseling process can be started. Assessment may have to be delayed if clients, families, or group members are in life-threatening situations. Based on behavior, observations, and incomplete information, the community mental health nurse may have to make a clinical decision about the following conditions: (1) whether a psychiatric emergency exists; (2) whether there is a high probability of harm to self or others by a client or clients; and (3) whether client or clients are unable to care for self. If any one of these three conditions are present, the community mental health nurse usually has a psychiatric and medical emergency at hand. The actions that the nurse takes in such situations involve obtaining psychiatric and medical assistance as rapidly as possible, protection of life of clients, self, others as best as can be devised, and call for immediate assistance from other persons who can provide support and psychiatric nursing care. Because many psychiatric emergencies are in fact medical emergencies, the community mental health nurse plays a vital role in recognizing life and death situations and providing emergency nursing care.

Generally, if there is not a medical or psychiatric emergency, the comprehensive community mental health nursing assessment usually requires a minimum of four sessions in order to obtain an adequate base for assessment. One of these sessions needs to be conducted in the family or primary group socialization setting in which clients reside. The remaining sessions may be conducted in organized care settings. The nurse also needs to locate data about the community of clients and, when needed, arrange to use special assessment strategies such as role playing and simulations to obtain data about work and school situations.

INITIAL ASSESSMENT COUNSELING SESSION

In the initial assessment counseling session, the assembling of a basic data base is started (see Appendix III for assessment format). In this session, the establishment of a sense of concern and caring between clients and nurse is very important. The community mental health nurse may also have to provide some interventions, such as lowering anxiety levels, so that families can provide data without too much discomfort and distortion. This session, like subsequent sessions, will have a distinct character. This is true because of the emergent feelings, actions, thoughts, and memories that remembering and recalling events, relationships, and situations in response to particular questions can evoke. There are patterns of interactions, coping, and thinking that are unfolding. At the same time there are recurring patterns of behaviors, thoughts, and actions that ensure continuity from one session to the next. These patterns serve as a basis for continuing a therapeutic relationship in order to examine and change behaviors as necessary.

Rather than conceiving of the initial assessment session as an "intake interview," it is conceived of as the beginning of a therapeutic relationship that has special characteristics. Families have an option about whether they wish to participate in the session and continue to participate in additional sessions. A decision to continue in the assessment counseling process depends in large part on the sense of *being cared about* and a *perception of competency* on the part of the nurse. In order to establish trust, caring, and competency, it is helpful to remember that in the initial session the nurse and family members do not have a common frame of reference on which to start a relationship such as would be the case if the situation involved a past acquaintance, friend, or kinsman. Furthermore, at this time, it is not known whether the session in progress will be the only one but this possibility should always be kept in mind. This means that the nurse is responsible for achieving some closure about what has happened in each session before members depart. While recognizing the possibility that the family may not continue in counseling to the point of forming a therapeutic relationship, the nurse also needs to consider a related assumption that because a family has sought help it will continue in counseling if members believe they can obtain assistance.

In the first session, the assessment counseling process is initiated by establishing a frame of reference in which to collect needed information and to use interactive data as part of the data base. Auger (1976) described this part of the nurse–patient relationship as a composite of initial and extended interaction. Initial interactions are usually based on existing behavioral patterns and extended interactions expand from this foundation.

In general, the aim of the first session is to obtain basic information about families, members, or clients and to establish a sense of trust between the nurse and family members or clients. Basic information includes biographical, coping, social, and interactional data as well as a beginning evaluation of family strengths and mental health by interrelationships and mental health indicators of family or primary socialization group systems. The emotional and mental health concerns of members are important to identify and hear about in this session. To this end, the community mental health nurse:

1. Establishes a sense of caring and competency with clients by applying principles of nursing, community mental health nursing, and therapeutic use of self.
2. Obtains basic biographical information about clients relating to physical, personal, social, familial, and community relationships, problems, and experiences.
3. Obtains information about patterns of behavior used to handle stressful, unstressful, and crisis relationships and events relating to physical, mental, and emotional health and illness behaviors and identification of the situational contexts in which such patterns are used.
4. Establishes the identity of significant groups and community networks about which more information may be needed.
5. Identifies strengths, potential, concerns, and problems being experienced by members and what effects they are perceived as having on family and daily living activities, roles, relationships, and responsibilities.
6. Obtains definitions from members of family problem situations and information about how these have been handled and how they might be more effectively handled.
7. Reviews with clients their perceptions of what has gone on in the session to determine whether any new ideas or suggestions have evolved as a result of discussions and interactions.
8. Orients clients to information that will be needed and arranges for a visitation in the home or other domiciliary setting.
9. Informs clients of the possibility for referral to other mental health professionals if major problems are identified.

In the initial assessment session, information is obtained in ways that the session does not become a structured question-and-answer format. Rather, clients are provided with opportunities to respond to questions in ways that allow them to test their perceptions of what is being asked. Information about relationships and events in social contexts in which they have occurred has to be explored. When this approach is used, data are provided that give a wholeness to experiences rather than responses to specific questions. People usually know what brought them to a mental health professional, and if given the chance will provide significant kinds of information. Specific questions telegraph a message that the information being sought is important. When used to excess, specific questioning may send a message to clients that the problems and concerns they have do not seem as important as those which the questions posed by the nurse address. If the session is too structured, there will be too few opportunities for interactions to occur. In this circumstance, it would be difficult for the nurse to get a sense of how clients relate to others, or whether repetitive thoughts, feelings, and actions are expressed, or what the feelings are that are associated with different kinds of events and information.

As soon as possible in the assessment counseling process, families need to be oriented to the kinds of information the nurse needs. This orientation usually provides the opening for helping members to start participating in the assessment counseling session. In the first session, it is important that clients be helped to understand that family functioning, whatever its level, involves significant others, community and social networks, and daily living groups and activities. The purpose is to establish a frame of reference for assessment counseling that includes both the family and the groups in which living, working, and playing take place. Families are encouraged on the first visit to begin participation in problem solving by enlisting their assistance in planning the next counseling session, which may include significant others.

Sometimes an entire family will come or call for assistance with a mental health problem. When this happens, the community mental health nurse has to be concerned about the group both as an interacting social unit and as a source of obtaining information that all the members of the family may not be able to provide or need to know, particularly if some of the members are small children. In such a case, the nurse may elect to see the entire family initially and observe the interactions that emerge, get a sense of the roles of the adults and children, and hear what or who has been defined as the family's problem. It may be necessary to obtain more specific information from adult family members, particularly about marital and sexual relationships. However, before the family leaves the session, it is important to have all members assemble with the nurse to review their experience and decide how to proceed. During this review, additional information can be obtained about the expectations now held by the family and whether the things that the family wanted to have covered have been identified. This is an important part of the session for both the family and the nurse. The family has to make a commitment to continue into a therapeutic relationship if that seems necessary. The nurse has to convey her or his caring concern and orient the family to the additional information needed as well as convey the professional competency to conduct a relationship with the family that has the potential for helping the family.

Comprehensive mental health nursing assessments cannot be made on the basis of data collected in only one assessment counseling session. Such an assessment requires data from home visitation, community observation and information, participation of members in interaction, and peer group functioning. These data provide the base from which the community mental health nurse begins to get a picture of how members function in natural social, cultural, and community settings and daily living groups. Data about school and employment settings and peer group relationships are areas that have to be tactfully and carefully handled. In this respect, indirect approaches may be used because of the potential for creating labels of mental illness or emotional problems with peers, employers, and school personnel. For example, one indirect approach that is useful is to structure a peer group similar to one at work that a working member finds supportive and one that causes stress and frustration. Such sessions are often quite revealing about the kinds of relationships that affect families in positive and negative ways. Role playing and simulations of game playing may also be used to collect data about experiences in these settings.

The comprehensive mental health nursing assessment also needs to use the data about the "mental health" of the community in which families reside. Information is needed about participation in community activities and the kind and quality of life experiences provided by the community for children and adults to meet basic social, recreational, and health needs. The general economic status of the community, the primary social groups in which clients participate, the concerns held by people in the community, and the distribution of patterns of behavior as reflected by violence, apathy, and hopelessness have to be considered. The presence or absence of involvement of citizens in activities that might make the community a safer and better place to live provides an idea of how the community is perceived by people. The possibility of obtaining community involvement through support systems and activities needs to be explored.

A comprehensive mental health nursing assessment is ongoing and an update is done in each subsequent session. Although the first three or four assessment counseling sessions focus on the comprehensive assessment, counseling is always an integral part of this process.

Before the family and the community mental health nurse end the initial assessment counseling session, a considerable amount of basic biographical and interactive data will have been obtained. There is the need to establish rapport and obtain a commitment from members that they are interested in continuing the therapeutic process that has been established. Families need to understand that the assessment counseling process takes several sessions and that they will participate in making a decision about whether they want to establish a longer relationship.

SECOND ASSESSMENT COUNSELING SESSION

Before the first assessment counseling session draws to a close, the nurse summarizes major and minor events, relationships, strengths, and any problems that have been identified. The strengths of the family or primary socialization group and its members are important for the group to know and have validated. The nurse clarifies the need to meet in the home and makes the necessary arrangements for assessment to continue in this setting.

The second assessment counseling session is usually conducted in a natural social setting such as the home or wherever the primary socialization group resides. This part of the assessment counseling process is conducted when all members are present. Usually the best time to do this is in the late afternoon or on a weekend day.

The purpose of moving the assessment to the natural setting is to minimize the influence of new situations and settings on patterns of interactions used by people in order to get a sense of the usual roles, responsibilities, relationships, and communications. Smoyak (1975), in describing the psychiatric nurse as a family therapist, noted that because human beings are socialized within family systems to play their future societal roles, it is necessary to seek an understanding of the various styles and workings of these intricate systems as they affect the cognitive and emotional development of members. Smoyak considers the family's home the logical place for a first visit and very often uses this as the place of choice for subsequent therapy.

In general, the aim of the second assessment counseling session is to get a sense of how members function in family systems in their usual roles, responsibilities, and how

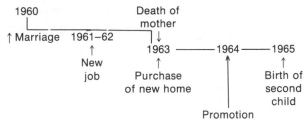

Figure 9.1
Social history: Significant events

patterns of communication evolve in the home setting. The nurse continues to develop trust and a sense of caring with clients as well as demonstrating her or his expertise and professional competency.

To achieve the objectives for the second assessment counseling session, the community mental health nurse:

1. Obtains a picture of the family or primary socialization group's social systems in interaction in the natural social setting.
2. Identifies some of the stated and unstated rules, norms, patterns of communication, and interrelationships that reflect the ways in which the family or primary socialization group functions.
3. Uses indicators of mental health to obtain information about specific relationships and roles between siblings and siblings and parents, particularly those in which members identify satisfaction as well as strain.
4. Obtains information on the community resources the family or primary socialization group may call on and the social networks in which they participate.
5. Maps the family system to get a clear picture of where all members "fit" in the age–role structure.
6. Obtains information about how the family or primary socialization group views its milieu in terms of safety, the availability of the necessities of life, and the resources that may be called on in times of increased need and support.
7. Judges overall family functioning in terms of potential for providing a milieu for emotional, cognitive, and social development of members.

The kind of information that the community mental health nurse finds useful is explained to the family in general terms. The indicators of mental and emotional health provide a guide to the kinds of information that are needed. Smoyak (1975) provided an account of how she approaches the family, obtains basic information, and draws inferences from the kinds of interactions that occur in the process of responding to questions.

Sedgwick (1981) used a more structured and traditional approach to interviewing families. She described an approach for organizing social and personal history events as data on them are obtained. A chronological social history diagram is constructed on which critical events, year of occurrence, and family members most involved are cited. Arrows that point upward indicate the events that family or a member identify as positive, whereas arrows turned downward show those experiences thought to be negative. An illustrative example of a map of significant events is shown in Figure 9.1.* The

* The figure is reprinted with permission from Rae Sedgwick. *Family Mental Health: Theory and Practice.* St. Louis: C. V. Mosby, 1981, p. 176.

schema lends itself quite readily to having family members construct a chronological social history for themselves. The nurse may ask the family as a group or as individual members to prepare a history and bring it to the third assessment counseling session.

THIRD ASSESSMENT COUNSELING SESSION

In the third assessment counseling session, the nurse reviews previous agreements and gets feedback about what has been happening with members. In this review process, information that has been remembered or developed since the previous session is considered. During the discussion that ensues, the nurse can usually get a good idea of whether members have been thinking about strengths, issues, concerns, or problems that were identified in previous sessions. There may have already been attempts to enhance strengths or modify and solve some of the concerns.

Over the time that will have elapsed between the first and third sessions, the family has usually "chewed over" the kinds of information they have provided and may be viewing relationships and roles in a different way. This reflection process, or "talking-back-to-self" phenomenon, can be used to determine how members now define the situation that motivated them to participate in an assessment. It is not surprising to find that in a relatively short time this inner dialogue with self and interactive exchanges with significant others may have resulted in some startling new ways of looking at situations. Families quite often identify certain actions that might be taken that would reduce strain, frustration, or produce a different way of handling relationships and suggest ways of using family strengths to better advantage.

In the interval between the first and third assessment counseling session, the community mental health nurse will have secured demographic data about the community in which the family lives. Such data is generally available from health systems agencies, health departments, mental health and health centers, and area health education centers. One reason why such data is generally available today is that they are part of required need assessments for new programs and grant applications. By the time of the third session, the nurse should have a reasonably good picture of the demographic, physical, social, and economic aspects of the community.

The general aim of the third assessment counseling session is to obtain additional data to round out the comprehensive data base and to determine the climate in the family or primary socialization group for making changes that are mutually agreed on as being desirable. To achieve objectives for the third assessment counseling session, community mental health nurse:

1. Validates with members their definition of the situation as it has evolved over the past two sessions.
2. Determines whether any actions have been taken to address the problematical or stressful situations uncovered in the assessment counseling process.
3. Obtains additional data that is needed for the comprehensive assessment on the basis of the nurse's review and indicate to members any referrals that the nurse thinks would provide additional data and information.
4. Continues interactions with the family in order to get a sense of how reality is tested in living and working situations.
5. Identifies repetitive coping patterns that are used to try to handle usual and crisis situations.

6. Identifies significant others who seem to be central to the strengths, concerns, and anticipated changes or problems in the family.
7. Makes a judgment about level of family functioning and mental and emotional health status of members as a basis for an appropriate plan of recommendations.
8. Assesses the strengths and potential of the family and its members to make changes in relationships, roles, and responsibilities that would promote and maintain the emotional and mental health of members.

One of the objectives of the comprehensive community mental health nursing assessment is to use the process itself in a therapeutic way. In the third session, the effects of this process can provide a considerable amount of information to the nurse. Such information ranges from an informal estimate of the commitment of clients to participate in a therapeutic relationship to one of how reality in the first and second sessions has been perceived by participants. These perceptions can be compared with the reality perceived by the nurse in order to arrive at a measure of congruence. For example, is there distortion or failure on the part of the family to acknowledge some of the verifiable things that have occurred in interactions? If so, the nurse may develop a tentative hypothesis that adaptive behaviors and coping strategies are stressed or that a persistent distortion seems to be related to certain relationships or situations. On the other hand, the assessment counseling process itself may have been adequate to help concerned families establish a perspective and balance and proceed to a more effective level of functioning. This kind of situation is not at all unusual today because of the willingness of people to accept that stress is a valid human experience and to seek counseling before major disruptive problems occur.

In the third assessment counseling session, the community mental health nurse orients the family to basic indicators of emotional and mental health for the families with adaptive functioning and for individuals. Because the indicators point to areas of emotional involvement and commitment about others, this assessment counseling session may be more unsettling to members than the ones in which basic biographical data were obtained.

In the third session, there may be changes in the interactions between the nurse and clients. Pent-up feelings may be expressed by various members that may come as a surprise to all concerned. What happens is that the inclusion of the community mental health nurse in the usual system of roles, responsibilities, and rules changes these enough to alter communication and interrelationship patterns and make these more open to a consideration of new aspects that members either could not or would not consider before. New information thus obtained can be used to get a different perspective on family interrelationships or primary social group system functioning and their potential for contributing to the emotional and mental health of members.

By the end of the third assessment counseling session, the community mental health nurse should have a fairly comprehensive data base about clients, their strengths and problems, their social and familial or group situation, and the socialization process as these relate to the stabilization of adult personalities and socialization of the young. The nurse reviews with the family its perceptions and evaluations of the assessment and counseling process.

Between the third and fourth assessment counseling sessions, the nurse has to pause in order to study the data, confer with others, and plan for the fourth session. Since a considerable amount of data will have been collected over the three assessment counseling sessions, these data must now be more completely organized by using the conceptual framework, and judgments must be made. This process is necessary in order to understand the problems, issues, and potential of the family to carry out its functions for its members. Use of the conceptual framework will also help the nurse make clinical decisions about recommendations.

The social psychological framework of mental health and mental illness helps in the organization of data. It focuses attention on primary socialization systems and daily living groups and their potential for providing growth and development across the life span for members. Special attention has to be paid to the development and maintenance of the emotional and mental health of individual members as they cope in family and daily living groups. Appropriate age–phase developmental and maturational tasks, basic social competencies and problem-solving skills, cognitive development, and the conduciveness of highly intense milieus to promote, develop, and maintain the mental and emotional health of members are major considerations. The models of adaptive, stressed, and distressed family profiles are also useful in organizing assessment data in order to make clinical judgments and decisions. The clinical organizing framework in which key interrelationships are specified is also used.

During the assessment process, the community mental health nurse encodes diverse kinds of information obtained from the family and its members. That is to say, the nurse converts very rapidly bits and pieces of information, feelings that seemed to be associated with different experiences, communication patterns, and information about interactions that occurred during the counseling assessment into working hunches and tentative conclusions as the assessment counseling process proceeded. An integral part of this pulling together is that the nurse has to include her or his own interactions and feelings as part of the therapeutic process.

During the encoding process, the nurse must make instantaneous decisions about what seem to be the key pieces of information, crucial experiences, and feelings and provide some direction to the members about additional information needed. This includes how members perceive what is happening to them and how they experience such happenings. This very complex and rapidly unfolding process requires competency and ability on the part of the community mental health nurse. Effectiveness in this therapeutic process is similar to that described by Benner (1982) for clinical practice at an expert level. At this level of competence, the nurse grasps situations as wholes, focuses accurately on problems, and operates from a deep understanding of the situation being described. It is recognized that students new to community mental health nursing cannot be expected to hold this level of clinical competence; however, faculty should be able to model such behavior and be able to assist students to evaluate their level of practice and progress to a higher one.

After each assessment counseling session, the community mental health nurse must organize the data as much as possible. In the pause between the third and fourth session, data have to be organized and evaluated in more depth. Themes have to be identified, patterns of communication and behavior recognized, and interrelationships studied. Clinical judgments based on examination of the data may be somewhat different from the rapidly formulated ones that were made during assessment. These judgments and hunches now have to be considered in terms of the conceptual framework and related to data. The framework helps the nurse to focus on key systems, behaviors, and relationships with the family system and between this system and other community contacts.

A useful way of sorting out assessment data and relating it to theory is to follow a set procedure, for example:

1. State concisely the conceptual framework used to guide the collection of data in the assessment

2. Organize data by using sets of essential relationships in whatever system is the focus; identify patterns of interaction, communications, and recurring events and experiences as well as usual patterns of coping

3. Identify themes that tie recurring experiences and patterns of interaction together and note if and how these change for handling unusual experiences

4. Organize the themes into related clusters of experiences, all of which have something in common

5. Relate the clusters of experiences to whatever theories of community mental health nursing, mental health, and family functioning are being used by the nurse.

6. Identify gaps in information and secure additional data as necessary

7. State evaluation of family functioning, strengths, and potential for promotion of mental and emotional health of members; support with assessment data from family, school, work, and community interrelationships and patterns of coping

8. Predict what you think will happen to the primary socialization system if concerns, issues, or problems identified are not addressed

9. Decide on appropriate nursing approach, that is, whether prevention, intervention, or referral is most appropriate; review appropriate strategies if the nurse is to provide clinical management

10. Validate with family your evaluation, clinical judgments, and recommendations

11. Determine whether family wants to continue to enhance strengths and release potentials, describe strategies and evaluation

12. Continue in a therapeutic relationship until goals are reached.

When preventions or interventions with family systems are indicated, the community mental health nurse needs to schedule further counseling sessions preferably in the natural family system setting. If referral is indicated, the nurse facilitates this process.

Some care needs to be exercised by the nurse so as to schedule mental health counseling sessions far enough apart that dependence on the nurse for answers and as an "on-call" source of support does not develop to any extent. In this kind of counseling, the approach is to foster independence and autonomy; the nurse facilitates the family handling their own concerns and problems. Although there is no set rule for how frequently mental health counseling should occur, sessions scheduled each week will probably create too much emotional intensity and foster dependence on the nurse. Just how frequently to meet with families is a clinical judgment the community mental health nurse has to make. It should be noted that the assessment counseling sessions are usually scheduled quite close together—as much as three times in one week—to complete the comprehensive assessment process. The nurse should be sensitive to the responses of families during this intense interaction period and note whether dependency behaviors start to develop. The assessment counseling experience may provide the best data about how frequent subsequent sessions need to be scheduled.

Once the data have been organized, the community mental health nurse enlists the suggestions and opinions of the mental health team as well as makes clinical decisions and recommendations about therapeutic nursing actions. Such recommendations may be either preventions or therapeutic interventions. After the mental health team has rendered their recommendations, the community mental health nurse decides on the therapeutic plan that is reviewed with families in the fourth counseling session.

FOURTH ASSESSMENT COUNSELING SESSION

The fourth session is essentially a counseling session. The general aim is to review with the family the results of the assessment, to determine areas of concern about which there may be a need for preventions or interventions, and to present recommendations for therapeutic activities.

In this session, it is not unusual to find that a considerable amount of problem-solving has been under way. Adaptive and stressed families may have already worked out a number of things for themselves and are in the process of making changes.

Ideally, this session should be relaxed with information sharing and a general feeling of trust. Everyone's contributions should be acknowledged and respected. During this session the community mental health nurse points out the strengths of family functioning. Examples of such strengths may be given so that the family can link this general concept to specific instances of behavior. The nurse may also give examples of how functions, roles, and relationships relate to the emotional and mental health of all members in primary group systems. The climate should be one in which strains of various kinds can be identified without undue blaming or scapegoating of any one member at the expense of another.

Before the session ends, the community mental health nurse finds out from members how they have defined the assessment process and counseling experience. There is a need to ascertain whether questions or anxieties have been raised that have not been sufficiently addressed. The nurse also needs to find out whether the family wants to continue in counseling to work through any specific problems or concerns that have come to light during the previous sessions. If this approach is desired, then arrangements are made and objectives for the next counseling session discussed.

The comprehensive community mental health nursing assessment is both an assessing and a counseling process blended into one. In families or primary socialization groups that have a tremendous potential for influencing the mental and emotional health of members and recognizing problematical situations, the process, in and of itself, is a therapeutic one. The one advantage to this approach of assessment is that it uses the unique characteristics of nursing practice and makes available to clients the professional expertise and special roles and functions that society and law have mandated as the province of professional nursing practice.

SUMMARY

The comprehensive community mental health nursing assessment is a special nursing activity. It is implemented through a process that combines assessment and counseling and the therapeutic use of self by the community mental health nurse. The assessment provides both basic information about the mental health of families, groups, communities, and clients and the essential information needed to formulate preventions and interventions for applications in community mental health nursing practice.

The comprehensive community mental health nursing assessment is based on a general theory of community mental health nursing. This theory emphasizes a social psychological perspective leading the nurse to focus on small groups in daily living situations as systems in which the promotion and maintenance of mental health can be addressed through preventions for children and adults across the life span.

One goal of community mental health nursing is to help keep healthy families healthy, to decrease the chance of significant mental and emotional problems developing in members. Adaptive family functioning is known to release the potential of family systems to provide environments conducive to development of positive mental health. With stressed family systems, the goal of community mental health nursing is to provide interventions that reduce risk factors; with distressed families, the goal is to address specific emotional problems and pathologies. Referrals are made as needed to clinical nurse specialists.

The community mental health nursing assessment is a therapeutic process in its own right. The community mental health nurse establishes in this process a professional presence that demonstrates caring and competence. The assessment is organized and implemented through the use of a problem-solving approach that fosters independence and autonomy on the part of families and their members. At no time is the sick role with its attendant dependency characteristics used in community mental health nursing practice.

REFERENCES

Auger, Jeanine R. *Behavioral Systems and Nursing*. Englewood Cliffs, NJ: Prentice-Hall, 1976, chapters 7 and 8.

Barker, R. G. *Ecological Psychology: Concepts and Means for Studying the Environments of Human Behavior*. Palo Alto, CA: Stanford University Press, 1968.

Benner, Patricia. From novice to expert. *American Journal of Nursing* 82:402–407, 1982.

Francis, Gloria, M., and Munjas, Barbara A. *Manual of Socialpsychologic Assessment*. New York: Appleton-Century-Crofts, 1976, pp. 3–10.

Fromm, Erich. *The Sane Society*. New York: Rinehart, 1955.

Hume, Nicholas, O'Conner, William A., and Lowery, Carol R. Family, adjustment, and the psychosocial ecosystem. *Psychiatric Annals* 7:32–49, 1977.

Jahoda, Marie. *Current Concepts of Positive Mental Health*. New York: Basic Books, 1958, pp. 104–106.

Lewis, Jerry M. Family matrix in health and disease. In Hofling, Charles, and Lewis, Jerry, eds. *The Family: Evaluation and Treatment*. New York: Brunner/Mazel, 1980, pp. 5–44.

Reiss, David. Pathways to assessing the family: Some choice points and a sample route. In Hofling, Charles, and Lewis, Jerry, eds. *The Family: Evaluation and Treatment*. New York: Brunnel/Mazel, 1980, pp. 86–121.

Sedgwick, Rae. *Family Mental Health: Theory and Practice*. St. Louis: C. V. Mosby, 1981, chapters 13–16.

Smoyak, Shirley. *The Psychiatric Nurse As a Family Therapist*. New York: John Wiley & Sons, 1975, pp. ix–xiv.

CHAPTER 10 | COMMUNITY MENTAL HEALTH NURSING: PREVENTIONS

INTRODUCTION

Community mental health nursing increasingly has to expand its scope of practice by providing various kinds of primary preventions in mental health. Emphasis must be placed on promoting and maintaining the healthy functioning of families and other kinds of primary socialization groups in order for them to fulfill their unique functions and aid their members to fulfill their social roles and responsibilities. Achievement of these basic functions in such systems requires that they establish climates or milieus that have an organization and structure promoting the development of positive mental health of members. Positive mental health is reflected by a person's acquisition of a sense of autonomy; mastery; a positive self-identity; selfhood; essential social, cognitive, and personal competencies; and an attitude of openness toward living and people, leading to a process of growth throughout the various phases of life.

A holistic conception of the functioning of families or groups organized to function like families is essential in order to assess the complementarity of the various dimensions involved in family system interaction (Pless & Satterwhite, 1973). Family functioning is defined as the give and take of daily living, that is, the ways in which members interact as a unit to manage the various aspects of living that daily arise. In this respect, such functioning is multidimensional and requires the consideration of more than one or two features of functioning. For example, social structural features that are characteristically included in assessment of family systems are marital status, birth order, number and sex of children, and age of members. Information about these and other such factors have at times been used to make various kinds of judgments about level and adequacy of functioning. However, judgments about family system functioning need to have a data base broader than structural aspects. Information about basic interrelationships in primary socialization systems is needed, particularly when the data are to be used for clinical decisions and applications of preventions in mental health.

Primary prevention in mental health has been described by Cowen (1977) as a "glittering, diffuse, and thoroughly abstract term." He pointed out that different people tend to use different language to define primary prevention, particularly in mental health, and noted that quite often what is called primary prevention is not primary prevention at all. He further noted that mental health professionals have so long and so singularly come from the therapeutic–restorative side of services that it is difficult for them to make the needed and refined discriminations between primary and secondary preventions. He also noted that the distinctions between true primary preventions and anything else that the mental health fields have done, or are currently doing, are enormous. Goldston (1977) emphasized that primary preventions in mental health are *specific acitions* directed at *specific populations* for *specific purposes* to prevent the development of mental and emotional problems.

As previously noted, preventions of a primary nature are nursing actions that are provided before the occurrence of events, behaviors, repetitive responses, conditions, or interactions that are likely to create emotional and mental stress and to promote the learning of ineffective coping responses. Preventions use a number of strategies that are useful for the promotion of mental health. With adaptative or healthy families, prevention activities include those that focus on threats or risks to mental and emotional health and on health promotion. Health-promoting activities include mental health education, problem solving as an integral mental health competency, values clarification, and understanding the conditions and resources needed in families to promote the emotional and mental health of family members. Pender (1982) defined health-promoting activities as those directed toward developing the resources of clients that maintain and enhance well-being. Primary prevention activities are defined as those activities that seek to protect clients from potential or actual health threats and their harmful consequences.

Vaughan and co-workers (1975) pointed out an obvious but sometimes blurred fact, namely, that primary prevention programs are oriented toward health rather than illness. There are no designated patients. No stigmatic labels related to mental illness are affixed to persons and families participating in such programs. The focus is on relationships and interactions in the family system and between families and the communities in which they live. Clinical emphasis is on how to potentiate the strengths of family and community to increase the level of competence of family functioning. In this process, consideration needs to be given to the identification of basic problem-solving skills that people need for relating to one another, for defining and coping with situations, and for achieving goals, all of which relate to positive health and mental health.

The need for primary preventions in relation to mental and emotional health has long been recognized. One problem in providing primary prevention programs and services has been the difficulty of implementing them by using traditional public health models, concepts, and principles. By and large, these models have been developed for disease prevention, environmental sanitation, and public health safety and have been and continue to be based on medical, biological, physical, and environmental sciences, whereas mental and emotional problems are primarily based on social, cultural, familial, psychological, and psychiatric sciences. A second problem of note is the continued emphasis in mental health on illness rather than health. This emphasis continues to foster systems and services of care that for the most part reduce mental and emotional illness to psychopharmacological and somatic medical problems. Models for primary prevention of mental and emotional problems and mental health promotion are not easy to develop or implement in established systems of mental health care that are oriented to quite different kinds of services.

There is a major reason why community mental health nursing needs to focus on primary socialization systems, particularly families, to provide preventions in mental health. Evolutionary changes have occurred in families in a relatively short span of time. During and following World War II, family systems underwent many changes that altered the structure and organization of the nuclear family. Changes occurred in role, responsibilities, and patterns of relationships in families, between families, and in social and kin networks. The ability to maintain community roots and neighborhood relationships and to retain strong family identity and cohesion became difficult. Other changes include increased mobility and upheavals that changed places of residence and the role of women in the home and in the world of work, emergence of different conceptions about the rights and needs of children in families and different views about premarital sex and intimate living arrangements, having children before marriage, having children late in marriage, and not having children at all. Concomitant with such changes, research on family life and living has provided new information about the influence of family and community milieus on both children and adults. The organization of family functioning, roles, and relationships and the social climates in families has increasingly been related to its influence on emotional and mental health, cognitive development, patterns of coping, and physical growth and development of members.

Perez (1979) pointed out that so much ferment in families about family life and norms in such a short time presented a powerful message to parents: *Do not parent the way you were parented.* At the same time, new concepts about parenting were never made clear and did not describe new approaches in ways that parents could understand and adopt them. Parents have not been fully helped to understand relationships between the need to create family social environments that are conducive to promotion and maintenance of mental, emotional, physical, and social health and development of self-hood and self-actualization for themselves and their children.

In mental health, the prevailing view has long been that mental illness and emotional problems are primarily individual in nature. This strong belief has been a major factor in delaying the development of mental health models focusing on preventions directed to other than the individual level of functioning. Furthermore, it has delayed the development and adoption of new and modified approaches to parenting and the continued socialization of adults across the life span.

The social psychological model of mental health provides a conceptual community mental health nursing framework that is useful for developing and implementing primary preventions and health-promoting activities. This specialty area of practice has a major role in the field of mental health for providing leadership in the development and implementation of therapeutic activities designed primarily for prevention of emotional problems and mental illnesses in small-group behavior settings. Since the turn of the century, nurses have been leaders in providing health services to people in community settings. Such contributions to the health care of citizens have been directed toward the prevention of illness and promotion of health. The modification and application of such experiences to mental health is an exciting challenge for community mental health nursing.

LEVEL OF ORGANIZATION FOR PREVENTIONS

Small-group settings are a major level of organization for application of prevention concepts and strategies. Such settings have long been used in mental health for various kinds of therapeutic interventions and are equally as important for applying preventions. Small-group settings for preventions include natural and adoptive families, surrogate families, and family-like groups organized as homes for children and adults. These groups are all *primary socialization systems.*

Peer groups in school, work, and community settings are also small-group settings contributing to the socialization of people across the life span; however, these groups are organized for reasons other than to promote the primary socialization of people. Peer groups of various kinds do provide a great deal of the social and psychological support that people need for promoting and maintaining emotional and mental health. Mental health preventions may be applied in these systems, as, for example, prevention programs that have been conducted in school settings for a number of years. However, primary socialization systems are key ones in the application of preventions because of their central role in socialization, their universality, and their accessibility.

In primary socialization systems, such as famlies, preventions have the potential for setting into motion multiplier effects that may be transmitted from one generation to another. When children in healthy functioning families become adults, establish their own families, and become parents, they use knowledge and understanding gained from personal experiences to establish socioemotional climates in family settings that incorporate new ideas about familial relationships, traditions, roles, responsibilities, and functions. More enlightened attitudes, beliefs, and parenting practices are used that encourage the development of opportunities promoting positive mental and emotional health. Such practices include a variety of living and learning experiences in which children and adults develop essential social, cognitive, and interpersonal competencies relevant to specific developmental phases and that foster the development of selfhood. Such a transmittal process includes the inculcation of beliefs and practices about the need for primary socialization systems to be more conscious of their influence on members and responsible for helping them to prepare for diverse roles, to be comfortable in relationships, and to develop a positive sense of self.

It is possible to place "boundaries" around primary socialization systems so as to identify key interrelationships and interactions, roles, responsibilities, the ways in which the system is organized, the kinds of socioemotional climates that prevail, relationships with community and social groups and networks, and relationships with the work place and schools. These interrelationships may then be assessed in the context of the system's interactions and interrelationships in order to get a picture of how some of the mutual influences interact on the mental health of members and affect the level of functioning.

Primary socialization systems, such as families, are naturally organized and easily accessible. They are the systems in which nursing has for years had experiences in providing health promotion and supervision for both adults and children. In mental health, the purpose of preventions shifts in emphasis from environmental and physical care to include relationships, roles, and ways of coping that do not have direct and precise causal relationships to emotional and mental health. Furthermore preventions in mental health are mostly actions that try to achieve small, even subtle, changes in behavior and attitudes, none of which are easily measured by usual epidemiological standards but which have a multiplier effect on the system and its members.

In adaptive family systems, preventions are most effective when used in anticipation of changes in human experiences and events that will occur as a result of normal developmental and maturational processes. Such experiences, in conjunction with situational and individual experiences, are known to generate stress, even crises. Changes in roles and status of family members at any stage and phase of development have the potential to cause temporary imbalances, strains in family system functioning, and changes in family structure. Such changes are an integral part of living and closely related to the two basic functions of the family in contemporary society: socialization of the young and the stabilization of adult personalities across the life span.

THERAPEUTIC PROCESSES

Therapeutic processes are integral to the effectiveness of prevention counseling. These are clinical actions that are used to encourage the development over time of behaviors in people in order to gain some desired outcome. One important therapeutic process is expectation, particularly that which is held by the nurse about the family's role and function in counseling. Expectations about what is expected of clients shape the role of the nurse in the counseling process and the strategies selected to achieve goals. Expectations are often, unknowingly, translated into interactions and interrelationships in the counseling process, through which the nurse, as an expert mental health professional, expresses herself or himself.

Another important therapeutic process that needs to be addressed any time it can be done in a timely and appropriate way is the encouragement of families and their respective members to assume responsibility for their health, for promoting mental and physical health, and for using health-protective behaviors. This responsibility can be somewhat alarming to many people because, for so long, mental health and health professionals have adopted a view that they are the custodians of health and mental health. Each person and each family have to recognize and accept the responsibility for their own health in all its dimensions. Professional mental health workers and physicians cannot and should not assume this important familial and personal responsibility.

The inculcation of the idea that families and their members have to "tend" to family health is another therapeutic process important in mental health. In order for the family to maintain and use its strength and potential to promote and maintain emotional and mental health, all members have to realize how this can be accomplished. Too often, families do not appreciate the importance of the family setting as a highly intense learning and support milieu. Furthermore, family members may not recognize that many essential tasks, competencies, and relationships cannot be learned in alternative settings as well as they can in family systems. In this respect, there is a need to foster the idea that the promotion and maintenance of mental health require preventions on a continuing basis. Such an approach is essential to the use of preventive health behaviors in mental health.

In prevention counseling, families and members have to be active. This expectation may be somewhat disquieting to clients because of stereotypes about psychiatric treatments and therapeutic activities in mental health, many of which depict patients as recipients of a talking cure therapy. Prevention counseling also requires people to be involved in active learning and problem-solving situations.

To implement the idea of active participation, the community mental health nurse may use validation as an integral part of the therapeutic process. In this approach, the nurse and family members periodically review an evaluation the nurse makes about family functioning, potential strengths and problems, and observations about family interactions. Family members then provide their evaluation and cover the same ground. Once both evaluations are on the table, discussion about each one takes place to arrive at a consensus or an agreement to disagree about the evaluation in whole or part. This process actively involves clients in examining what changes have been achieved in counseling and how such changes are being experienced. It also establishes opportunities to check assessment and monitoring skills. Collaboration with an authority figure (the nurse) is an important learning opportunity in which conflicting views can be accorded respect and considered without demeaning the persons holding them.

THERAPEUTIC USE OF SELF

The therapeutic use of self by the nurse in prevention counseling requires the use of many subroles in the clinical role of community mental health nurse. This clinical role includes the idea of the nurse as a caring, competent, and concerned mental health professional and the use of self in the subroles of counselor, mental health educator, facilitator, co-problem solver, teacher, role model, and advocate. Each of these subroles requires the use of self in ways that promote the development and maintenance of wellness behaviors in clients and help them to assume responsibility for their own health. A nurse's use of subroles that do not "provide care to" someone and minimize the technical aspects of nursing may create a sense of role reversal for the nurse. Nursing and other mental health disciplines continue to heavily socialize their members to use approaches and therapy models that encourage clients to adopt sick roles and related dependency behaviors.

Prevention counseling requires clinical nursing competencies that are quite varied. Such competencies use principles of learning, principles of nursing, and relevant principles from the psychological, social psychological, educational, and psychiatric sciences. Therapeutic use of self and strategies in prevention counseling differ in several ways from those used in traditional mental health therapy models. Traditional approaches tend to have prescribed roles and behaviors that are based on conceptual frameworks developed for mental and emotional illnesses. Conceptual frameworks that foster prevention counseling in mental health are developed from nursing concepts of positive mental health, holistic concepts of mind and body, the social and cultural aspects of mental health in interaction with psychological factors, and the role of socialization in emotional and mental health.

CLINICAL ORGANIZING FRAMEWORK: STRUCTURE

The clinical organizing framework for community mental health nursing is used to structure clinical practice for preventions relating to promotion and maintenance of positive mental health. This framework is used to identify strategies by which theory may be applied and makes up the clinical plan of action.

One part of the framework is a set of general goals that is derived from the set of basic interrelationships associated with primary socialization groups in general and family systems in particular. Activities that are useful to achieve goals are identified. Once this part of the clinical plan is established, it becomes an important part of the basic structure used to organize and guide community mental health nursing in prevention counseling. This structure may be modified as needed to meet the specific concerns and needs of particular families during the course of the counseling.

General goals related to positive mental health are used to organize the emergent and ongoing interactional data as they are generated in counseling sessions. On one hand, these goals provide enough structure to give sessions purpose, direction, and a clinical process that is consistent with prevention counseling; on the other hand, the goals have to be general and flexible so that the nurse can modify them and related activities and strategies on the basis of interactional data. Interactional data contain specific and unique concerns, views, and particular needs of families as these evolve in each counseling session.

A second part of the clinical organizing framework consists of the strategies, or methods, that the nurse uses in prevention counseling to achieve both general goals and behavioral changes. Specifically, counseling strategies are used to alter or modify existing behaviors, attitudes, views, and changes in family systems and in individual behaviors. At present, there are no specific strategies that can be designated solely as "prevention strategies." Rather, there are a number of strategies that facilitate changes in behavior that have proven to be useful in prevention counseling. These strategies have been developed in a number of professional disciplines and are generalizable to community mental health nursing.

In addition to goals, activities, and strategies, the clinical organizing framework has other aspects of structure that need to be attended in each session. They include a review of (1) the general understanding that the family has about what went on in previous sessions; (2) the overall prevention plan; (3) the family's responsibility and commitment to learning how to promote positive mental and emotional health; (4) a determination of concerns that the family thinks needs be addressed; (5) a statement about how specific family and member strengths and concerns relate to overall goals and the identification of additional ones as necessary; and (6) a specification of desired changes in family functioning and how these may be evaluated.

Data from families will include information about stable experiences that recur over time, place, and situation. Data will also be available about how infrequent or unusual experiences are handled in response to unanticipated events, situations, or sudden changes in roles and relationships of members. Characteristic patterns of coping for different kinds of experiences can usually be identified from both assessment data and interactions that occur during prevention counseling sessions. Although characteristic patterns may be effective during certain phases of development of a family system and its individual members, they may become less so as changes occur in ages, interests, psychological and social needs, and the world views of members as a result of growth and maturation. In adaptive, or healthy, functioning families, strengths and potential for addressing the changing roles and developmental needs of members need to be made explicit so that they can be used during counseling.

Modifications in the structure and process of the clinical organizing framework are not difficult to make. The part of the structure that cites the general goals and related activities represents the advanced knowledge, research, and experiences about mental health that the nurse brings to the counseling process. This body of knowledge and experience, used in the implementation of the clinical nursing process, is linked to the social psychological concepts of behavior from which the clinical framework evolves. The part of the structure that relates to data specific to particular needs of families is expected to require modification over a series of counseling sessions in order to accommodate strengths, concerns, and problems.

In prevention counseling with adaptive, or healthy, functioning families, the data base is expected to have characteristic patterns of interactions, roles, relationships, communications, marital relationships, parent–child relations, family cohesion, and world views. These patterns are consistent with research that shows that such behaviors are found in family systems functioning at a high level of competency. Such patterns are expected to show *small variations in family functioning* rather than easily discernible maladaptations or pathological patterns of functioning. Effective patterns of coping are to be expected in healthy functioning family systems because, by definition, they would be assessed as such only when there are no major problems in system function or in coping and adaptation of individual members.

CLINICAL ORGANIZING FRAMEWORK: DIRECTION AND PROCESS

The process of prevention counseling in community mental health nursing proceeds along two pathways at the same time. On one pathway, direction comes from general goals known to be associated with positive mental health. On the second pathway, direction comes from data provided by clients in the counseling process.

The two kinds of information have to be integrated by the community mental health nurse in order to achieve in counseling both the general goals of positive mental health and the specific goals that address the particular concerns and needs of individual families. To achieve these goals, there is continuing need to integrate old knowledge and experiences with new ones as these evolve in the counseling process and new learning takes place with family members. This ongoing process makes it necessary to validate the various perceptions and connections that are made between people, relationships, events, and situations in order to understand the meanings that members attribute to them. Furthermore, there is a need to have members define situations as they see them and consider ways in which such definitions influence present behavior, attitudes, and expectations about behavior for individual family members.

The fifth counseling session is usually the one in which prevention counseling begins to be more directly addressed. It is organized to start the program of preventions. Sessions are rather open in both structure and process. Because of this openness, the community mental health nurse has to provide the leadership to see that enough structure is present to ensure that counseling goals can be achieved.

The prevention counseling process requires careful encoding and decoding of data by the nurse as they evolve in the ongoing session. After discussing the general structure that will be used to organize the session, the nurse has to make some clinical judgments in rapid order as the session starts. First, specific areas of concern identified by the family have to be considered in the context of theoretical and clinical frameworks in order to provide direction. Next, appropriate prevention strategies have to be decided on. Then, the nurse has to make a decision about therapeutic use of self. All of these decisions are made in the context of an assessment of the family's readiness to participate in the prevention counseling process.

A clinical decision-making process about use of self, prevention strategies, and readiness of the family occurs anew in each prevention counseling session. This is necessary because of the openness of the structure of the counseling session and the active participation of family members. The nurse has to get as good a "fit" as possible between strengths and concerns of the family, readiness to participate, therapeutic use of self, and activities and strategies that may be used to achieve goals. For example, if patterns of interaction within the family system have been selected as the area of family functioning in which recurrent strains and tensions occur, the nurse may decide to be a passive yet acutely interested listener as family members describe their perceptions of family roles and interactions. Such descriptions would include information about both effective and less than effective efforts to handle tension-producing situations. The nurse notes the things that seem to trigger tenseness in interactions as well the roles that family members play in such encounters. While listening to such descriptions, the nurse notes the content and observes the group process in interaction. She or he may become more active when it is necessary for commitments and expectations to be made explicit so that they do not become obscured as more concrete concerns are dealt with.

At some point in counseling, the community mental health nurse may recognize that family members have developed a pattern of reactions to certain kinds of interactions. Even where such reactions are ineffective, they may continue to be used because they have not been made explicit and evaluated as to their effectiveness. Such responses do not handle interactional situations effectively except temporarily to relieve anger, frustration, and anxiety. Connections between past and present actions and reactions are not integrated in ways that the need to explore alternatives is indicated. In such instances, the nurse will have to help the family make some connections between the kinds of events that are tension-producing, the responses that such events characteristically elicit from members, and the effectiveness of such responses. Once this has been done, the family can usually examine interactions, events, and roles of members and arrive at alternative ways of coping and interacting.

The direction and intensity of prevention counseling change as different concerns are dealt with and as the family becomes more knowledgeable about participation and problem solving. In this changing situation, the role of the nurse may frequently shift and require the use of the array of clinical competencies brought to the counseling process. The establishment of a comfortable working relationship between the community mental health nurse and the family is an important goal in this process.

Once a plan for prevention counseling has been established, counseling sessions are usually less frequent than when the comprehensive community mental health nursing assessment was being conducted. Families need time to try out competencies and changes in behavior in the family living situation. If crises or special needs arise, more frequent sessions may be needed for a while. In general, the nurse and family will have to make a judgment about the frequency of sessions based on what needs to be done and the rapidity with which the family learns to use the knowledge about preventions.

In prevention counseling, changes in behavior, attitudes, and outlook will in all likelihood be characterized by small variations that are neither dramatic nor easily observed. In fact, changes may be experienced before they are noticed. Because of this, the nurse needs to be very careful that an impression is not conveyed that "quick fixes" will result from prevention counseling.

Goals related to adaptive responses in healthy families have to be established for counseling sessions. Having made this statement, it should be emphasized that care needs to be taken to see that the goals do not inadvertently become the major organizing focus of the prevention counseling process rather than the growth and development of family members and family potential. It is helpful to remember that prevention counseling to promote and maintain positive mental health is relatively new. Therefore, the imposition of clinical, educational, and behavioral models of change with related goals and objectives on the delicate and complex caring process of prevention counseling has to be approached with care. Until more definitive prevention models evolve from clinical nursing practice and research, a balance has to be maintained between too much structure and too little structure and appropriate use of models of behavioral change.

In general, prevention counseling for positive mental health means that the community mental health nurse has to help others recognize the need for change in their usual ways of coping in the primary socialization systems in which they spend a great deal of time and have emotional investments and accept responsibility for their mental and emotional health. There is an essential need to incorporate problem solving in this process.

Once a family has recognized its strengths and discussed how these may be potentiated, the concept of responsibility for promotion and maintenance of positive mental health is well on its way to being accepted as an essential part of preventive health. Mental health as a general concept becomes anchored to specific concerns, related behaviors, and indicators of health and family and individual functioning, thus eliminating much of the concern that seems to be associated with this aspect of health.

In prevention counseling it is important for the nurse to remember that the general aim is to keep healthy families healthy. In such families, there are always events, experiences, and relationships that cause some stress and concern. It is the potential for stresses and tensions to persist, develop in intensity, and create problems at some future date that is the major concern of prevention counseling. In this respect, families have to learn to handle "normal problems of daily living" before these develop a life of their own. Satisfactory resolutions have to be developed to prevent the build-up of accumulative effects that influence in negative ways the growth, development, achievement of self-identity, and selfhood of family members.

CLINICAL ORGANIZING FRAMEWORK: APPLICATIONS

The clinical organizing framework includes general goals that relate to positive mental health. As noted, these come from the body of research, knowledge, and experiences that have been accumulated by the mental health and related disciplines. More specifically, goals are anchored to conceptions of mental health and how it is promoted and maintained and to the basic interrelationships found in all primary socialization groups in one form or another.

One of the first goals related to prevention in mental health concerns the need to help the family identify its strengths and potential. This area needs to be addressed as soon as possible in the counseling process because it sets a climate and a base that the family can understand in terms of healthy family functioning. The family needs to know explicitly what it as a system does to achieve and promote positive mental health for its members. In the process of identifying what such factors are, the family usually strengthens its commitment to understand more clearly its functioning and to accept more consciously responsibility for promoting and maintaining its emotional and mental health. Equally important, a distinction between mental health and mental illness develops. Over time, it is expected that this awareness will have the outcome of decreasing the stigma associated with activities related to mental health.

In the first prevention counseling session, it usually becomes evident to the nurse that a great deal of information evolves about family interactions as families participate in the counseling process. For example, if there are difficulties completing activities that require members to develop a consensus or to collaborate, the nurse is alerted that there may be tensions relating to authority, competition, giving up or sharing control of situations or relationships, or understanding communications that are not clear in either intent or content. Further observations would, of course, be needed to validate such observations and impressions.

In the process of obtaining clarifications and definitions of situations, different views are expressed by various members. If such views are not readily accepted, disputed, or cut off, such interactions alert the nurse to the tolerance level of the family about the acceptance of differences of opinion and willingness to look at alternatives. If the family views its functioning and identifies its world view much the same at the end of a number of prevention counseling sessions as it did at the beginning, this suggests that information, discussions, and definitions of situations are not being synthesized and reconceived to bring about changes in perceptions, attitudes, and behaviors related to family functioning.

The community mental health nurse, in conjunction with the family, has to judge when members are ready to move from one goal to another. The family does need to achieve the first general goal relating to family strengths and potential before moving to consider other aspects of its functioning. If this groundwork is not laid, it may be difficult for a family to consider other concerns because the collective knowledge and experience base about its own functioning is not clear. Such incompleteness makes it difficult for prevention counseling to proceed with any effectiveness.

Other general mental health goals are developed from the set of basic interrelationships that are characteristically found in primary socialization systems and from information provided by particular family systems. The needs and concerns of individual families differ and these specific aspects have to be integrated into the clinical organizing framework of positive mental health.

GOAL RELATING TO PRIMARY SOCIALIZATION SYSTEM STRENGTHS AND POTENTIAL

A goal relating to the strength and potential of primary socialization systems is basic for all prevention counseling in mental health. Attending to this goal with families and family-like systems at the outset of counseling sets a focus on mental health rather than on psychiatric problems and illnesses.

> *Goal: To help adaptive functioning family systems recognize what they do to create healthy environments that promote and maintain positive mental health of members and identify areas of functioning that may be strengthened.*

Activities Relative to Goal Achievement

1. Share characteristic patterns of family system functioning developed from the comprehensive assessment data and obtain the family perception about the effectiveness of its functioning, strengths, cohesion, and world view.
2. "Fit" the family system profile to the model of adaptive family functioning in order to provide a perspective of the family as an interacting unit.
3. State areas of functioning that may not be functioning up to potential and identify any changes that may be expected as a result of age, status, and developmental or maturational changes in one or more of family members.
4. Select with the family members the concern(s) they want to focus on in counseling sessions and place these in the context of the basic interrelationships that are to be found in all primary socialization systems.

Strategies Useful for Achieving Goal

Obtaining Perceptions of Family Functioning

This strategy involves *obtaining perceptions* from family members of how they view the family system in terms of its strengths, cohesion, and identify. Views are also needed about how well members achieve their interests and goals; how support is provided; the potential of the family to help members achieve autonomy, independence, and selfhood; the world view held by the family; and identification of concerns. Data from the perceptions that families hold about themselves as a system provide the community mental health nurse with specific, possibly unique, information about the family as an interacting unit.

This strategy requires the participation of family members and the information generated is usually known to family members but never before expressed in this kind of framework. It is not unusual for family members to be quite surprised about the perceptions various members hold as they realize the extent of differences in views and perspectives. Use of this strategy early in prevention counseling sets the stage for the expectation that family members will be active participants. Its use also sends a powerful message to all family members that their input into the prevention counseling process is essential. This is a time when members can be asked to identify the strengths of the family, how such strengths might be potentiated to the advantage of members in terms of growth and development, and how family interactions might promote and enhance the mental health of the family as a unit.

Sharing Information and Obtaining Descriptions

Sharing information, as opposed to giving information, and *obtaining complete and accurate descriptions* of family functioning, member behavior, interactions, and interrelationships are necessary so that the family members and community mental health nurse share a common information base. This strategy helps to obtain more complete descriptions of experiences and facilitates the organization of bits and pieces of data about experiences into a more complete picture in which connections can be made and meanings more clearly understood.

This strategy may be used in several ways. One way is to ask members to identify experiences related to specific concerns or situations in daily living that have recently occurred and that caused changes in roles and relationships, or that aroused strong emotions of one kind or another in one or more members. The nurse may have to encourage the expression of feelings, particularly anger, in relation to such experiences. Members may need assistance in describing experiences. It is important for the nurse to make a clinical judgment about the adequacy of the descriptions of experiences early in the prevention counseling process because conclusions may be made from incomplete experiences and information.

Often, few connections have usually been made by family members between recurring experiences that arouse frustration by the feeling of "here we go again." Adequate descriptions facilitate the identification of patterns of interactions and interrelationships. However, descriptive data alone are not enough. Experiences have to be connected in terms of their impact, the emotions associated with them, and the meanings attributed to them. The process of helping families make such connections usually requires some assistance from the nurse. The integration of fragments of experiences is necessary if closure is to be achieved about them and resulting conclusions validated.

Clarification

Clarification involves a process in which the explicit and implicit aspects of communications are made more precise and clear. It helps to make more understandable information and experiences in terms of their content, intent, and the feelings attached to them. Clarification of communications is an essential part of understanding messages. Literally, the clarification process tries to make things more "pure" by making sure the intent and content of messages are as free as possible from distortion.

Defining Situations

Obtaining *definitions of situations* is a strategy that encourages the family to consider social, environmental, and situational factors as well as personal and familial ones. The nurse tries to obtain both subjective and objective definitions because both contribute to the development of perceptions of reality. It is not surprising to find that subjective and objective definitions of situations use different observations and arrive at quite different conclusions. When such differences are evident, the nurse needs to explore the bases for these.

The definition of a situation that a person holds is reality for that person and serves as the basis for actions and related feelings. This holds true irrespective of whether the definition is true or distorted. Only by making definitions of situations explicit and providing for validation is there a possibility of correcting incomplete, erroneous, or distorted information.

Constructing the Family Strength Ladder

The construction of a *family strength ladder* helps the family to identify family strengths and potential. This is a powerful strategy in that it enhances positive thoughts and feelings about the family as an entity and members as part of this entity. Developing the ladder usually creates a receptive climate for the discussion of areas in which improvement in family relationships may be useful or for preparing for anticipated changes in family roles or relationships.

The family strength ladder may be used in many ways, and when kept updated, provides an account of changes in the assessment of family functioning over time. When and if the family becomes discouraged about achieving some desired change, the ladder may be used to review strengths and potential, to reassure members, and to provide some ideas about why dificulties are being encountered.

The family develops a ladder on which its greatest strength is placed on the top rung; at least five additional strengths are placed on descending rungs. A similar ladder is developed alongside in which areas are identified in which the family strengths and potential could be enhanced. When placed side by side, a clear record of strengths and potential is available for discussion and consideration of actions.

Making the Family Wish

The *family wish* is a nonthreatening strategy providing a format for obtaining information about some of the inner wishes, visions, even fantasies, that members would like to have happen to the family. Families are asked to take two or three minutes to come up with the family wish and identify why it is important and what actions the family needs to take in order to make the wish come true.

In the process of deciding on a common family wish, the community mental health nurse has an opportunity to observe how the family reaches a consensus, who served as the leader in this effort, what member, if any, dominated the selection, and how competing wishes other than the one selected were handled.

Cognitive Restructuring

Cognitive restructuring is a process through which concepts, particular relationships, fellings, roles, situations, and experiences are organized to arrive at perspectives and conclusions different from the ones held before restructuring. Cognitive restructuring comes about as a result of new information, more complete information from a different point of view, or a rethinking about the meanings given to certain phenomena. Oddly enough, verbal statements by people of different views about a particular thing may be enough to bring about restructuring. The process of actually hearing a statement of views and perspectives and revealing feelings about these can bring about sudden insight and realizations. For example, it is not uncommon for a person to be describing an experience as it was experienced and, suddenly, a "light dawns" as different connections and conclusions are made. Such changes in the structure of thinking about experience can usually be seen by the expression on the person's face. When the person is questioned about this, she or he usually acknowledges that such a change has occurred. Of course, not all cognitive restructuring occurs in such a dramatic fashion. Many times, and perhaps most often, people tend to think about and mull over old and new information and undergo a more gradual change in what they think, believe, and feel.

Cognitive restructuring is a strategy that has been widely used in rational–emotive therapy (Ellis & Greiger, 1977). Following this orientation, Pender (1982) described cognitive restructuring as an individual's response that is made on the basis of both the actual situation and what the person says to herself or himself before and during target events. This self-statement is a covert verbalization that elicits emotional reactions and influences restructured cognitions.

Bracketing

Bracketing is a strategy that allows one to bring an experience into clearer focus by isolating related experiences or segments of such experiences. Bracketing permits the examination of a limited aspect of reality while holding other aspects in abeyance. This is a useful strategy when there is value in examining some particular experience in depth. It is useful for helping people express their feelings about the "set-off," or bracketed, experience because it is possible to control and direct these experiences to some extent. Oiler (1982) described bracketing as an approach in which people are asked to lay aside what they think they know about a particular experience and allow themselves to wonder, to feel, to be uncertain and puzzled, and to ask for different opinions from others in order to broaden their perspective. Both approaches are useful in primary prevention counseling.

Analysis

Analysis involves a process that breaks experiences into small parts so that they may be more closely examined and aspects of these experiences made more explicit. In this process, connections and interactions between parts of experiences can be identified. A final step is to consider the experiences being analyzed as a whole. Analysis helps one to make distinctions between similarities and differences about experiences in part and in whole.

Mental Health Education

Mental health education involves the acquisition of information about mental and emotional health, what it is, how it may be supported, and the role of families in this effort. Educational materials may also be used to disseminate information.

Mental health education used in prevention counseling is quite varied. This is true because the knowledge that people have about mental health is incomplete and incorrect. Too often, information consists mainly of stereotypes, information about specific kinds of bizarre mental illnesses, accounts of mental and emotional problems as told by friends and family members, and, possibly, experiences with a person who has had mental and emotional problems.

Mental health education is an important strategy in prevention counseling. The President's Commission on Mental Health Prevention Task Force *Panel Reports* (1978) cited it as the most promising and powerful tool of prevention in mental health. In prevention counseling settings, new and different ideas can be presented in ways that favorably compete with older notions of mental health and mental illness, thus new ideas have a good chance of being accepted. Educational materials may be used as appropriate; however, more effective learning usually occurs if such information can be integrated into the context of the counseling process.

GOAL RELATING TO FAMILY SYSTEM INTERACTIONS, COHESION, IDENTITY, AND POSITIVE MENTAL HEALTH

Six of the basic interrelationships common to all primary socialization systems concern interactions between emotional, mental, personal, and social development of family members and the relationships between these and selected aspects of the family as an interacting system. This emphasis is needed because families and other kinds of primary socialization groups are the milieus in which preventions are effective. A general goal that addresses these areas of family functioning needs to be included in the clinical organizing framework.

> *Goal: To help family systems identify themes in family interactions and interrelationships that influence the development of family cohesion and identity, caring attitudes about others, and individual identity, autonomy, and selfhood of members.*

Activities Related to Goal Achievement

1. Describe at least one experience that the family does as a group each week that makes members feel close to each other and as members of a family.
2. Share perceptions of positive events, relationships, and experiences that parents, or parent surrogates, do to encourage growth and development within the family system and outside of the family.
3. Identify one experience outside of the family occurring weekly that encourages development of individual interests of members with friends and peers and participation in community activities and relationships.
4. Discuss how experiences in which disagreements occur between family views, expectations, and standards, or individual behavior, views, and interests are handled.
5. Share some family experiences that make members feel a part of the family, self-worth, and respect as a member of the family.

Strategies Useful for Achieving Goal

Constructing the Family Experience Calendar

The *family experience calendar* is a good strategy to use in prevention counseling when there is a need for the family to focus on the diversity and frequency of certain kinds of experiences. Family members are asked to identify some experiences during a specified time frame in which the family participated as a group and some in which individual members initiated experiences to meet their own needs and interests.

There is a human tendency to remember very enjoyable and very unenjoyable experiences, both of which may infrequently occur. The generalization of such memories to other experiences makes it difficult to sort out where fact ends and idealization begins. Fairly recent and accurate information about family experiences is needed. It is known that a variety of experiences in different social and interpersonal contexts that require meeting and relating to people in diverse roles, relationships, and positions helps people develop the essential personal and social competencies that are used in human relationships and builds self-confidence and self-reliance. All of these are related to social adjustment, which in turn is related to behaviors associated with positive mental health.

As the family prepares the experience calendar, the nurse has an opportunity to observe the ways in which the family organizes for such a task, the participation of members, their roles and contributions, and how well individual needs and opinions are met in the discussion process. These data help the nurse to get a good idea about such things as the kind and diversity of activities that the family as a whole participates in and whether any one member exerts influence to the extent that his or her views are accepted by the family as a group.

Feuding, Fussing, and Fighting Slate of Action

The *feuding, fussing, and fighting slate of action* is a very good strategy for getting a family to examine experiences that are tension-producing. It is a format in which emotionally charged experiences can be brought out in the open. The format makes possible the injection of humor in such situations.

In tension-producing experiences, the arousal of negative emotions is most likely to occur. Awareness of these emotions sometimes makes a family feel uncomfortable. Use of this strategy is a way of establishing a framework in which such experiences can be examined and discussed. Humor can be used to great advantage to deflect emotional tension. Tension may also be handled through use of analogous situations or by identification of roles played by television or comic figures in tension-producing situations.

Ventilation, or the expression of feelings associated with relationships and experiences, may be used to relieve tensions. Such expressions may be hurtful for other family members so the community mental health nurse has to make sure that other members have opportunities to express their views and feelings. Some closure about such expressions needs to be achieved by members by reestablishment of interactions that accept the feelings expressed but go beyond to find common grounds for future interactions now that feelings have been stated and acknowledged.

Therapeutic fighting, direct verbal assaults about grievances, hurts, and behaviors that are used by people in close relationships followed by compromise or contracts to alter certain kinds of behavior, is used by some counselors as a way of handling hostile feelings in family and marital situations. For the nurse who may not be experienced in this technique, a modified form of therapeutic fighting can be established by creating conflict situations in role play.

Role Playing and Role Restructuring

Role playing and *role restructuring* are invaluable strategies when there is a need to examine ongoing familial interactions. In role play, there are many techniques that may be used to consider interactions. For example, one may "stop the clock," a play in which action is frozen at some particular point and members are asked to discuss their perceptions and feelings about what is happening in the situation. Many of the techniques developed in encounter groups may be useful for structuring different kinds of role-play contexts. If facilities are available, video taping is of value and can be used in a number of ways for immediate feedback or held for a later date and be used for comparisons.

Role restructuring can be managed in several ways. The major principle in this strategy is to set up situations in which certain roles can first be played as they actually happened and then to establish a situation in which these same roles can be restructured in a different way. Members may be asked to restructure a role as they would have liked it to have occurred, or if the situation occurred again, what could be different about the role that might make a different outcome occur.

Family members can usually identify major patterns of interactions by the time they have examined certain kinds of experiences. After identification of these, the nurse can move the counseling process toward helping members make important connections between roles and relationships and how these influence and promote positive mental health. Every opportunity that arises needs to be used to establish the idea that families can monitor aspects of family functioning for themselves and may use the strategies that they are learning in prevention counseling to improve family relationships and functioning.

Argyle (1980) developed a social skills training program that may be used to teach or improve the basic social competencies that people need to function in daily living and work relationships and activities. He found role play to be one of the most effective strategies for this type of training. In his work, he developed the following sequence of activities to facilitate effective role playing and learning:

1. instruction and modeling—by demonstration and film
2. role playing with other trainees or role partners for 5 minutes to 8 minutes
3. feedback—verbal comments from trainer and playback from video recorders
4. repeated role playing

Video Feedback Analysis

This strategy involves the use of feedback from video recording. Video feedback may take several directions. Portions of sessions may be recorded and used immediately for analysis of family interactions or other kinds of behaviors. Recordings may also be used to provide feedback for learning particular kinds of behaviors and the account on tapes serves as a form of supervision. The use of *video feedback analysis* allows the family to stand back somewhat from their own behavior and examine it from the stance of observer rather than participant.

Video feedback analysis is a powerful learning tool and therapeutic strategy (Alger, 1969). Care needs to be taken to ensure that opportunities are provided for analysis in a supportive atmosphere because the impact of seeing oneself acting apart from oneself, so to speak, can sometimes be an overwhelming experience. It is a time when the perceptions people hold about themselves in terms of how they act, talk, and relate collide with the reality of actual behavior. Video feedback analysis may be used in conjunction with many other strategies. It is the one strategy that has the capability to capture a total situation: verbal and nonverbal communication, body language, the sequence and flow of interactions, and physical placement of persons in groups. The use of video recordings requires the availability of technical equipment, technicians, and facilities. The value of using this strategy is so great that efforts should be made to incorporate its use at least on a selected basis in prevention counseling.

Interactional Analysis

Interactional analysis involves an examination of the flow of interactions and sequences that occur as the family participates in the prevention counseling process. In effect, this type of analysis tries to capture the ongoing life of the family as a group as it unfolds. This strategy provides information about how the family usually interacts. Data may show that there are times when members enter into unspoken agreements that something is not to be discussed or considered. Analysis shows something of the shifts back and forth in the family as a system in reference to communications, changes in topics, and member participation.

Nurses are familiar with collecting interactional data by process recordings. If this approach is used, it would be necessary to have someone outside of the family conduct the recording. Another method of getting the kind of data that is needed for interactional analysis is from video taping of actual counseling sessions. Audio-tape recordings may be used to capture the communication patterns; however, this approach loses much of the data that are useful for interactional analysis. There are a number of interaction rating scales available that may be used either by an observer recording for the group or by group members conducting self-ratings.

Participation

Participation in the prevention counseling process means that members have to be involved in group interactions and activities and have a commitment to help to achieve the goals that the family decides on. Members also have to assume, through participation, the responsibility for making the counseling process a highly intense learning milieu.

Participation means to partake of and share with others. Learning how to participate may be a part of the competencies that have to be enhanced in the counseling process. Teachers have long had to cope with students who excused themselves from participation in class discussions and other learning opportunities on the grounds that they really had nothing to say that had not already been said. Furthermore, these students claimed that when they had something important to say, they would make a contribution at that time. Family members who adopt this approach need to be helped to understand that they are depending on others to establish ideas and events to which they respond or react. They take no risk in having ideas rejected or subjected to critical examination. What is more important is that persons who characteristically use this approach do not gain self-confidence in presenting their ideas and views. They also minimize experiences in which they hear themselves "talk" in order to get a sense of the clarity and adequacy of their presentation. People who do not participate fail to experience the joy of sharing a wild idea with others and partaking of what others have to offer to develop something useful and innovative.

Reframing

Reframing is when particular experiences, events, feelings, or ideas are placed in a different perspective or situation in ways that change roles, relationships, and meanings originally associated with these. In the reframing process, experiences may be "re-peopled," that is, the people in major roles, relationships, and experiences are changed in order to think about experiences rather than the people originally involved.

In using this strategy, the community mental health nurse usually asks family members to identify experiences or events that have a significance—in different ways—for members. Once this identification process is completed, different settings and situations may be devised for the experience or event and members are asked to consider their feelings in relation to this new arrangement. Or, the situation, setting, or event may be held constant while the same people are established in roles and relationships with feelings explored on an "as if" basis. In a general sense, reframing is a focused form of boundary setting in relation to fairly specific experiences and contexts.

Formulation and Reformulation

The strategy of *formulation* involves stating in a systematic way an account of relationships, events, experiences, interactions, and feelings that identify the family's formula for handling these. *Reformulation* involves going another step to ask questions about what one wishes to get out of experiences and out of life and how to make experiences more meaningful by rewriting the original formulation. Through reformulation, it is possible to make more explicit some of the aspects of experiences that might be improved or restructured.

It should be noted that the strategies identified thus far may be used not only with the particular goal cited but also with other goals as they seem appropriate. Many of the strategies may be formalized by presenting them in a format that requires the use of questionnaires or other kinds of instruments. Such a formalization and mechanization of the counseling process is not particularly recommended for at least two reasons. First, adaptive and healthy functioning families can take an idea and do a great deal of the structuring that may be needed to make a particular strategy an effective learning experience. It is quite informative for the community mental health nurse to observe the ways in which such families organize, and quite often, recast a given strategy into something more creative. Second, the use of testing formats creates the possibility of making counseling sessions too structured and causing a focus to be placed on the completion of tests rather than on active problem solving, growth, and self-discovery.

GOAL RELATING TO FAMILY ORGANIZATION, STRUCTURE, AND INTERRELATIONSHIPS

A general goal that relates four of the interrelationships common to all primary socialization groups concerns family structure, organization, and interrelationships. The activities that are useful for achieving this goal tend to evoke curiosity about the "inner workings" of the family. Once family members recognize the strengths and potentials of their family, they are usually willing to find out more about how they function as a family system. Curiosity and interest are generated and serve as motivating factors. Often, without quite realizing what is happening, families learn to make judgments about the effectiveness of family functioning and to make connections between this and the mental and emotional health of their members.

> *Goal: To help family systems identify their basic organization characteristic patterns of interactions, communications, and major value and belief systems and relate these to the support and strengths that are used to promote personal development of members in personal, social, and work roles and relationships.*

Activities Related to Goal Achievement

1. Plot the basic family system in terms of the structure of the family and the perceptions held by members about who is the "boss" in the family, who makes decisions, the

roles of adults and children in the family, interaction patterns, cliques or best pal in the family or who can be "counted on" in a crunch, and the ways in which communications flow in the family system.

2. Identify three or four of the most important values, beliefs, and standards of conduct that the family uses to guide members in daily living, in family life and related activities, at work, and in community activities.

3. Cite some examples of how the family organization supports individual members to seek novel and risk-taking experiences in order to advance personal growth and career interests and expand their views about the ways in which the world functions.

4. Discuss several kinds of competencies learned in the family that have helped members to become more autonomous and independent in personal behavior and to gain the freedom to be different.

5. State views of members about family potential and strengths that may be used in different ways or more effectively to help members learn additional competencies as maturational needs and personal interests and career goals of members change.

Strategies Useful for Achieving Goal

Family Mapping

Family mapping is a strategy that involves the development of a map of the basic structure of the family by identifying members of the family by their age, sex, and birth order. Toman (1976) placed considerable importance on the relationship between birth order of members and the roles they hold in the family system. He suggested a number of relationships that relate birth order and roles. On the other hand, Lewis (1980) found that in competent functioning families, differences in the roles of children seemed to be more a function of the sex of the child than the order of birth.

No doubt different interpretations can be made about the relationships between age, birth order, sex, and roles. What is more important in prevention counseling is for the community mental health nurse to help the family map out the family system in order to obtain a picture of the family structure. Once this picture has been drawn, it can be used in many different ways in counseling including the development of working hypotheses about the relationships between birth order and role behavior.

Role Mapping

Role mapping is a strategy by which information about roles can be obtained to enhance the picture of family structure and organization. This strategy focuses on the identification of roles that are commonly used in daily living activities, at work, and in community activities and relationships. It may include some of the perceptions that members hold about these roles. The nurse may have to help start the mapping of roles by giving illustrative examples. Role mapping may show that relatively few roles are used in the different aspects of family life, work relationships, and community activities and relationships. On the other hand, role mapping may show that a wide variety of roles are used, depending on the situations and settings in which actions and activities take place.

Members may be asked to imagine how roles would need to change in relation to anticipated changes in family structure, organization, or relationships. Examples of such changes might be the arrival of a new child, the last child going off to college, the loss of employment by the spouse who is the chief breadwinner, a mother who usually stays at home but has to go to work, and the onset of teenage or widowhood. Another event that has many implications for the family is when drastic changes in careers or career goals of parents occur. Usually discussions about possible changes in family roles and functions indicate some areas in which anticipatory guidance may be helpful.

Sociogramming

Sociogramming is a strategy that charts the pathways of social and interpersonal relationships of people in groups. This is particularly useful in prevention counseling with families because it is another way of obtaining information about family interaction patterns, the flow of interactions, and the placement of family members in the family group as they gather for family counseling. With experience, the community mental health nurse almost automatically notes how members arrange themselves, the flow of interactions, who is the "star" of the group, who sits where and by whom, and who makes contributions and takes risks. Changes in the sociogram of family groups may be the first indicator that roles and relationships between family members are undergoing change.

Genogramming

Genogramming is the mapping of aspects of family structure across generations of family systems. This mapping may also include characteristics of family members that have been transmitted either socially or genetically from one generation to another.

Genogramming can get rather involved; however, there are excellent detailed instructions available about the use of this strategy (Smoyak, 1982; Starkey, 1981, Guerin, 1972). It does reveal patterns of behavior and certain characteristics such as recurring illnesses and certain kinds of deviant responses to life across generations that are difficult to identify when only the present family system is considered. It is not uncommon in mental health for very cursory data to be collected about grandparents and relatives. The use of genogramming is a systematic way by which such data can be collected and organized to show interrelationships across intergenerational lines.

Sculpting

Sculpting is a strategy that allows feelings to be expressed in actions without any verbalizations. This strategy is useful in counseling when different dimensions of family interactions need to be explored.

As a counseling strategy, sculpting is relatively nonthreatening to participants, yet quite revealing in showing how relationships between family members are perceived by members. In effect, one member is asked to act out his or her perceptions of the relationships in the family by creating a "picture of the family." No words are spoken as members assume positions showing the relationships of members to each other and to the member who is sculpting the family portrait. Sculpting helps each member look through the eyes of another member in reference to unstated relationships within a family system (Perez, 1979; Duhl et al., 1973).

Repeopling

Repeopling is a strategy that places different people in relationships, events, or situations when the actual participants are emotionally involved and having difficulty sorting out "the forest from the trees." Situations may then be considered on an "as if" basis, that is, the experience can be examined as if the persons actually involved in the experiences were not involved.

To organize experiences by use of repeopling, the community mental health nurse asks the members who occupied the roles in the acutal experience to enact these. Then, one-by-one the roles are repeopled by other members. After roles have been assigned to new role occupants, it is usually possible to role play and discuss aspects of the experiences from different perspectives. A final part of this strategy is to reconstitute the experience by placing members back in their original roles one by one until all the roles are filled. Usually by the time this is completed the original occupants of roles are able to view experiences in quite different ways. Repeopling is a strategy that has the capability to develop insight fairly rapidly and to change behavior.

Anticipatory Guidance

Anticipatory guidance is an educational and counseling strategy used in many kinds of prevention activities. In effect, it is guidance that is provided on the basis of events or relationships that are anticipated and in which people need advance preparation so that they can cope in ways that they are not overwhelming.

The community mental health nurse uses his or her knowledge of growth and development across the life span to plan anticipatory guidance in relation to maturational and developmental events. Unanticipated events and changes in roles and relationships may also be handled by helping members identify similar experiences that they have handled successfully. Members can be helped to do some problem solving about unexpected situations that suddenly face the family.

Demonstrations

The use of *demonstrations* in prevention counseling is very effective for portraying certain kinds of roles and experiences or teaching certain kinds of competencies. This strategy may also be used to present actual situations of family living in which family strengths can be attached to experiences. Demonstrations may also be used to have members portray examples of relationships or situations that they find uncomfortable or not supportive in achieving some of their needs.

The use of demonstrations is an active strategy. It requires a considerable amount of participation on the part of members and the nurse. Of course, return demonstrations may be part of this strategy, particularly in attempts to change behaviors, where coaching and practice are useful.

Calling Attention to Mind Reading

Mind reading is a form of interaction in which one person completes sentences for another, thus intruding on the thought processes and chain of communication of the person trying to communicate. This kind of interaction is common in family and other social relationships. Irrespective of when such interactions occur, mind reading establishes unsatisfactory communications for both the person trying to state his or her thoughts and for the person who becomes so anxious or impatient at any delay in this process that he or she moves to shape the content of the message for the other person.

Oddly enough, this kind of interaction is often not recognized by either party or it may be recognized by the person who is not allowed by other people to express his or her thoughts without assistance. People who mind read almost always hold their breaths at the delay in expression of communication and are usually relieved when they can intervene to complete a communication. The community mental health nurse may have to use other strategies to show this process in action if calling attention to it does not create enough sensitivity to alter behavior.

Mind reading has the capability of generating anger in people who are on the receiving end of this kind of interaction. Eventually, they wonder whether something is wrong with them. In such instances, there is often a lack of sensitivity and recognition of the effect of slow and incomplete communications on both the sender and listener. The sender does not realize that a delay in the communication process causes listeners considerable anxiety, until a point is reached where they leap in to help out by completing the communication. The sender, groping for words to express, may be unaware that the flow of communication has altered to the extent that the process has become more important than the content of the message.

Successful communications are closely related to how a person feels about self and they are necessary for satisfying relationships with others. The ability to express clear and concise communications is a basic competence that is essential for personal growth and social relationships, thus has a direct relationship to mental health.

Clarification through Feedback

This strategy is a basic one in prevention counseling as it is designed to validate communications, thoughts, feelings, and actions by getting clarifications until everyone is satisfied that a picture is complete and the messages understood. On the basis of validation, restatements of communications, the intent of these, and associated feelings encourage reactions and openness in responses. Often, an account of an experience is set forth and in this process, members become aware that there are gaps and incompleteness about the episode. If clarifications are not sought, the person telling the account will think that the message imparted is correct and understood. *Clarifications through feedback* assist in the cognitive restructuring process and help to bring into focus aspects of experiences that may not have been thought of very clearly.

In counseling, care should be used to ensure that clarifications are based on accurate data. Although one would not expect unwitting distortions in accounts of experiences provided by members in adaptive and healthy functioning families, this strategy is also used for counseling families and individuals who are experiencing psychiatric problems. Nurses and other mental health helpers sometimes unknowingly support clarifications of experiences when they know that such accounts are bizarre and untrue. Such clarifications from people who think rationally in support of obviously irrational ideas and experiences must really make mentally ill persons very frightened as reality is not being presented to them in ways that help get their thoughts better organized and straightened out.

Calling Attention to Repetitive Patterns of Communication

Calling attention to repetitive patterns of communication is a strategy that is useful when people repeat the same thing over and over and the person does not use information provided by others to alter communications. In mentally healthy people, this kind of communication is usually the result of habits they may not even be aware of. For example, the patterned use of "you know" as a substitute for clear communications is a common practice. Excessive use of "you know" implies that the listener can fill gaps. It also assumes the listener knows the thoughts and messages that the person is ineffectively communicating. Extensive use of repetitive patterns of communication has an effect of causing a listener's attention to focus on this phenomenon rather than on the content and intent of the communication.

Pinpointing

Pinpointing is a strategy that allows one to bring into sharp focus limited aspects of experiences, communications, feelings, or situations in order to examine these in depth and to determine what learning can be generalized to other situations and experiences.

Pinpointing is a form of boundary setting. As a counseling strategy, it is useful for holding the larger contexts of experiences and relationships in abeyance so that more limited parts of the experience can be examined and analyzed. In effect, pinpointing examines a micro experience under powerful lenses, so to speak, in order to bring the salient features to the fore. A determination then has to be made about whether these features can be generalized to whole experiences or used to understand particular ones.

Values Clarification

Values clarification is a most useful strategy when information is needed about the value system that families hold and that has great influence on parenting, family, and individual behavior, roles, and family organization and function. Values held by families and their respective members tend to be inculcated in both subtle and direct ways in the process of socialization.

Values are acquired in large part by subtle and indirect means. These include non-verbal communication, behavior observed and associated with particular situations and relationships, congruences and incongruences between what parents or significant others may state are values for conduct and the behavior actually used or condoned, feelings that may be incongruent with behavior, and rewards provided by significant others for certain kinds of behavior. Learning by indirection often leaves people with an incompleteness about the relationship between particular values and behavior. It is not surprising to find that families may never have made explicit the value system that they try to live by and inculcate in their members.

A first step in the use of this strategy is to have the family identify values that the family holds. Next, clarification of these values is needed because members usually have different interpretations attached to values, particularly when a number of "if's" are involved. Then, family members can be asked to identify some situations in which values were difficult if not impossible to hold to as a guide for behavior. In this process, it usually becomes evident that there are some values that families will uphold even great cost, while others may be relative to particular relationships and situations. This knowledge makes it possible to clarify the ranking of values in terms of their importance and absoluteness. The important point in values clarification is to make more explicit just what the family's set of values consists of and the relative importance of these. Through such clarification, values tend to distill to some basic essences and these are the base for the family's set of values. They are very important in understanding the family system functioning and individual behavior of members.

All of the strategies discussed in relation to this goal have the capability to obtain data that is useful for examining family interactions, relationships, organization, and structure. Some strategies are more effective for some things than for others. The community mental health nurse will have to exercise judgment about the best strategies to use for particular purposes.

GOAL RELATING TO FAMILY ORGANIZATION FOR HANDLING DAILY LIVING RELATIONSHIPS AND ACTIVITIES

A fourth general goal that needs to be included in the clinical organizing framework in prevention counseling is one that focuses on the organization and functioning of the family system in relation to coping and managing in both daily living and crises situations. One of the basic interrelationships common to primary socialization groups concerns the interrelationship between family organization and functioning and the mental health of family members.

Daily living includes the relationships and internal family arrangements of roles and division of labor that are necessary for the system to be dynamic. Such relationships include coping with daily problems, satisfying and frustrating experiences, and recurring experiences that require time, energy, and emotional investment. Some of these types of experiences may be satisfying to some people and quite frustrating to others. For example, the tasks that are required to maintain a house, provide support, and rear children are experienced by people in quite different ways.

Family systems also have to cope with unexpected events, some of which may be crises of one kind or another. The organization and strengths of the family as a system have a direct bearing on the ability of the family to cope under such circumstances without considerable stress being experienced by the family as a unit and by individual members. Usual methods of coping may prove to be inadequate or have to be modified in crisis situations or when unexpected events of some magnitude occur.

Family organization also concerns the way in which members are encouraged to use their time and energy, to avail themselves of different kinds of activities, and to seek relationships outside the family. At both the family and individual levels of organization, competencies have to be learned in daily living that make it possible to handle expected and crisis events. Development of self-confidence in family members is usually enhanced by participation in diverse experiences in which social, interpersonal, and problem-solving competencies are learned. These competencies need to include learning how to handle conflicting relationships and situations, collaboration with others, opportunities to practice the art of compromise, and learning how to function in groups.

There are some basic competencies that are best learned in environments that have a high intensity of concern, emotional involvement, and closeness between members in the system. Such environments usually have cohesion, an intimate knowledge of members, and conflicts and agreements of various kinds; in them, adults have distinct roles, functions, and authority. Behavior and values learned in these environments are governed for the most part by norms and standards set by the adults and are enforced on their authority. Competencies have to be general enough to be useful in both primary socialization groups and social settings in quite different contexts.

An integral part of the family organization that relates to daily living is the set of attitudes and behaviors held about health in both its mental and physical aspects. Belloc and Breslow (1977) suggested a lifetime health monitoring program to increase longevity and prevent illness. The exact linkages that exist between physical and mental health continue to be difficult to isolate; however, clinical observations and experiences suggest that such connections do exist.

Examination of family functioning in daily living situations usually evokes some anxiety, guilt, and blame placing. It is important for the nurse to realize this will occur and to recognize such responses for what they are: reactions associated with the discomfort of looking at relationships between people who care about each other and wonder whether they have been adequate in fulfilling roles and responsibilities for themselves and family members. So it is not surprising to find that an inquiry in this area tends to be emotionally arousing. Parents may feel somewhat threatened and anxious and experience anger because they relate such observations to the adequacy of their parenting. It is just as well to get these emotionally charged feelings in the open and help members to recognize them as valid. An attitude of acceptance on the part of the nurse usually goes a long way toward establishing the idea that such feelings are not "sick," are not abnormal, and are not something about which one should feel a need to accept blame.

> *Goal:* To help family systems identify how they are organized to cope in daily living and crisis situations and promote mental and physical health of members.

Activities Related to Goal Achievement

1. Identify characteristic patterns of coping in the family system in relation to daily living relationships and activities; specify how these patterns enhance or create difficulties in coping for members.
2. Describe some crisis situations that the family has recently dealt with looking at the roles, responsibilities, and coping actions that were used by the family as a system and by individual members.
3. Compare the ways in which the family as a unit copes in daily living situations and in crisis situations.
4. Discuss the effectiveness of coping in daily living and crisis situations and identify areas in which additional education and different kinds of approaches might be more useful in efforts to promote and maintain mental and physical health.
5. Discuss the family's plan for health promotion and maintenance for both mental and physical health.

Strategies Useful for Achieving Goal

Coping Pattern Identification
Coping pattern identification is a strategy that is used to identify the ways in which families organize the various dimensions of family living in order to survive and achieve some measure of satisfaction. Such patterns are primarily developed by experience, through observations of parents and significant others, and from educational and media sources.

Coping patterns may be identified by having the family provide detailed descriptions of selected daily living situations and how these were managed. It is helpful to get accounts of experiences that have the potential for showing diversity in coping. For example, family living situations that cover breakfast and getting children off to school and adults to work and those that cover the dinner and after-dinner hours are two such experiences. Other situations would be when baby-sitters cannot come at the last minute; the illness of a child, particularly when both parents work; unexpected car troubles; or sudden unexpected responsibilities at work or with the family that demand a temporary change in roles, responsibilities, or residence. Information also needs to be obtained about how the family provides private time for its members and uses its leisure time.

Coping patterns can be mapped out for both crisis and noncrisis situations. This mapping process consists of identifying the steps and actions that were taken as the daily living events or the crisis unfolded. The sequence of actions needs to be placed in a framework of time, whether by hours, days, or weeks, depending on what is relevant. Outcomes of the various steps can be noted as far as they are known. As the coping process is broken down in sequential steps, data are usually secured about the feelings of members and the kinds of things that led them from one step to the next.

This analysis will indicate whether families are using their potential for effective coping. It will also provide information about the use of the problem-solving approach, particularly in situations in which the usual coping dialogue was not effective or adequate.

Problem Solving

Problem solving as a strategy is used systematically to examine problems of various kinds. The process is a series of steps organized to build one on the other. It starts with a definition of a problem. Data are collected relating to the problem. An initial assessment may show the problem needs to be redefined as well as additional data collected. Data are organized to arrive at a tentative conclusion relating to the problem. This conclusion is considered or tested for plausibility. It may be necessary to reevaluate the data to arrive at other conclusions if the first conclusion does not produce the desired outcome. The overall sequence leads to the adoption of a conclusion on the basis of available data.

Problem solving as a counseling strategy is essential for eliciting participation from clients and helping them to learn to use a more rational approach to understanding how they function. It also helps members to develop one of the basic cognitive competencies that supports the development of selfhood and self-identity, both of which are related to positive mental health.

Problem solving in prevention counseling is important for another reason. Many experiences that are family-related involve current members of a family and have strong emotional feelings attached to them. This often makes it difficult to move beyond such feelings in order to examine other aspects of experiences. Problem solving provides a structure or another frame of reference in which such examinations may occur.

Development of Alternative Strategies

This strategy meets the need for families to expand their perceptions about different ways of perceiving relationships, events, and achieving goals. It is important to assist families to think about and develop alternative strategies, particularly when coping patterns and characteristic responses to situations are restrictive.

The *development of alternative strategies* can be promoted by asking families to develop different ways of handling situations that they have already experienced. Alternative approaches may be demonstrated and compared with the actual strategies that were used in order to assess their effectiveness.

The strategy of developing alternative strategies is an indirect way of helping families determine whether the usual coping dialogues and patterns are too restrictive and repetitive. In this situation, a milieu is provided in which evaluation can be recognized and accepted. This kind of participation is a challenge to families to use their strengths and potential to develop and try out alternative approaches of coping.

Exploring Person–Environment "Fit"

This strategy is used to help families recognize the interrelationship between the environment, or milieu, created in the family system and the "fit" it has for developing the kind of learning and experiences desired for family members. The family environment tends to reflect the values and beliefs held by the family, both of which influence the ways in which families provide for its members essential relationships, support, and experiences.

One part of the American myth is that people can be anything they choose to be by individual effort and hard work. This myth about individual efforts has obscured the importance of families and their role in helping members to achieve their goals and develop selfhood. It is not surprising to find that families often do not realize the extent of their role in the individual development of their members and the importance of the family milieu as a unique, highly intense learning environment.

The first step in *exploring person–environment fit* is to obtain from the family selected dimensions of family life and living they emphasize and hold expectations about in terms of behavior and attitudes of members. For example, the religious dimension may be the major organizing force in the family. Such an emphasis creates certain expectations for family members in terms of their commitments to others and to community, the use of appropriate actions and behaviors, the organization of family living, the kind of milieu established in the home, and the opportunities provided members for their growth and development. Next, members consider how these dimensions are expressed in family living and in what ways they impact on each member. Finally, some expressions of how the family environment fits individual members are obtained if at all possible. Such statements may cause anguish to parents if a child does not regard the family environment as positively as they do.

Analysis of Winning and Losing Processes and Attitudes

The *analysis of winning and losing processes and attitudes* as they are expressed in families provides information that is different from that generated by other strategies. Winning and losing have different consequences for the family and each of its members and involve family and individual identities, values, and ethics. The chances of winning or losing mean there is competition for some particular thing or goal. Competition involves striving, vying, and seeking some goal or benefit against some kind of opposing force. It is the importance attached to competing and winning and the processes that are established for competition that are of concern in prevention counseling.

Labels of winners or losers may be attached to individuals as well as to families, and they have a relationship to positive mental health. All of us have heard someone referred to as "a born winner" or "a born loser." Like all such labels, these tend to become part of a self-fulfilling prophecy for the person so labeled. Gradually, behavior associated with such labels becomes incorporated as an integral part of the organization of the self.

The analysis in counseling is started by asking family members to indicate how they view their family: as a winner or loser. Next, information is obtained about the importance of winning and being winners. Usually, the discussion that occurs suggests some of the values that govern competition and the importance of winning. For example, a value that may be expressed by families is that members adhere to fair play—as long as they win. Other families may say that it is not the outcome of competition that is important but whether the game is played by the rules with both winners and losers accorded respect for good sportsmanship and effort.

An analysis of winning and losing attitudes and processes is important because competition is involved in most of the relationships and activities that make up personal and social life. A problem arises when the need to compete and win becomes a major part of relationships and goal attainment. In such cases, the community mental health nurse has to help to reconceive such relationships in different frames of reference.

Developing a Plan for Health-Protective Behaviors

An important strategy in prevention counseling in mental health is to help families identify their plan for health maintenance and illness prevention. Such a plan needs to include protective behaviors that address both mental and physical health.

It is not unusual for families to indicate that they have no plan for preventions relating to mental health and that members go to the family physician for physical checkups as needed or for medical care when illness occurs. Health education about the importance of a more systematic approach to the prevention of mental, physical, and emotional health problems is usually needed.

The community mental health nurse can teach the family to use certain kinds of health-protective behaviors (Sommers & Breslow, 1977; Belloc & Breslow, 1972). Such things as periodic checks on the vital signs, particularly blood pressure, obtaining immunizations, using proper nutrition, having a regular exercise program, and maintaining proper weight are the responsibility of the family to its members. They are also part of *developing a plan for health-protective behaviors*. The nurse can provide current information about the need for frequency of certain kinds of preventive health behaviors. These include such things as annual physicals, Pap tests, breast examinations, various kinds of blood and urine examinations, and stress and cardiac tests. Health-protective behaviors to prevent emotional and mental problems include using stress reduction exercises; learning how to express emotions, particularly anger; learning how to be active in decision making through assertive training; and using laughter as a therapeutic activity for wellness. People can be sensitized to recognize behaviors that indicate undue stress, anxiety, or depression so that professional assistance is sought before these become too serious. Mental health checkups are just as important as physical ones. Such a checkup includes a review of behaviors associated with positive mental health, effective coping, and identification of concerns about growth and development.

Anxiety Management

Anxiety management is a strategy in which the community mental health nurse needs to have clinical expertise. The management of anxiety, that is, an uncomfortable, vague, and tension-producing feeling, is necessary in all kinds of counseling. In prevention counseling, it is especially important because of the active participation of families in problem-solving and learning experiences that relate to personal and sensitive relationships.

Anxiety has many dimensions, two of which are useful in its management. First, there is the experience of feeling uncomfortable, of being anxious, of having vague feelings of dread. Second, there are behaviors that most poeple use that indicate anxiety. In individuals, these behaviors vary from person to person; however, some common ones are lacing and unlacing of fingers or rhythmically swinging a limb, perspiration, tenseness of the body, body movements of various sorts, paleness, wandering attention, not feeling well in the stomach, and attempts to cut off, divert, or ignore communications that are anxiety-producing.

Management of anxiety in individuals first involves recognition by the nurse of what is happening. This includes making a judgment about when anxious behaviors first appear and what was happening in the counseling process at the time. Then, the nurse may observe that counseling sometimes causes people to feel anxious and wonder aloud whether this is happening in the family. Usually, this is enough to make the admission and discussion of anxiety acceptable. Some connections have to be made between the feelings of anxiousness, the behaviors through which these feelings are expressed, and the experiences that trigger both feelings and behavior. It usually rests on the judgment of the nurse to determine when the family is ready for this kind of learning. Sometimes, a linkage between the feelings and behavior can be made while the linkage to experiences are held in abeyance.

The idea that feelings are expressed by behaviors is quite novel to many people and needs to be thought about and other examples considered. Sometimes, it is possible to have members take on an assignment of identifying their own anxious behaviors. In this process, they become sensitive to both feeling and behavioral cues that can alert them when they are becoming anxious.

Anxiety in groups may be managed by getting the groups to pinpoint what they think is making them anxious. In groups, the feeling of being anxious has a contagious effect and can be transmitted to members quite rapidly, thus some members may have no idea of what is happening that makes them feel so uncomfortable. Once some pinpointing has been done, it is then possible to get the group to do some problem solving in order to get a better picture of the anxiety-producing experience or relationship. Once such a data base is available, the group can decide on what, if any, actions they want to take.

Anxiety management in a group setting provides some opportunities for positive learning experiences. It also requires members to assume part of the responsibility for group actions and reach a consensus on some common goals. Members have to be concerned about the consequences of actions on the group itself and on its individual members.

GOAL RELATING TO FAMILY SYSTEM AND COMMUNITY INTERRELATIONSHIPS

The last basic interrelationship common to primary socialization groups that needs to be addressed in prevention counseling concerns the linkages between family systems and community systems of activities and networks. Such linkages or interrelationships include activities, friendship and support groups, and various kinds of networks and service organizations, all of which provide essential and enhancing services to people in the community. All of these systems and services interrelate directly and indirectly to the mental health of families and the mental health of the community.

> *Goal: To help family systems identify and recognize the importance of interrelationships between their mental health and the mental health of communities.*

Activities Useful for Achieving Goal

1. Identify some of the indicators that are considered to be evidence of the mental health of a community.
2. Specify some of the linkages between family systems and the community that affect the mental health of both.
3. List some of the community activities in which families participate that help members learn essential social and interpersonal competencies related to social adjustment and satisfying relationships.
4. Obtain definitions of community that are held by families and of the responsibilities they assume for the general good of the community and its people.

Strategies Useful for Achieving Goal

Defining the Community

The strategy of having families define what their community means to them is a first step toward emphasizing the importance of the community to their mental health. Furthermore, this activity highlights the intertwining of factors that link the mental health of families and individuals and the mental health of communities.

Family and individual mental health have social and cultural aspects as well as interpersonal and psychological ones. Many of the social, cultural, and interpersonal aspects of mental health are embedded in community living. The extent and kind of essential social experiences and support networks available in a community are important for positive mental health.

Defining the community may have several dimensions. It is helpful to have families discuss some of these dimensions because they set a frame of reference about the community in a way that may never have been considered before. Although there are many ways of approaching the defining of one's community, the dimensions identified in earlier concepts have been found to be effective for this purpose. First is the dimension known as the *emotional community*. How does a family define this, that is, where is the place that they have a sense of belonging, an attachment, a feeling of roots? Another dimension is the *structural community*. It concerns the kind and frequency of relationships the family has with other primary groups on a continuing basis. What community does the family feel responsibility for? What kinds of patterns of health and illness exist in the boundaries of the defined community? Next, does the family have an identifiable *functional community*? That is, does the family participate in various groups that have common interests and concerns about the community and work toward enhancement of the quality of life? Or bring about change in the community? In the process of developing such definitions, families come to acquire a broader concept of community. They also realize that the community is a living entity and must receive attention for its health and well-being because of the relationship to the quality of life and health of its people.

Development of a Profile of Indicators of Community Mental Health

In prevention counseling, it is necessary for families to acquire some specific ideas about the so-called indicators of community mental health. Mental health is an abstract term and means many things. It gets even more abstract when applied to another abstraction like the community. Therefore, in order to discuss the mental health of a community, some concrete things have to be identified that indicate examples of community mental health.

In the *development of a profile of indicators of community mental health*, the nurse may use several approaches, two of which will be mentioned. The first one consists of the nurse presenting information about selected indicators and followed by discussion. A second approach involves the identification of indicators and then asking members to use these to collect and organize information about the community. There may also be a combination of the two approaches. Selected community indicators usually include the following:

1. the extent that the community provides for experiences for its children and adults that are essential for positive health and mental health across the life span

2. the extent that resources are provided so that families may experience satisfying and growth-promoting personal, interpersonal, and group relationships
3. the extent to which the community has high-risk populations that live in poverty and are prone to the development of major social, health, and mental health problems
4. the extent to which social and community networks link families, primary groups having diverse interests, and community resources and activities
5. the extent to which the community's population enjoys mental wellness and is enlightened about mental health and mental illness
6. the presence of kin and friend networks and community resources that can be called on in case of need or crisis
7. the extent that the community provides essential services for survival to populations who are homeless, friendless, and penniless
8. the extent that the community provides cultural and recreational programs as well as special programs that recognize people in the community and their contributions

Assessment of Community Participation

Community participation is necessary for adaptive and healthy functioning families. As a counseling strategy, families need to conduct an assessment of such participation. It is not unusual for such participation to be limited in scope though adequate in number. Participation may be primarily in recreational activities or clustered around some other kind of activity. The assessment may also show that community participation is primarily for meeting the needs of individual family members with little contribution to the common good of the community.

The assessment consists of asking each family member and the family as a whole to identify activities in which they have participated over some particular period of time. The kinds of activities are identified and information obtained about whether the same or different persons were involved. This data base gives a good idea of the nature of interrelationships that exist between the family and the community.

In the prevention counseling process, a milieu can be established in which active participation can be used to establish powerful learning experiences. Prevention counseling establishes a frame of reference in which mental health education and principles of positive mental health can be experienced and incorporated in the systems of values, attitudes, and behaviors held by families and members.

The clinical organizing framework for prevention counseling in community mental health nursing is a way of planning and using both concepts of mental health and nursing to promote and improve the mental health of families and communities. Prevention in mental health is at the heart of what has been described as a bold new approach in this field.

SUMMARY

An approach to prevention in community mental health nursing is to focus on counseling with primary socialization systems. Prevention counseling for positive mental health emphasizes a holistic concept of health and an assumption of responsibilities by people for promoting, maintaining, and monitoring the mental health of themselves, their families, and the communities in which they live.

Primary socialization groups such as families are key systems of interaction in which concepts of mental health and principles of prevention for emotional and mental health may be applied directly by use of prevention activities and strategies. A clinical organizing framework organizes and integrates theory, research, and prevention strategies. This framework combines the general goals of mental health and the specific goals for mental health for individual families. Indicators of mental health for families and communities provide referents that are based on experiences and may be attached to behavior.

Community mental health nursing, by providing leadership and new approaches to promote and maintain positive mental health, enhances the profession's traditional emphasis in this area of public health. It is an approach that expands and extends the contributions of psychiatric and mental health nursing that has traditionally focused on stressed and psychiatrically ill people and families.

REFERENCES

Alger, I. Therapeutic use of video-tape play back. *Journal of Nervous Disorders* 148:430–436, 1969.

Argyle, Michael. Interaction skills and social competence. In Feldman, Philip, and Orford, John, eds. *Psychological Problems: The Social Context.* New York: John Wiley & Sons, 1980, pp. 132–150.

Belloc, Nedra B., and Breslow, Lester. Relationship of physical health status and health practices. *Preventive Medicine* 1(3):409–421, August, 1972.

Cowen, Emory L. Baby-steps toward primary prevention. *American Journal of Community Psychology* 5:1–22, 1977.

Duhl, F. T., Kantor, D., and Duhl, B. S. Learning, space and action in family therapy: A primer of sculpture. In Blick, D. A., ed. *Techniques of Family Psychotherapy: A Primer.* New York: Grune and Stratton, 1973, p. 60.

Ellis, Albert, and Greiger, R. *Handbook of Rational–Emotive Therapy.* New York: Springer, 1977.

Goldston, Stephen E. An overview of primary prevention programming. In Klein, Donald C., and Goldston, Stephen E., eds. *Primary Prevention: An Idea Whose Time Has Come.* Washington, DC: National Institute of Mental Health, 1977, pp. 23–40.

Guerin, Philip. Study your own family. In Ferber, A., Mendelsohn, M., and Napier, A., eds. *The Book of Family Therapy.* Boston: Houghton Mifflin, 1972, pp. 449–457.

Lewis, Jerry M. Family matrix in health and disease. In Hoflinger, Charles, ed. *The Family: Evaluation and Treatment.* New York: Brunner/Mazel, 1980, pp. 199–217.

Oiler, Carolyn. The phenomenological approach in nursing research. *Nursing Research* 31(3):178–181, May/June, 1982.

Pender, Nola J. *Health Promotion and Nursing Practice.* Norwalk, CT: Appleton-Century-Crofts, 1982, pp. 2 and 213–216.

Perez, Joseph. F. *Family Counseling.* New York: Van Nostrand Reinhold, 1979, pp. 1–3.

Pless, I. B., and Satterwhite, B. A measure of family functioning and its application. *Social Science and Medicine* 7:613–621, 1973.

President's Commission on Mental Health Prevention Task Force. *Task Panel Reports Submitted to the President's Commission on Mental Health,* vol. 4 (No. 040-000-00393-2). Washington, DC: Government Printing Office, 1978, pp. 1822–1863.

Smoyak, Shirley. Family Systems: Use of genograms As an assessment tool. In Smoyak, Shirley, ed. *Family Therapy: A Nursing Perspective.* New York: John Wiley & Sons, 1982, pp. 245–250.

Sommers, Anne, and Breslow, Lester. The lifetime health monitoring program: A practical approach to preventive medicine. *New England Journal of Medicine* 296(11):601–608, March 17, 1977.

Starkey, Penny J. Genograms: A guide to understanding one's own family system. *Perspectives in Psychiatric Care* 19(6):164–173, September–December, 1981.

Toman, Walter. *Family Constellation,* 3rd ed. New York: Springer, 1976, Chapter 16.

Vaughan, Warren T., Huntington, Dorothy S., Samuels, Thomas E., Bilnes, Murray, and Shapiro, Marvin I. Family mental health maintenance: A new approach to primary prevention. *Hospital and Community Psychiatry* 26(8):503–508, 1975.

I | MESSAGE FROM THE PRESIDENT OF THE UNITED STATES RELATIVE TO MENTAL ILLNESS AND MENTAL RETARDATION

February 5, 1963: Referred to the Committee on Interstate and Foreign Commerce and ordered to be printed

To the Congress of the United States:
It is my intention to send shortly to the Congress a message pertaining to this Nations's most urgent needs in the area of health improvement. But two health problems—because they are of such critical size and tragic impact, and because their susceptibility to public action is so much greater than the attention they have received—are deserving of a wholly new national approach and a separate message to the Congress. These twin problems are mental illness and mental retardation.

From the earliest days of the Public Health Service to the latest research of the National Institutes of Health, the Federal Government has recognized its responsibilities to assist, stimulate, and channel public energies in attacking health problems. Infectious epidemics are now largely under control. Most of the major diseases of the body are beginning to give ground in man's increasing struggle to find their cause and cure. But the public understanding, treatment, and prevention of mental disabilities have not made comparable progress since the earliest days of modern history.

Yet mental illness and mental retardation are among our most critical health problems. They occur more frequently, affect more people, require more prolonged treatment, cause more suffering by the families of the afflicted, waste more of our human resources, and constitute more financial drain upon both the Public Treasury and the personal finances of the individual families than any other single condition.

There are now about 800,000 such patients in this Nation's institutions—600,000 for mental illness and over 200,000 for mental retardation. Every year nearly 1,500,000 people receive treatment in institutions for the mentally ill and mentally retarded. Most of them are confined and compressed within an antiquated, vastly overcrowded, chain of custodial State institutions. The average amount expended on their care is only $4 a day—too little to do much good for the individual, but too much if measured in terms of efficient use of our mental health dollars. In some States the average is less than $2 a day.

The total cost to the taxpayers is over $2.4 billion a year in direct public outlays for services—about $1.8 billion for mental illness and $600 million for mental retardation. Indirect public outlays, in welfare costs and in the waste of human resources, are even higher. But the anguish suffered both by those afflicted and by their families transcends financial statistics—particularly in view of the fact that both mental illness and mental retardation strike so often in childhood, leading in most cases to a lifetime of disablement for the patient and a lifetime of hardship for his family.

This situation has been tolerated far too long. It has troubled our national conscience—but only as a problem unpleasant to mention, easy to postpone, and despairing of solution. The Federal Government, despite the nationwide impact of the problem, has largely left the solutions up to the States. The States have depended on custodial hospitals and homes. Many such hospitals and homes have been shamefully understaffed, overcrowded, unpleasant institutions from which death too often provided the only firm hope of release.

The time has come for a bold new approach. New medical, scientific, and social tools and insights are now available. A series of comprehensive studies initiated by the Congress, the executive branch, and interested private groups have been completed and all point in the same direction.

Governments at every level—Federal, State, and local—private foundations and individual citizens must all face up to their responsibilities in this area. Our attack must be focused on three major objectives:

First, we must seek out the causes of mental illness and of mental retardation and eradicate them. Here, more than in any other area, "an ounce of prevention is worth more than a pound of cure." For prevention is far more desirable for all concerned. It is far more economical and it is far more likely to be successful. Prevention will require both selected specific programs directed especially at known causes, and the general strengthening of our fundamental community, social welfare, and educational programs which can do much to eliminate or correct the harsh environmental conditions which often are associated with mental retardation and mental illness. The proposals contained in my earlier message to the Congress on education and those which will be contained in a later message I will send on the Nation's health will also help achieve this objective.

Second, we must strengthen the underlying resources of knowledge and, above all, of skilled manpower which are necessary to mount and sustain our attack on mental disability for many years to come. Personnel from many of the same professions serve both the mentally ill and the mentally retarded. We must increase our existing training programs and launch new ones, for our efforts cannot succeed unless we increase by severalfold in the next decade the number of professional and subprofessional personnel who work in these fields. My proposals on the health professions and aid for higher education are essential to this goal, and both the proposed youth employment program and a national service corps can be of immense help. We must also expand our research efforts if we are to learn more about how to prevent and treat the crippling or malfunction of the mind.

Third, we must strengthen and improve the programs and facilities serving the mentally ill and the mentally retarded. The emphasis should be upon timely and intensive diagnosis, treatment, training, and rehabilitation so that the mentally afflicted can be cured or their functions restored to the extent possible. Services to both the mentally ill and to the mentally retarded must be community based and provide a range of services to meet community needs.

It is with these objectives in mind that I am proposing a new approach to mental illness and to mental retardation. This approach is designed, in large measure, to use Federal resources to stimulate State, local, and private action. When carried out, reliance on the cold mercy of custodial isolation will be supplanted by the open warmth of community concern and capability. Emphasis on prevention, treatment, and rehabilitation will be substituted for a desultory interest in confining patients in an institution to wither away.

In an effort to hold domestic expenditures down in a period of tax reduction, I have postponed new programs and reduced added expenditures in all areas when that could be done. But we cannot afford to postpone any longer a reversal in our approach to mental affliction. For too long the shabby treatment of the many millions of the mentally disabled in custodial institutions and many millions more now in communities needing help has been justified on grounds of inadequate funds, further studies, and future promises. We can procrastinate no more. The national mental health program and the national program to combat mental retardation herein proposed warrant prompt congressional attention.

I. A NATIONAL PROGRAM FOR MENTAL HEALTH

I propose a national mental health program to assist in the inauguration of a wholly new emphasis and approach to care for the mentally ill. This approach relies primarily upon the new knowledge and new drugs acquired and developed in recent years which make it possible for most of the mentally ill to be successfully and quickly treated in their own communities and returned to a useful place in society.

These breakthroughs have rendered obsolete the traditional methods of treatment which imposed upon the mentally ill a social quarantine, a prolonged or permanent confinement in huge, unhappy mental hospitals, where they were out of sight and forgotten. I am not unappreciative of the efforts undertaken by many States to improve conditions in these hospitals, or the dedicated work of many hospital staff members. But their task has been staggering and the results too often dismal, as the comprehensive study by the Joint Commission on Mental Illness and Health pointed out in 1961. Some States have at times been forced to crowd five, ten, or even fifteen thousand people into one large understaffed institution. Imposed largely for reasons of economy, such practices were costly in human terms, as well as in a real economic sense. The following statistics are illustrative:

> Nearly one-fifth of the 279 State mental institutions are fire and health hazards; three-fourths of them were opened prior to World War I.
> Nearly half of the 530,000 patients in our State mental hospitals are in institutions with over 3,000 patients, where individual care and consideration are almost impossible.
> Many of these institutions have less than half the professional staff required— with less than 1 psychiatrist for every 360 patients.
> Forty-five percent of their inmates have been hospitalized continuously for 10 years or more.

But there are hopeful signs. In recent years the increasing trend toward higher and higher concentrations in these institutions has been reversed—by the use of new drugs, by the increasing public awareness of the nature of mental illness, and by a trend toward the provision of community facilities, including psychiatric beds in general hospitals, day care centers, and outpatient psychiatric clinics. Community general hospitals in 1961 treated and discharged as cured more than 200,000 psychiatric patients.

I am convinced that, if we apply our medical knowledge and social insights fully, all but a small portion of the mentally ill can eventually achieve a wholesome and constructive social adjustment. It has been demonstrated that two out of three schizophrenics—our largest category of mentally ill—can be treated and released within 6 months, but under the conditions that prevail today the average stay for schizophrenia is 11 years. In 11 States, by the use of modern techniques, 7 out of every 10 schizophrenia patients admitted were discharged within 9 months. In one instance, where a State hospital deliberately sought an alternative to hospitalization in those patients about to be admitted, it was able to treat successfully in the community 50 percent of them. It is clear that a concerted national attack on mental disorders is now both possible and practical.

If we launch a broad new mental health program now, it will be possible within a decade or two to reduce the number of patients now under custodial care by 50 percent or more. Many more mentally ill can be helped to remain in their own homes without hardship to themselves or their families. Those who are hospitalized can be helped to return to their own communities. All but a small proportion can be restored to useful life. We can spare them and their families much of the misery which mental illness now entails. We can save public funds and we can conserve our manpower resources.

1. Comprehensive Community Mental Health Centers

Central to a new mental health program is comprehensive community care. Merely pouring Federal funds into a continuation of the outmoded type of institutional care which now prevails would make little difference. We need a new type of health facility, one which will return mental health care to the main stream of American medicine, and at the same time upgrade mental health services. I recommend, therefore, that the Congress (1) authorize grants to the States for the construction of comprehensive community mental health centers, beginning in fiscal year 1965, with the Federal Government providing 45 to 75 percent of the project cost; (2) authorize short-term project grants for the initial staffing costs of comprehensive community mental health centers, with the Federal Government providing up to 75 percent of the cost in the early months, on a gradually declining basis, terminating such support for a project within slightly over 4 years; and (3) to facilitate the preparation of community plans for these new facilities as a necessary preliminary to any construction or staffing assistance, appropriate $4.2 million for planning grants under the National Institute of Mental Health. These planning funds, which would be in addition to a similar amount appropriated for fiscal year 1963, have been included in my proposed 1964 budget.

While the essential concept of the comprehensive community mental health center is new, the separate elements which would be combined in it are presently found in many communities: diagnostic and evaluation services, emergency psychiatric units, outpatient services, inpatient services, day and night care, foster home care, rehabilitation, consultative services to other community agencies, and mental health information and education.

These centers will focus community resources and provide better community facilities for all aspects of mental health care. Prevention as well as treatment will be a major activity. Located in the patient's own environment and community, the center would make possible a better understanding of his needs, a more cordial atmosphere for his recovery, and a continuum of treatment. As his needs change, the patient could move without delay or difficulty to different services—from diagnosis, to cure, to rehabilitation—without need to transfer to different institutions located in different communities.

A comprehensive community mental health center in receipt of Federal aid may be sponsored through a variety of local organizational arrangements. Construction can follow the successful Hill-Burton pattern, under which the Federal Government matches public or voluntary nonprofit funds. Ideally, the center could be located at an appropriate community general hospital, many of which already have psychiatric units. In such instances, additional services and facilities could be added—either all at once or in several stages—to fill out the comprehensive program. In some instances, an existing outpatient psychiatric clinic might form the nucleus of such a center, its work expanded and integrated with other services in the community. Centers could also function effectively under a variety of other auspices: as affiliates of State mental hospitals, under State or local governments, or under voluntary nonprofit sponsorship.

Private physicians, including general practitioners, psychiatrists, and other medical specialists, would all be able to participate directly and cooperatively in the work of the center. For the first time, a large proportion of our private practitioners will have the opportunity to treat their patients in a mental health facility served by an auxiliary professional staff that is directly and quickly available for outpatient and inpatient care.

While these centers will be primarily designed to serve the mental health needs of the community, the mentally retarded should not be excluded from these centers if emotional problems exist. They should also offer the services of special therapists and consultation services to parents, school systems, health departments, and other public and private agencies concerned with mental retardation.

The services provided by these centers should be financed in the same way as other medical and hospital costs. At one time, this was not feasible in the case of mental illness, where prognosis almost invariably called for long and often permanent courses of treatment. But tranquilizers and new therapeutic methods now permit mental illness to be treated successfully in a very high proportion of cases within relatively short periods of time—weeks or months, rather than years.

Consequently, individual fees for services, individual and group insurance, other third-party payments, voluntary and private contributions, and State and local aid can now better bear the continuing burden of these costs to the individual patient after these services are established. Long-range Federal subsidies for operating costs are neither necessary nor desirable. Nevertheless, because this is a new and expensive undertaking for most communities, temporary Federal aid to help them meet the initial burden of establishing and placing centers in operation is desirable. Such assistance would be stimulatory in purpose, granted on a declining basis and terminated in a few years.

The success of this pattern of local and private financing will depend in large part upon the development of appropriate arrangements for health insurance, particularly in the private sector of our economy. Recent studies have indicated that mental health care—particularly the cost of diagnosis and short-term therapy, which would be major components of service in the new centers—is insurable at a moderate cost.

I have directed the Secretary of Health, Education, and Welfare to explore steps for encouraging and stimulating the expansion of private voluntary health insurance to include mental health care. I have also initiated a review of existing Federal programs, such as the health benefits program for Federal personnel, to determine whether further measures may be necessary and desirable to increase their provisions for mental health care.

These comprehensive community mental health centers should become operational at the earliest feasible date. I recommend that we make a major demonstration effort in the early years of the program to be expanded to all major communities as the necessary manpower and facilities become available.

It is to be hoped that within a few years the combination of increased mental health insurance coverage, added State and local support, and the redirection of State resources from State mental institutions will help achieve our goal of having community-centered mental health services readily accessible to all.

2. Improved Care in State Mental Institutions

Until the community mental health center program develops fully, it is imperative that the quality of care in existing State mental institutions be improved. By strengthening their therapeutic services, by becoming open institutions serving their local communities, many such institutions can perform a valuable transitional role. The Federal Government can assist materially by encouraging State mental institutions to undertake intensive demonstration and pilot projects, to improve the quality of care, and to provide inservice training for personnel manning these institutions.

This should be done through special grants for demonstration projects for inpatient care and inservice training. I recommend that $10 million be appropriated for such purposes.

3. Research and Manpower

Although we embark on a major national action program for mental health, there is still much more we need to know. We must not relax our effort to push back the frontiers of knowledge in basic and applied research into the mental processes, in therapy, and in other phases of research with a bearing upon mental illness. More needs to be done also to translate research findings into improved practices. I recommend an expansion of clinical, laboratory, and field research in mental illness and mental health.

Availability of trained manpower is a major factor in the determination of how fast we can expand our research and expand our new action program in the mental health field. At present manpower shortages exist in virtually all of the key professional and auxiliary personnel categories—psychiatrists, clinical psychologists, social workers, and psychiatric nurses. To achieve success, the current supply of professional manpower in these fields must be sharply increased—from about 45,000 in 1960 to approximately 85,000 by 1970. To help move toward this goal I recommend the appropriation of $66 million for training of personnel, an increase of $17 million over the current fiscal year.

I have, in addition, directed that the Manpower Development and Training Act be used to assist in the training of psychiatric aids and other auxiliary personnel for employment in mental institutions and community centers.

Success of these specialized training programs, however, requires that they be undergirded by basic training programs. It is essential to the success of our new national mental health program that Congress enact legislation authorizing aid to train more physicians and related health personnel. I will discuss this measure at greater length in the message on health which I will send to the Congress shortly.

II. A NATIONAL PROGRAM TO COMBAT MENTAL RETARDATION

Mental retardation stems from many causes. It can result from mongolism, birth injury or infection, or any of a host of conditions that cause a faulty or arrested development of intelligence to such an extent that the individual's ability to learn and to adapt to the demands of society is impaired. Once the damage is done, lifetime incapacity is likely. With early detection, suitable care and training, however, a significant improvement is social ability and in personal adjustment and achievement can be achieved.

The care and treatment of mental retardation, and research into its causes and cure, have—as in the case of mental illness—been too long neglected. Mental retardation ranks as a major national health, social and economic problem. It strikes our most precious asset our children. It disables 10 times as many people as diabetes, 20 times as many as tuberculosis, 25 times as many as muscular dystrophy, and 600 times as many as infantile paralysis. About 400,000 children are so retarded they require constant care or supervision; more than 200,000 of these are in residential institutions. There are between 5 and 6 million mentally retarded children and adults—an estimated 3 percent of the population. Yet, despite these grim statistics, and despite an admirable effort by private voluntary associations, until a decade ago not a single State health department offered any special community services for the mentally retarded or their families.

States and local communities spend $300 million a year for residential treatment of the mentally retarded, and another $250 million for special education, welfare, rehabilitation, and other benefits and services. The Federal Government will this year obligate $37 million for research, training and special services for the retarded and about three times as much for their income maintenance. But these efforts are fragmented and inadequate.

Mental retardation strikes children without regard for class, creed, or economic level. Each year sees an estimated 126,000 new cases. But it hits more often—and harder—at the underprivileged and the poor; and most often of all—and most severely—in city tenements and rural slums where there are heavy concentrations of families with poor education and low income.

There are very significant variations in the impact of the incidence of mental retardation. Draft rejections for mental deficiency during World War II were 14 times as heavy in States with low incomes as in others. In some slum areas 10 to 30 percent of the school-age children are mentally retarded, while in the very same cities more prosperous neighborhoods have only 1 or 2 percent retarded.

There is every reason to believe that we stand on the threshold of major advances in this field. Medical knowledge can now identify precise causes of retardation in 15 to 25 percent of the cases. This itself is a major advance. Those identified are usually cases in which there are severe organic injuries or gross brain damage from disease. Severe cases of mental retardation of this type are naturally more evenly spread throughout the population than mild retardation; but even here poor families suffer disproportionately. In most of the mild cases, although specific physical and neurological defects are usually not diagnosable with present biomedical techniques, research is rapidly adding to our knowledge of specific causes: German measles during the first 3 months of pregnancy, Rh blood factor incompatibility in newborn infants, lead poisoning of infants, faulty body chemistry in such diseases as phenylketonuria and galactosemia, and many others.

Many of the specific causes of mental retardation are still obscure. Socioeconomic and medical evidence gathered by a panel which I appointed in 1961, however, shows a major causative role for adverse social, economic, and cultural factors. Families who are deprived of the basic necessities of life, opportunity, and motivation have a high proportion of the Nation's retarded children. Unfavorable health factors clearly play a major role. Lack of prenatal and postnatal health care, in particular, leads to the birth of brain-damaged children or to an inadequate physical and neurological development. Areas of high infant mortality are often the same areas with a high incidence of mental retardation. Studies have shown that women lacking prenatal care have a much higher likelihood of having mentally retarded children. Deprivation of a child's opportunities for learning slows development in slum and distressed areas. Genetic, hereditary, and other biomedical factors also play a major part in the causes of mental retardation.

The American people, acting through their Government where necessary, have an obligation to prevent mental retardation, whenever possible, and to ameliorate it when it is present. I am, therefore, recommending action on a comprehensive program to attack this affliction. The only feasible program with a hope for success must not only aim at the specific causes and the control of mental retardation but seek solutions to the broader problems of our society with which mental retardation is so intimately related.

The panel which I appointed reported that, with present knowledge, at least half and hopefully more than half, of all mental retardation cases can be prevented through this kind of "broad spectrum" attack—aimed at both the specific causes which medical science has identified, and at the broader adverse social, economic, and cultural conditions with which incidence of mental retardation is so heavily correlated. At the same time research must go ahead in all these categories, calling upon the best efforts of many types of scientists, from the geneticist to the sociologist.

The fact that mental retardation ordinarily exists from birth or early childhood, the highly specialized medical, psychological, and educational evaluations which are required, and the complex and unique social, educational, and vocational lifetime needs of the retarded individual, all require that there be developed a comprehensive approach to this specific problem.

1. Prevention

Prevention should be given the highest priority in this effort. Our general health, education, welfare, and urban renewal programs will make a major contribution in overcoming adverse social and economic conditions. More adequate medical care, nutrition, housing, and educational opportunities can reduce mental retardation to the low incidence which has been achieved in some other nations. The recommendations for strengthening American education which I have made to the Congress in my message on education will contribute toward this objective as will the proposals contained in my forthcoming health message.

New programs for comprehensive maternity and infant care and for the improvement of our educational services are also needed. Particular attention should be directed toward the development of such services for slum and distressed areas. Among expectant mothers who do not receive prenatal care, more than 20 percent of all births are premature—two or three times the rate of prematurity among those who do receive adequate care. Premature infants have two or three times as many physical defects and 50 percent more illnesses than full-term infants. The smallest premature babies are 10 times more likely to be mentally retarded.

All of these statistics point to the direct relationship between lack of prenatal care and mental retardation. Poverty and medical indigency are at the root of most of this problem. An estimated 35 percent of the mothers in cities over 100,000 population are medically indigent. In 138 large cities of the country an estimated 455,000 women each year lack resources to pay for adequate health care during pregnancy and following birth. Between 20 and 60 percent of the mothers receiving care in public hospitals in some large cities receive inadequate or no prenatal care—and mental retardation is more prevalent in these areas.

Our existing State and Federal child health programs, though playing a useful and necessary role, do not provide the needed comprehensive care for this high-risk group. To enable the States and localities to move ahead more rapidly in combating mental retardation and other childhood disabilities through the new therapeutic measures being developed by medical science, I am recommending:

a. A new 5-year program of project grants to stimulate State and local health departments to plan, initiate, and develop comprehensive maternity and child health care service programs, helping primarily families in this high-risk group who are otherwise unable to pay for needed medical care. These grants would be used to provide medical care, hospital care, and additional nursing services, and to expand the number of prenatal clinics. Prenatal and post partum care would be more accessible to mothers. I recommend that the initial appropriation for this purpose be $5 million, allocated on a project basis, rising to an annual appropriation of $30 million by the third year.

b. Doubling the existing $25 million annual authorization for Federal grants for maternal and child health, a significant portion of which will be used for the mentally retarded.

c. Doubling over a period of 7 years the present $25 million annual authorization for Federal grants for crippled children's services.

Cultural and educational deprivation resulting in mental retardation can also be prevented. Studies have demonstrated that large numbers of children in urban and rural slums, including preschool children, lack the stimulus necessary for proper development in their intelligence. Even when there is no organic impairment, prolonged neglect and a lack of stimulus and opportunity for learning can result in the failure of young minds to develop. Other studies have shown that, if proper opportunities for learning are provided early enough, many of these deprived children can and will learn and achieve as much as children from more favored neighborhoods. This self-perpetuating intellectual blight should not be allowed to continue.

In my recent message on education, I recommended that at least 10 percent of the proposed aid for elementary and secondary education be committed by the States to special project grants designed to stimulate and make possible the improvement of educational opportunities particularly in slum and distressed areas, both urban and rural. I again urge special consideration by the Congress for this proposal. It will not only help improve educational quality and provide equal opportunity in areas which need assistance; it will also serve humanity by helping prevent mental retardation among the children in such culturally deprived areas.

2. Community Services

As in the case of mental illnesses, there is also a desperate need for community facilities and services for the mentally retarded. We must move from the outmoded use of distant custodial institutions to the concept of community-centered agencies that will provide a coordinated range of timely diagnostic, health, educational, training, rehabilitation, employment, welfare, and legal protection services. For those retarded children or adults who cannot be maintained at home by their own families, a new pattern of institutional services is needed.

The key to the development of this comprehensive new approach toward services for the mentally retarded is twofold. First, there must be public understanding and community planning to meet all problems. Second, there must be made available a continuum of services covering the entire range of needs. States and communities need to appraise their needs and resources, review current programs, and undertake preliminary actions leading to comprehensive State and community approaches to these objectives. To stimulate public awareness and the development of comprehensive plans, I recommend legislation to establish a program of special project grants to the States for financing State reviews of needs and programs in the field of mental retardation.

A total of $2 million is recommended for this purpose. Grants will be awarded on a selective basis to State agencies presenting acceptable proposals for this broad interdisciplinary planning activity. The purpose of these grants is to provide for every State an opportunity to begin to develop a comprehensive, integrated program to meet all the needs of the retarded. Additional support for planning health-related facilities and services will be available from the expanding planning grant program for the Public Health Service which I will recommend in my forthcoming message on health.

To assist the States and local communities to construct the facilities which these surveys justify and plan, I recommend that the Congress authorize matching grants for the construction of public and other nonprofit facilities, including centers for the comprehensive treatment, training, and care of the mentally retarded. Every community should be encouraged to include provision for meeting the health requirements of retarded individuals in planning its broader health services and facilities.

Because care of the mentally retarded has traditionally been isolated from centers of medical and nursing education, it is particularly important to develop facilities which will increase the role of highly qualified universities in the improvement and provision of services and the training of specialized personnel. Among the various types of facilities for which grants would be authorized, the legislation I am proposing will permit grants of Federal funds for the construction of facilities for (1) inpatient clinical units as an integral part of university-associated hospitals in which specialists on mental retardation would serve; (2) outpatient diagnostic, evaluation, and treatment clinics associated with such hospitals, including facilities for special training; and (3) satellite clinics in outlying cities and counties for provision of services to the retarded through existing State and local community programs, including those financed by the Children's Bureau, in which universities will participate. Grants of $5 million a year will be provided for these purposes within the total authorizations for facilities in 1965 and this will be increased to $10 million in subsequent years.

Such clinical and teaching facilities will provide superior care for the retarded and will also augment teaching and training facilities for specialists in mental retardation, including physicians, nurses, psychologists, social workers, and speech and other therapists. Funds for operation of such facilities would come from State, local, and private sources. Other existing or proposed programs of the Children's Bureau, of the Public Health Service, of the Office of Education, and of the Department of Labor can provide additional resources for demonstration purposes and for training personnel.

A full-scale attack on mental retardation also requires an expansion of special education, training, and rehabilitation services. Largely due to the lack of qualified teachers, college instructors, directors, and supervisors, only about one-fourth of the 1,250,000 retarded children of school age now have access to special education. During the past 4 years, with Federal support, there has been some improvement in the training of leadership personnel. However, teachers of handicapped children, including the mentally retarded, are still woefully insufficient in number and training. As I pointed out in the message on education, legislation is needed to increase the output of college instructors and classroom teachers for handicapped children.

I am asking the Office of Education to place a new emphasis on research in the learning process, expedite the application of research findings to teaching methods for the mentally retarded, support studies on improvement of curriculums, develop teaching aids, and stimulate the training of special teachers.

Vocational training, youth employment, and vocational rehabilitation programs can all help release the untapped potentialities of mentally retarded individuals. This requires expansion and improvement of our vocational education programs, as already recommended; and, in a subsequent message, I will present proposals for needed youth employment programs.

Currently rehabilitation services can only be provided to disabled individuals for whom, at the outset, a vocational potential can be definitely established. This requirement frequently excludes the mentally retarded from the vocational rehabilitation program. I recommend legislation to permit rehabilitation services to be provided to a mentally retarded person for up to 18 months, to determine whether he has sufficient potential to be rehabilitated vocationally. I also recommend legislation establishing a new program to help public and private nonprofit organizations to construct, equip, and staff rehabilitation facilities and workshops, making particular provision for the mentally retarded.

State institutions for the mentally retarded are badly underfinanced, understaffed, and overcrowded. The standard of care is in most instances so grossly deficient as to shock the conscience of all who see them.

I recommend the appropriation under existing law of project grants to State institutions for the mentally retarded, with an initial appropriation of $5 million to be increased in subsequent years to a level of at least $10 million. Such grants would be awarded, upon presentation of a plan meeting criteria established by the Secretary of Health, Education, and Welfare, to State institutions undertaking to upgrade the quality of residential services through demonstration, research, and pilot projects designed to improve the quality of care in such institutions and to provide impetus to inservice training and the education of professional personnel.

3. Research

Our single greatest challenge in this area is still the discovery of the causes and treatment of mental retardation. To do this we must expand our resources for the pursuit and application of scientific knowledge related to this problem. This will require the training of medical, behavioral, and other professional specialists to staff a growing effort. The new National Institute of Child Health and Human Development which was authorized by the 87th Congress is already embarked on this task.

To provide an additional focus for research into the complex mysteries of mental retardation, I recommend legislation to authorize the establishment of centers for research in human development, including the training of scientific personnel. Funds for 3 such centers are included in the 1964 budget; ultimately 10 centers for clinical, laboratory, behavioral, and social science research should be established. The importance of these problems justifies the talents of our best minds. No single discipline or science holds the answer. These centers must, therefore, be established on an interdisciplinary basis.

Similarly, in order to foster the further development of new techniques for the improvement of child health, I am also recommending new research authority to the Children's Bureau for research in maternal and child health and crippled children's services.

But, once again, the shortage of professional manpower seriously compromises both research and service efforts. The insufficient numbers of medical and nursing training centers now available too often lack a clinical focus on the problems of mental retardation comparable to the psychiatric teaching services relating to care of the mentally ill.

* * *

We as a Nation have long neglected the mentally ill and the mentally retarded. This neglect must end, if our Nation is to live up to its own standards of compassion and dignity and achieve the maximum use of its manpower.

This tradition of neglect must be replaced by forceful and far-reaching programs carried out at all levels of government, by private individuals and by State and local agencies in every part of the Union.

We must act—

to bestow the full benefits of our society on those who suffer from mental disabilities;

to prevent the occurrence of mental illness and mental retardation wherever and whenever possible;

to provide for early diagnosis and continuous and comprehensive care, in the community, of those suffering from these disorders;

to stimulate improvements in the level of care given the mentally disabled in our State and private institutions, and to reorient those programs to a community-centered approach;

to reduce, over a number of years, and by hundreds of thousands, the persons confined to these institutions;

to retain in and return to the community the mentally ill and mentally retarded, and there to restore and revitalize their lives through better health programs and strengthened educational and rehabilitation services; and

to reinforce the will and capacity of our communities to meet these problems, in order that the communities, in turn, can reinforce the will and capacity of individuals and individual families.

We must promote—to the best of our ability and by all possible and appropriate means—the mental and physical health of all our citizens.

To achieve these important ends, I urge that the Congress favorably act upon the foregoing recommendations.

John F. Kennedy

The White House, *February 5, 1963*

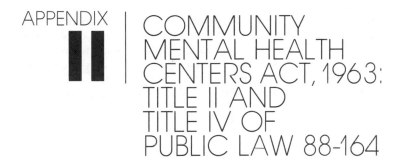

APPENDIX **II** | COMMUNITY MENTAL HEALTH CENTERS ACT, 1963: TITLE II AND TITLE IV OF PUBLIC LAW 88-164

An Act* to provide assistance in combating mental retardation through grants for construction of research centers and grants for facilities for the mentally retarded and assistance in improving mental health through grants for construction of community mental health centers, and for other purposes.

Be it enacted by the Senate and House of Representatives of the United States of America in Congress assembled, That this Act may be cited as the "Mental Retardation Facilities and Community Mental Health Centers Construction Act of 1963."†

TITLE I—CONSTRUCTION OF RESEARCH CENTERS AND FACILITIES FOR THE MENTALLY RETARDED

TITLE II—CONSTRUCTION OF COMMUNITY MENTAL HEALTH CENTERS

Short Title

Sec. 200. This title may be cited as the "Community Mental Health Centers Act."**

Authorization of Appropriations

Sec. 201. There are authorized to be appropriated, for grants for construction of public and other nonprofit community mental health centers. $35,000,000 for the fiscal year ending June 30, 1965, $50,000,000 for the fiscal year ending June 30, 1966, and $65,000,000 for the fiscal year ending June 30, 1967.

Allotments to States

Sec. 202. (a) For each fiscal year, the Secretary shall, in accordance with regulations, make allotments from the sums appropriated under section 201 to the several States on

* 77 Stat. 282.
† Mental Retardation Facilities and Community Mental Health Centers Construction Act of 1963.
** Citation of title.

the basis of (1) the population, (2) the extent of the need for community mental health centers, and (3) the financial need of the respective States; except that no such allotment to any State, other than the Virgin Islands, American Samoa, and Guam, for any fiscal year may be less than $100,000. Sums so allotted to a State for a fiscal year and remaining unobligated at the end of such year shall remain available to such State for such purpose for the next fiscal year (and for such year only), in addition to the sums allotted for such State for such next fiscal year.

(b) In accordance with regulations of the Secretary, any State may file with him a request that a specified portion of its allotment under this title be added to the allotment of another State under this title for the purpose of meeting a portion of the Federal share of the cost of a project for the construction of a community mental health center in such other State. If it is found by the Secretary that construction of the center with respect to which the request is made would meet needs of the State making the request and that use of the specified portion of such State's allotment, as requested by it, would assist in carrying out the purposes of this title, such portion of such State's allotment shall be added to the allotment of the other State under this title to be used for the purpose referred to above.

(c) Upon the request of any State that a specified portion of its allotment under this title be added to the allotment of such state under part C of title I and upon (1) the simultaneous certification to the Secretary by the State agency designated as provided in the State plan approved under this title to the effect that it has afforded a reasonable opportunity to make applications for the portion so specified and there have been no approvable applications for such portion or (2) a showing satisfactory to the Secretary that the need for facilities for the mentally retarded in such State is substantially greater than for community mental health centers, the Secretary shall, subject to such limitations as he may by regulation prescribed promptly adjust the allotments of such State in accordance with such request and shall notify such State agency and the State agency designated under the State plan approved under part C of title I, and thereafter the allotments as so adjusted shall be deemed the State's allotments for purposes of this title and part C of title I.

Regulations

Sec. 203. Within six months after enactment of this Act, the Secretary shall, after consultation with the Federal Hospital Council (established by section 633 of the Public Health Service Act*) and the National Advisory Mental Health Council (established by section 217 of the Public Health Service Act†), by general regulations applicable uniformly to all the States, prescribe—

1. the kinds of community mental health services needed to provide adequate mental health services for persons residing in a State;
2. the general manner in which the State agency (designated as provided in the State plan approved under this title) shall determine the priority of projects based on the relative need of different areas, giving special consideration to projects on the basis of the extent to which the centers to be constructed thereby will, alone or in conjunction with other facilities owned or operated by the applicant or affiliated or associated with the applicant, provide comprehensive mental health services (as

* 60 Stat. 1048. 42 USC 291k.
† 64 Stat. 466. 42 USC 218.

determined by the Secretary in accordance with regulations, for mentally ill persons in a particular community or communities or which will be part of or closely associated with a general hospital;

3. general standards of construction and equipment for centers of different classes and in different types of locations and

4. that the State plan shall provide for adequate community mental health centers for people residing in the State, and shall provide for adequate community mental health centers to furnish needed services for persons unable to pay therefore. Such regulations may require that before approval of an application for a center or addition to a center is recommended by a State agency, assurance shall be received by the State from the applicant that there will be made available in such center or addition a reasonable volume of services to persons unable to pay therefor, but an exception shall be made if such a requirement is not feasible from a financial viewpoint.

State Plans

Sec. 204. (a) After such regulations have been issued, any State desiring to take advantage of this title shall submit a State plan for carrying out its purposes. Such State plan must—

1. designate a single State agency as the sole agency for the administration of the plan, or designate such agency as the sole agency for supervising the administration of the plan;

2. contain satisfactory evidence that the State agency designated in accordance with paragraph (1) hereof will have authority to carry out such plan in conformity with this title;

3. provide for the designation of a State advisory council which shall include representatives of nongovernment organizations or groups, and of State agencies, concerned with planning, operation, or utilization of community mental health centers or other mental health facilities, including representatives of consumers of the services provided by such centers and facilities who are familiar with the need for such services, to consult with the State agency in carrying out such plan;

4. set forth a program for construction of community mental health centers (A) which is based on a statewide inventory of existing facilities and survey of need; (B) which conforms with the regulations prescribed by the Secretary under section 203(1); and (C) which meets the requirements for furnishing needed services to persons unable to pay therefor, included in regulations prescribed under section 203(4);

5. set forth the relative need, determined in accordance with the regulations prescribed under section 203(2), for the several projects included in such programs, and provide for the construction, insofar as financial resources available therefor and for maintenance and operation make possible, in the order of such relative need;

6. provide such methods of administration of the State plan, including methods relating to the establishment and maintenance of personnel standards on a merit basis (except that the Secretary shall exercise no authority with respect to the selection, tenure of office, or compensation of any individual employed in accordance with such methods), as are found by the Secretary to be necessary for the proper and efficient operation of the plan;

7. provide minimum standards (to be fixed in the discretion of the State) for the maintenance and operation of centers which receive Federal aid under this title;

8. provide for affording to every applicant for a construction project an opportunity for hearing before the State agency;

9. provide that the State agency will make such reports in such form and containing such information as the Secretary may from time to time reasonably require, and will keep such records and afford such access thereto as the Secretary may find necessary to assure the correctness and verification of such reports; and

10. provide that the State agency will from time to time, but not less often than annually, review its State plan and submit to the Secretary any modifications thereof which it considers necessary.

(b) The Secretary shall approve any State plan and any modification thereof which complies with the provisions of subsection (a). The Secretary shall not finally disapprove a State plan except after reasonable notice and opportunity for a hearing to the State.

Approval of Projects

Sec. 205. (a) For each project for construction pursuant to a State plan approved under this title, there shall be submitted to the Secretary through the State agency an application by the State or a political subdivision thereof or by a public or other nonprofit agency. If two or more such agencies join in the construction of the project, the application may be filed by one or more of such agencies. Such application shall set forth—

1. a description of the site for such project;

2. plans and specifications therefor in accordance with the regulations prescribed by the Secretary under section 203(3);

3. reasonable assurance that title to such site is or will be vested in one or more of the agencies filing the application or in a public or other nonprofit agency which is to operate the community mental health center;

4. reasonable assurance that adequate financial support will be available for the construction of the project and for its maintenance and operation when completed;

5. reasonable assurance that all laborers and mechanics employed by contractors or subcontractors in the performance of work on construction of the project will be paid wages at rates not less than those prevailing on similar construction in the locality as determined by the Secretary of Labor in accordance with the Davis-Bacon Act, as amended (40 U.S.C. 276a—276a-5*); and the Secretary of Labor shall have with respect to the labor standards specified in this paragraph the authority and functions set forth in Reorganization Plan Numbered 14 of 1950 (15 F.R. 3176; 5 U.S.C. 133z–15†) and section 2 of the Act of June 13, 1934, as amended (40 U.S.C. 276c**); and

6. a certification by the State agency of the Federal share for the project.

The Secretary shall approve such appliction if sufficient funds to pay the Federal share of the cost of construction of such project are available from the allotment to the State, and if the Secretary finds (A) that the application contains such reasonable assurance

* 49 Stat. 1011.
† 64 Stat. 1267.
** 53 Stat. 108.

as to title, financial support, and payment of prevailing rates of wages and overtime pay; (B) that the plans and specifications are in accord with the regulations prescribed pursuant to section 203; (C) that the application is in conformity with the State plan approved under section 204 and contains an assurance that in the operation of the center there will be compliance with the applicable requirements of the State plan and of the regulations prescribed under section 203(4) for furnishing needed services for persons unable to pay therefor, and with State standards for operation and maintenance; (D) that the services to be provided by the center, alone or in conjunction with other facilities owned or operated by the applicant or affiliated or associated with the applicant, will be part of a program providing, principally for persons residing in a particular community or communities in or near which such center is to be situated, at least those essential elements of comprehensive mental health services for mentally ill persons which are prescribed by the Secretary in accordance with regulations; and (E) that the application has been approved and recommended by the State agency and is entitled to priority over other projects within the State in accordance with the regulations prescribed pursuant to section 203(2). No application shall be disapproved by the Secretary until he has afforded the State agency an opportunity for a hearing.

(b) Amendment of any approved application shall be subject to approval in the same manner as an original application.

Withholding of Payments

Sec. 206. Whenever the Secretary, after reasonable notice and opportunity for hearing to the State agency designated as provided in section 204(a) (1), finds—

1. that the State agency is not complying substantially with the provisions required by section 204 to be included in its State plan, or with regulations under this title;
2. that any assurance required to be given in an application filed under section 205 is not being or cannot be carried out;
3. that there is a substantial failure to carry out plans and specifications approved by the Secretary under section 205; or
4. that adequate State funds are not being provided annually for the direct administration of the State plan, the Secretary may forthwith notify the State agency that—
5. no further payments will be made to the State from allotments under this title; or
6. no further payments will be made from allotments under this title for any project or projects designated by the Secretary as being affected by the action or inaction referred to in paragraph (1), (2), (3), or (4) of this section,

as the Secretary may determine to be appropriate under the circumstances; and, except with regard to any project for which the application has already been approved and which is not directly affected, further payments from such allotments may be withheld, in whole or in part, until there is no longer any failure to comply (or to carry out the assurance or plans and specifications or to provide adequate State funds, as the case may be) or, if such compliance (or other action) is impossible, until the State repays or arranges for the repayment of Federal moneys to which the recipient was not entitled.

Nonduplication of Grants

Sec. 207. No grant may be made after January 1, 1964, under any provision of the Public Health Service Act,* for any of the three fiscal years in the period beginning July 1,

* 58 Stat. 42 USC 201 note.

1964, and ending June 30, 1967, for construction of any facility described in this title, unless the Secretary determines that funds are not available under this title to make a grant for the construction of such facility.

TITLE III—TRAINING OF TEACHERS OF MENTALLY RETARDED AND OTHER HANDICAPPED CHILDREN

TITLE IV—GENERAL

Definitions

Sec. 401. For purposes of this Act—

(a) The term "State" includes Puerto Rico, Guam, American Samoa, the Virgin Islands, and the District of Columbia.

(b) The term "facility for the mentally retarded" means a facility specially designed for the diagnosis, treatment, education, training, or custodial care of the mentally retarded, including facilities for training specialists and sheltered workshops for the mentally retarded, but only if such workshops are part of facilities which provide or will provide comprehensive services for the mentally retarded.

(c) The term "community mental health center" means a facility providing services for the prevention or diagnosis of mental illness, or care and treatment of mentally ill patients, or rehabilitation of such persons, which services are provided principally for persons residing in a particular community or communities in or near which the facility is situated.

(d) The terms "nonprofit facility for the mentally retarded", "nonprofit community mental health center", and "nonprofit private institution of higher learning" mean, respectively, a facility for the mentally retarded, a community mental health center, and an institution of higher learning which is owned and operated by one or more nonprofit corporations or associations no part of the net earnings of which inures, or may lawfully inure, to the benefit of any private shareholder or individual; and the term "nonprofit private agency or organization" means an agency or organization which is such a corporation or association or which is owned and operated by one or more of such corporations or associations.

(e) The term "construction" includes construction of new buildings, expansion, remodeling, and alteration of existing buildings, and initial equipment of any such buildings (including medical transportation facilities); including architect's fees, but excluding the cost of off-site improvements and the cost of the acquisition of land.

(f) The term "cost of construction" means the amount found by the Secretary to be necessary for the construction of a project.

(g) The term "title", when used with reference to a site for a project, means a fee simple, or such other estate or interest (including a leasehold on which the rental does not exceed 4 per centum of the value of the land) as the Secretary finds sufficient to assure for a period of not less than fifty years undisturbed use and possession for the purposes of construction and operation of the project.

(h) The term "Federal share" with respect to any project means—

1. if the State plan under which application for such project is filed contains, as of the date of approval of the project application, standards approved by the Secretary

pursuant to section 402 the amount determined in accordance with such standards by the State agency designated under such plan; or

2. if the State plan does not contain such standards, the amount (not less than 33⅓ per centum and not more than either 66⅔ per centum or the State's Federal percentage, whichever is the lower) established by such State agency for all projects in the State: *Provided*, That prior to the approval of the first such project in the State during any fiscal year such State agency shall give to the Secretary written notification of the Federal share established under this paragraph for such projects in such State to be approved by the Secretary during such fiscal year, and the Federal share for such projects in such State approved during such fiscal year shall not be changed after such approval.

(i) The Federal percentage for any State shall be 100 per centum less that percentage which bears the same ratio to 50 per centum as the per capita income of such State bears to the per capita income of the United States, except that the Federal percentage for Puerto Rico, Guam, American Samoa, and the Virgin Islands shall be 66⅔ per centum.

(j) (1) The Federal percentages shall be promulgated by the Secretary between July 1 and August 31 of each even-numbered year, on the basis of the average of the per capita incomes of the States and of the United States for the three most recent consecutive years for which satisfactory data are available from the Department of Commerce. Such promulgation shall be conclusive for each of the two fiscal years in the period beginning July 1 next succeeding such promulgation; except that the Secretary shall promulgate such percentages as soon as possible after the enactment of this Act, which promulgation shall be conclusive for the fiscal year ending June 30, 1965.

(2) The term "United States" means (but only for purposes of this subsection and subsection (i)) the fifty States and the District of Columbia.

(k) The term "Secretary" means the Secretary of Health, Education, and Welfare.

State Standards for Variable Federal Share

Sec. 402. The State plan approved under part C of title I or title II may include standards for determination of the Federal share of the cost of projects approved in the State under such part or title, as the case may be. Such standards shall provide equitably (and, to the extent practicable, on the basis of objective criteria) for variations between projects or classes of projects on the basis of the economic status of areas and other relevant factors. No such standards shall provide for a Federal share of more than 66⅔ per centum or less than 33⅓ per centum of the cost of construction of any project. The Secretary shall approve any such standards and any modifications thereof which comply with the provisions of this section.

Payments for Construction

Sec. 403. (a) Upon certification to the Secretary by the State agency, designated as provided in section 134 in the case of a facility for the mentally retarded, or section 204 in the case of a community mental health center, based upon inspection by it, that work has been performed upon a project, or purchases have been made, in accordance with the approved plans and specifications, and that payment of an installment is due to the applicant, such installment shall be paid to the State, from the applicable allotment of such State, except that (1) if the State is not authorized by law to make payments to the applicant, the payment shall be made directly to the applicant, (2) if the Secretary, after investigation or otherwise, has reason to believe that any act (or failure to act) has occurred requiring action pursuant to section 136 or section 206, as the case may be, payment may, after he has given the State agency so designated notice of opportunity for hearing pursuant to such section, be withheld, in whole or in part, pending corrective action or action based on such hearing, and (3) the total of payments under this subsection with respect to such project may not exceed an amount equal to the Federal share of the cost of construction of such project.

(b) In case an amentment to an approved application is approved as provided in section 135 or 205 or the estimated cost of a project is revised upward, any additional payment with respect thereto may be made from the applicable allotment of the State for the fiscal year in which such amendment or revision is approved.

Judicial Review

Sec. 404. If the Secretary refuses to approve any application for a project submitted under section 135 or 205, the State agency through which such application was submitted, or if any State is dissatisfied with his action under section 134(b) or 204(b) or section 136 or 206, such State, may appeal to the United States court of appeals for the circuit in which such State is located, by filing a petition with such court within sixty days after such action. A copy of the petition shall be forthwith transmitted by the clerk of the court to the Secretary, or any officer designated by him for that purpose. The Secretary thereupon shall file in the court the record of the proceedings on which he based his action, as provided in section 2112 of title 28, United States Code.* Upon the filing of such petition, the court shall have jurisdiction to affirm the action of the Secretary or to set it aside, in whole or in part, temporarily or permanently, but until the filing of the record, the Secretary may modify or set aside his order. The findings of the Secretary as to the facts, if supported by substantial evidence, shall be conclusive, but the court, for good cause shown, may remand the case to the Secretary to take further evidence, and the Secretary may thereupon make new or modified findings of fact and may modify his previous action, and shall file in the court the record of the further proceedings. Such new or modified findings of fact shall likewise be conclusive if supported by substantial evidence. The judgment of the court affirming or setting aside, in whole or in part, any action of the Secretary shall be final, subject to review by the Supreme Court of the United States upon certiorari or certification as provided in section 1254 of title 28, United States Code.† The commencement of proceedings under this section shall not, unless so specifically ordered by the court, operate as a stay of the Secretary's action.

Recovery

Sec. 405. If any facility or center with respect to which funds have been paid under section 403 shall, at any time within twenty years after the completion of construction—

1. be sold or transferred to any person, agency, or organization (A) which is not qualified to file an application under section 135 or 205, or (B) which is not approved as

---

* 72 Stat. 941.
† 62 Stat. 928.

a transferee by the State agency designated pursuant to section 134 (in the case of a facility for the mentally retarded) or section 204 (in case of a community mental health center), or its successor; or

2. cease to be a public or other nonprofit facility for the mentally retarded or community mental health center, as the case may be, unless the Secretary determines, in accordance with regulations, that there is good cause for releasing the applicant or other owner from the obligation to continue such facility as a public or other nonprofit facility for the mentally retarded or such center as a community mental health center,

the United States shall be entitled to recover from either the transferor or the transferee (or, in the case of a facility or center which has ceased to be public or other nonprofit facility for the mentally retarded or community mental health center, from the owners thereof) an amount bearing the same ratio to the then value (as determined by the agreement of the parties or by action brought in the district court of the United States for the district in which the center is situated) of so much of such facility or center as constituted an approved project or projects, as the amount of the Federal participation bore to the cost of the construction of such project or projects. Such right of recovery shall not constitute a lien upon such facility or center prior to judgment.

State Control of Operations

Sec. 406. Except as otherwise specifically provided, nothing in this Act shall be construed as conferring on any Federal officer or employee the right to exercise any supervision or control over the administration, personnel, maintenance, or operation of any facility for the mentally retarded or community mental health center with respect to which any funds have been or may be expended under this Act.

Conforming Amendment

Sec. 407. (a) The first sentence of section 633(b) of the Public Health Service Act* is amended by striking out "eight" and inserting in lieu thereof "twelve". The second sentence thereof is amended to read: "Six of the twelve appointed members shall be persons who are outstanding in fields pertaining to medical facility and health activities, and three of these six shall be authorities in matters relating to the operation of hospitals or other medical facilities, one of them shall be an authority in matters relating to the mentally retarded and one of them shall be an authority in matters relating to mental health, and the other six members shall be appointed to represent the consumers of services provided by such facilities and shall be persons familiar with the need for such services in urban or rural areas."

(b) The terms of office of the additional members of the Federal Hospital Council authorized by the amendment made by subsection (a) who first take office after enactment of this Act shall expire, as designated by the Secretary at the time of appointment, one at the end of the first year, one at the end of the second year, one at the end of the third year, and one at the end of the fourth year after the date of appointment.

Approved October 31, 1963, 10:07 A.M.

* 60 Stat. 1048. 42 USC 291k.

Legislative history: House Reports No. 694 (Comm. on Interstate & Foreign Commerce), No. 862 (Comm. of Conference). Senate Report No. 180 (Comm. on Labor & Public Welfare). Congressional Record, Vol. 109 (1963), May 27, considered and passed Senate; Sept. 10, considered and passed House, amended; Oct. 21, conference report agreed to in House and Senate.

COMPREHENSIVE COMMUNITY MENTAL HEALTH NURSING ASSESSMENT OF FAMILY FUNCTIONING

The comprehensive assessment of family functioning is an approach by which a data base can be obtained and clinical decisions made about the mental and emotional health of families and other kinds of primary socialization systems. The dimensions of family system functioning are reflected in characteristic response patterns. These patterns in turn may be used to make judgments about the potential of a family system for promoting and maintaining the mental and emotional health of its members.

A *high frequency of adaptive response patterns* in family systems suggests an excellent potential for development of positive mental and emotional health in members. A *moderate frequency of adaptive responses* suggests that the family system has a good potential for the development of behaviors and attitudes in members that are consistent with positive mental health and that a milieu is provided in which the essential competencies contributing to such behaviors are routinely learned. However, family systems with this level of response patterns experience recurring tensions, stresses, and relationship strains and problems. None of these is serious enough to be considered a frank familial pathology. Family systems with a moderate level of adaptive responses and tensions and problems that are not too serious are probably the normative pattern for family system interactions, interrelationships, and organization. A *low frequency of adaptive response patterns* in family systems suggests a distressed family system and the existence of pathologies and problems in many areas of family functioning. The potential of such family systems to promote and maintain the mental and emotional health of members and to maintain a milieu within the family system that provides for socialization and support of members to learn essential competencies that encourage members to develop selfhood is fair.

Profiles of adaptive, stressed, and distressed family systems are given in Chapter 7. Response patterns of behavior that characterize these family systems may be used as references for judging the dimensions of family functioning in terms of adaptiveness. The social psychological model of mental health and illness in Table 3.4 may also be used as an orientation for assessment of response patterns in primary socialization systems such as families. This model is an integral part of the conceptual framework for guiding clinical nursing practice in community mental health nursing.

Clinical judgements have to be made about the potential of any kind of family system to provide a milieu, relationships, and experiences that promote and maintain the mental and emotional health of members and maintain and sustain the family system itself. The frequency of occurrence of response patterns in relation to the various dimensions of family functioning is one such yardstick. In the assessment, the following guide may be used to organize the information required to make such judgements:

High Frequency of Responses	Responses occur repeatedly on most of the dimensions of family functioning. With this frequency of responses, functioning suggests adaptive response patterns with excellent or optimal potential for providing relationships, resources, support, and opportunities for learning in areas that foster and promote mental and emotional health of family members and maintain the family system for socialization and support of members.
Moderate Frequency of Responses	Responses occur in most of the dimensions of family functioning at least once during assessment. With this frequency of responses, characteristic response patterns may indicate strain, even stress, but overall the family system functions so that growth and development of members occurs and mental and emotional health is not imperiled, and the system itself remains organized and cohesive. The potential for promotion and maintenance of mental and emotional health is good. The majority of family systems probably function at this level, so assessment of the dimensions of family functioning provide needed information about areas in which prevention counseling is useful.
Low Frequency of Responses	Responses occur in less than one-half of the dimensions of family functioning infrequently or not at all during assessment. At this level of frequency, characteristic responses do not indicate adaptive functioning; rather, the response pattern indicates distress in roles, relationships, and family organization; problems are not being effectively handled. Potential for promotion and maintenance of emotional and mental health is fair. Generally, family systems functioning at this level of adaptation need therapy that addresses major system problems within the family as an interacting unit.

In conducting the community mental health nursing assessment, information may be obtained by perceptions and from observations and factual information provided by family members. Certain kinds of information may be obtained by using some of the strategies that are also used in prevention counseling in order to get families to interact, address various kinds of tasks, and provide data that may be difficult to obtain by discussion and questioning. A number of such strategies are described in Chapter 10.

FAMILY FUNCTIONING ASSESSMENT FORM

Part I. Information about Family and Its Members

To be completed by the family in the first assessment session:

1. Name

   Mother: _____ Last _____ First _____ Middle _____ Age _____ Birthplace

   Father: _____ Last _____ First _____ Middle _____ Age _____ Birthplace

2. Address _____ Street _____ City _____ State _____ Zip code

3. Phone _____ Home

4. Marital status _____ Mother's work place _____ Father's work place

   Single: Years _____ Married: Years _____ Divorced: Years _____ Separated: Years

5. Living situation _____ Alone _____ With parents _____ With friend(s) _____ With a partner

6. Religion _____ Mother _____ Father _____ Other members

7. Employer _____ Mother _____ Father _____ Other members

8. Position _____ Mother: How long? _____ Father: How long?

9. Check education

   Mother: _____ Grades 1–9 _____ 10–12 _____ BS or BA _____ MS or MA _____ Doctorate (kind)

   Father: _____ Grades 1–9 _____ 10–12 _____ BS or BA _____ MS or MA _____ Doctorate (kind)

10. Check family income

    Range: _____ $3000–5000 _____ $6000–8000 _____ $9000–11,000 _____ $12,000–15,000 _____ $16,000–20,000 _____ Above $20,000

11. Names, ages, sex, and school history of all children and names of any other family members:

	Name	Date of Birth	Sex	Grade in School
1st child				
2nd child				
3rd child				

299

4th child _____

5th child _____

Other family
members _____

12. Length of time in community _____
    Months/Years

13. How would your family rate the following resources in your community? (Please check appropriate column.)

	Excellent	Good	Poor	None
Schools				
Law enforcement				
Recreational activities				
Social services				
Church activities				
Community activities				
Library services				
Health and hospital services				

14. How would your family judge the extent to which it contributes to the needs and development of your community?
    ☐A great deal   ☐Now and then   ☐Hardly ever

15. Please identify what your family considers its greatest strengths. If there are problems or tensions within the family, please note the source of these.
    Strengths _____

    Tensions or problems _____

To be completed by the community mental health nurse:

Name of Family _____ Nurse _____

Session	Date	Place	Members Present
1			
2			
3			
4 (summary session)			

Part II. Primary Nursing Data Base

Instructions: Please assess each of the dimensions of family functioning by using observations, communications, and information provided by the family in the assessment interaction process. Some dimensions of functioning may not be evident in each session, however by the end of the third session, the nurse should be able to make clinical judgments about the various dimensions of family functioning in cooperation with the family. Please check the frequency that behaviors related to the various dimensions are observed or occur in the interaction process in the appropriate column.

High frequency: behavior observed repeatedly in most dimensions of family functioning during assessment
Moderate frequency: behavior observed in most dimensions of family functioning at least once during assessment
Low frequency: behavior observed infrequently or not at all or less than one-half of dimensions of family functioning during assessment

A. Dimension: Family Cohesion and Identity

Socioemotional climate is one that:

	Frequency of Behaviors		
	High	Moderate	Low
Promotes emotional closeness between members without any one member's losing a sense of personal self and identity.			
Encourages development of a family identity by members.			
Uses a set of values and standards of conduct to guide family functioning.			
Accepts individual members who have values and goals different from family expectations without negative valuation and/or punishment.			
Promotes and supports members' development of caring attitudes for others.			
Engages in relationships and activities that help others.			
Encourages members to accept responsibility for self, to become more autonomous and independent.			
Supports and maintains the family as a unit with each member contributing to this effort.			
Encourages members to develop relationships with peers in different kinds of settings and activities.			
Encourages development of respect for each member as a person and values his or her achievements.			
Patterns of responses by frequency of occurrence of behaviors:		Total checks	

301

B. Dimension: Family Organization, Structure, and Roles

The overall pattern is one that:

Defines roles and responsibilities of family members for conducting daily living activities.

Uses parental authority in a constructive manner.

Communicates messages clearly and explicitly within the family system to and between family members.

Provides opportunities for members to learn essential social, personal, and interpersonal competencies.

Provides opportunities for members to learn essential cognitive and problem-solving skills.

Provides opportunities for members to learn roles and relationships in the family setting that may be generalized to other settings, relationships, and situations.

Encourages participation in:

    Cultural activities.

    Intellectual pursuits.

    Recreational activities.

    Political activities.

    Religious activities.

    Social activities.

    School activities.

    Community projects and concerns.

Shows respect for standards and rules of family conduct in family interactions and in peer relationships.

Shows pride and respect for each member's contributions and achievements.

Shows support by spouses for each other to develop roles and identities other then the parental role.

Engages in family interactions and decision making without use of coalition formation.

	Frequency of Behaviors		
	High	Moderate	Low

Uses family's resources and strengths to meet the needs of members in ways that promote positive physical, emotional, and mental health.

Shows a clear sense of self in roles and relationships by parents.

Reports satisfaction in sexual intimacy by parents.

Pays attention to the "mental health" of the family as a system.

Indicates a "theme" that influences roles, relationships, and values.

Shows acceptance of members who deviate from family values, standards, and expectations.

Shows sharing of roles and responsibility by parents where both work or have outside-of-the-home responsibilities.

Shows willingness to work out conflicts in family around roles, relationships, work demands, and school commitments.

Encourages members to achieve potential in school.

Encourages participation in school, cultural, recreational, and athletic activities.

Provides a climate in which parents enjoy parental and work roles.

Provides opportunities for the developmental and maturational needs of members through changes in roles and expectations.

Provides learning opportunities for family members who have special educational, developmental, maturational, and health needs.

Pattern(s) of responses by frequency of occurrence of behaviors.   Total checks

C. Dimension: Organization of Family to Handle Daily Living Activities

The overall pattern is one that:

Delineates roles and responsibilities necessary for family living without undue stress and strain on any one member.

303

	Frequency of Behaviors		
	High	*Moderate*	*Low*

Organizes daily living activities without undue stress and strain on the family as an interacting system.

Provides for sharing by family members of the responsibility of "getting the family moving each day."

Provides leadership in crisis situations.

Tries out new ways of managing and making changes in family organization to more effectively manage both daily living and crisis situations.

Recognizes recurring problems in family that involve member(s), relationships, and situations and tries to more effectively handle these.

Considers the impact of daily stresses and strains on mental and emotional health of the family and its members and provides support to lessen impact.

Promotes positive feelings of self in members in their handling of daily and crisis situations.

Develops a support system that can be called upon in time of need.

Pattern(s) of responses by frequency of occurrence of behaviors: Total checks

D. Dimension: Interrelationship Between Family and Community

Overall pattern is one that:

Embodies acceptance of responsibility of family to contribute to the mental health of the community by involvement in community needs and concerns.

Contributes to community projects that address the needs of the community and special needs of groups within the community.

Provides for family members to participate on an ongoing basis in social networks that link the family and community groups.

Participates in groups to obtain essential school, health, social, and recreational services for the community.

Assists in development of friend, kin, and community networks to provide assistance to people in the community in time of need.

Contributes to the development of a sense of identity of community for the family as a vital part of the community.

Knows the key sources the family may call on to get assistance and resources in time of need.

Knows some of the patterns of health and illness in the community.

Recognizes a relationship between the emotional and mental health of the family and that of the community.

Uses the political and organizational resources of the community to help to organize groups to address particular problems and/or to develop needed projects.

Pattern(s) of responses by frequency occurrence of behaviors: Total checks

E. Dimension: Family Strengths

The overall strength of family system is one that:

Provides a milieu in which the emotional and mental health of members are considered as part of the health of the family system.

Provides a milieu in which family concerns can be identified and considered valid for the family problem-solving.

Provides a milieu in which stress is acknowledged and opportunities provided to find better ways of handling it.

Provides a milieu in which distresses (pathologies) can be made explicit and strategies for handling them mutually arrived at.

Provides a milieu in which professional help for mental and emotional problems is viewed as appropriate in the way that physical health problems are handled.

Provides a milieu in which family values are carried out in family interrelationships.

Provides a milieu in which members express caring and love for one another.

Provides a milieu in which all family members accept some responsibility for what happens to any one member.

	Frequency of Behaviors		
	High	Moderate	Low

Provides a milieu in which family strengths may be recognized.

Identifies family strengths:

1. _____
2. _____
3. _____
4. _____
5. _____

(Check the frequency of observed patterns of behavior which validate family strengths.)

Provides a milieu in which family concerns may be recognized.

Identifies current family concerns:

1. _____
2. _____
3. _____

(Check the frequency of observed patterns of behavior which validate family concerns.)

Provides a milieu in which sources of stress may be recognized.

Identifies at least three sources of stress within family system:

1. _____
2. _____
3. _____

(Check the validity through observations, synthesis of information, and use of perceptions.)

Provides a milieu in which distresses (pathologies in family interrelationships) may be pointed out and discussed.

Identifies family distresses, (if any:)

1. _____
2. _____
3. _____

(Check frequency of observed patterns of behavior that indicate familial pathologies may be developing or already exist)

Pattern(s) of responses by frequency of occurrence of behaviors: Total checks

Part III. Secondary Data Base: General Health Information

A. Dimension: Health-Protective Behaviors

	Actions Taken			
	Adults		Children	
	Yes	No	Yes	No
Have recommended immunizations				
Exercise at least three times a week				
Recommended weight maintained				
Diet has low fat foods				
Sleep 7–8 hours nightly				
No smoking				
Moderate or no drinking of alcoholic beverages				
Use stress management exercises on a regular basis				
Have medical check-ups as recommended				
Total checks				

Patterns of actions by frequency of responses:

Patterning:
Recurring health problem(s) of family members: _____

Circumstances associated with recurrence: _____

Impact on other family members: _____

Members who experience more intensely the impact of health problem of another member: _____

Family interrelationships most affected: _____
Family roles most affected: _____

Major disruptions in family organization and functioning when health problem: _____

B. Tensions or Problems
Identify any tensions or problems in communications, relationships, roles, and behaviors that have occurred over the past year in work, school, and family settings.

Member	Problem	Setting
1.		
2.		
3.		
4.		
5.		

Patterning:
Setting(s) in problem(s) occur: _____

Problems involving one or more of the same family members in recurring episodes: _____

Explicit efforts made to correct problems: _____

Family interrelationships most affected: _____
Family roles most affected: _____

Major disruptions in family organization and functioning: _____

Impact on harmony and cohesion of family: _____

Comments:

C. Dimension: Illness in Family

Identify illnesses of family members over past year.

Member	Nature of Illness
1.	
2.	
3.	
4.	
5.	
6.	
7.	

Patterning:
Times any one member has been ill: _____

Times any one type illness has occurred: _____

Situations associated with illnesses: _____

Family interrelationships most involved when illness has occurred: _____

Family roles most affected when illness has occurred: _____

Major disruptions in family organization and functioning during illnesses: _____

Identify present health problems if any.

Member	Health Problem
1.	
2.	
3.	

D. Dimension: Distress or Disruption in Family Functioning

Identify any major distressing situations or changes in roles and relationships that have disrupted family functioning over the past year:
1. _____

2. _____

3. _____

	Health Status		
	High	Moderate	Low

E. Dimension: Self-assessment by Family of Health Status

Family's assessment of their general health

Family's assessment of their emotional and mental health

Part IV. Summary of Assessment Data About Family Functioning

Instructions: Please bring forth the pattern of responses for the various dimensions of family functioning and place in appropiate column under appropiate dimension.

A. Dimensions of Family Functioning

	Frequency of Response Patterns		
	High	Moderate	Low
1. Family cohesion and identity			
2. Family organization, structure, and roles			
3. Organization of family to handle daily living			
4. Interrelationships between family and community			
5. Family strengths			
6. Use of health-protective behaviors			
7. Recurring tensions/emotional concerns over past year (frequency)			
8. Illnesses of members over past year (frequency)			
9. Disruptions in family functioning over past year (frequency)			
Total checks			

B. Overall Assessment by Nurse of Family Functioning

Instructions: Please check the box that best describes the characteristic response patterns of family functioning by frequency of occurrence of related behaviors during assessment.

☐ High = adaptive functioning

☐ Moderate = stressed functioning

☐ Low = distressed functioning

C. Recommendations

☐ Primary prevention counseling
☐ Prevention counseling combined with therapeutic interventions
☐ Family therapy
☐ Referral to _____

Source(s) _____

D. If Referral Is Made, Major Areas of Concern

1. _____
2. _____
3. _____
4. _____

E. If Prevention Counseling Is Recommended, Concerns by Priority

1. _____
2. _____
3. _____

F. Summary Prepared on _____ by _____
        Date   Name of nurse

311

INDEX